Computational Visualization:
Graphics, Abstraction, and Interactivity

Springer
*Berlin
Heidelberg
New York
Barcelona
Budapest
Hong Kong
London
Milan
Paris
Singapore
Tokyo*

Thomas Strothotte

Computational Visualization

Graphics, Abstraction, and Interactivity

Foreword by K. van Overveld

With the collaboration of

Oliver Deussen, Frank Godenschweger,
Jörg Hamel, Ralf Helbing, Axel Hoppe,
Kathrin Lüdicke, Maic Masuch,
Rainer Michel, Ian Pitt, Bernhard Preim,
Andreas Raab, Alf Ritter, Michael Rüger,
Jörg R. J. Schirra, Stefan Schlechtweg,
Martin Scholz, Kornelia Ullrich,
and Hubert Wagener

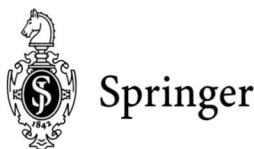

Springer

Prof. Dr. Thomas Strothotte
Otto-von-Guericke University of Magdeburg
Faculty of Computer Science
Universitätsplatz 2, D-39106 Magdeburg, Germany
E-mail: tstr@isg.cs.uni-magdeburg.de

With 214 Figures and 11 Tables

ISBN 3-540-63737-0 Springer-Verlag Berlin Heidelberg New York

ACM Computing Classification (1998): I.3, I.7.5, H.5.1-2, K.3, J.3

Library of Congress Cataloging-in-Publication Data
Computational Visualization: Graphics, Abstraction, and Interactivity/
Thomas Strothotte. p. cm. Includes bibliographical references and index.
ISBN 3-540-63737-0 (hardcover: alk. paper)
1. Computer graphics. 2. Abstraction. 3. Interactive computer systems.
I. Strothotte, Thomas, 1959-. T385.A273 1998 006.6-dc21 98-26278 CIP

This work is subject to copyright. All rights are reserved, whether the whole or part of the material is concerned, specifically the rights of translation, reprinting, reuse of illustrations, recitation, broadcasting, reproduction on microfilm or in any other way, and storage in data banks. Duplication of this publication or parts thereof is permitted only under the provisions of the German Copyright Law of September 9, 1965, in its current version, and permission for use must always be obtained from Springer-Verlag. Violations are liable for prosecution under the German Copyright Law.

© Springer-Verlag Berlin Heidelberg 1998
Printed in Germany

The use of designations, trademarks, etc. in this publication does not imply, even in the absence of a specific statement, that such names are exempt from the relevant protective laws and regulations and therefore free for general use.

Cover Design: Künkel + Lopka, Heidelberg
Typesetting: Camera-ready by authors
Printed on acid-free paper SPIN 10649026 45/3142 5 4 3 2 1 0

Dedicated to
Rul Gunzenhäuser
on the occasion of his
65th birthday in September, 1998

Thomas Strothotte

Foreword

Many computer applications deal with communication. Far over twenty years, the use of text processors has been common practice in office environments. The field of computer graphics, one of the dominant fields in computer science, deals with the role of computers in (visual) communication. The emphasis of much of this work has been on the techniques of image generation, and efficient graphical interaction for a variety of application domains. It is interesting to note that, in the computer science community, relatively little attention has been paid to the underlying semantics of the communicated pictorial messages. This may be partly understood from the fact that the semantics of a message, communicated by computers, is not very different from a similar message communicated without computer assistance. Semiotics[1] has developed largely as a separate discipline from computer science.

A second reason for the long-lasting mutual ignorance between computer science (and computer graphics in particular) and semiotics may be that it requires sophisticated computer algorithms to represent the semantics of images. Until quite recently, the algorithms of image generation in themselves were sufficiently challenging to absorb the majority of the efforts in the field. Also, computer architecture and programming sophistication were not sufficiently developed to deal with the complicated task of representing the *meaning* of the rendered images.

In the next few years there will be an ongoing research effort in mainstream computer graphics, focussing, e.g., on hardware architectures for real-time rendering and increasingly advanced paradigms for geometric modeling and virtual reality. However, there is also a relatively new trend within computer graphics in which visual communication and interaction are indeed tied in with an explicit attention for the *meaning* of the communicated images. This relatively young branch of computer science is called *Computational Visualistics*.

Background

In order to understand the necessity of linking the visual aspects of an image with its meaning, which is one of the starting points of computational visu-

---

1 Semiotics: "...the study of patterned [...] communication behavior, including [...] signs and symbols." [Web90]

alistics, it may be illustrative to study an example first. Let us look at the evolution of the Western alphabet. Although the alphabet developed separately from the notion of computers, it is instructive to become aware of some of the issues regarding the representation of meaning that underly (dealing with) images – even if these images are just the individual characters of the alphabet.

In the Western alphabet, every letter is a little drawing, a distribution of dark on a light background, the result of many centuries of gradual transformations and artistic font design originating in ancient pictograms. For instance, the "A" shape apparently originated in an Egyptian hieroglyph of an eagle (ahom) in cursive hieratic writing.

A naturalistic drawing of an eagle is capable of conveying many anatomical attributes of an individual bird. However, in some cases the drawing does not refer to an individual bird, but to the more abstract notion of "an eagle" in general, for instance in a pamphlet that has the purpose of instructing shepherds to watch out for eagles. Now the artist responsible for drawing this "generic eagle" faces a conceptual difficulty. Which instance of the class "eagle" should he choose? To give a full account of the potential danger of eagles for sheep, the artist really should refer to all possible eagles in all possible postures. But it is clearly impossible to render this multitude of drawings.

Interestingly, it is not only *impossible* to draw all individual postures of all possible eagles, it is also *unnecessary*. In virtue of a powerful but mysterious mental process in the observer's mind, a drawing of one particular eagle, in one particular posture will automatically associate with the class of all possible eagles[2] in all possible postures. This process, which we will call *implicit generalization* is a peculiar phenomenon. Implicit generalization is nothing that has to be negotiated between the artist and the observer. It occurs automatically, and it is probably one of the reasons that human beings do rather well in an environment where successful recognition and classification of similar, but different things (food, enemies, mates, etc.) is critical in order to survive.

In the case of pictorial artifacts, however, implicit generalization takes on more baroque forms. One reason for this is that not all artists are capable of the perfect impressions[3] we assumed above. And even a skilled artist is sometimes in a hurry. So undoubtedly, less perfect drawings of eagles have been around, some with wrong proportions, some with few details, indeed, some highly schematic.

Implicit generalization in the case of the pragmatic meaning of an eagle as a potentially dangerous large bird of prey may carry over to other species,

---

2 note: not only all existing eagles, but even all possible eagles!
3 We could call such impressions "photorealistic", although in this context the invention of photography was still some 3900 years in the future and the usage of the word "photorealistic" in the sense now used by computer graphics practitioners yet another hundred years later ...

such as falcons or buzzards. But there is a limit to the scope of this generalization. The abstraction will probably never include larks or blackbirds, or leopards or wolfs.

The implicit generalization of the pragmatic meaning of *pictures*, however, is much more "contagious". First, this may be due to the imperfection of the picture. If the artist leaves out sufficient details the observer may be able to make a successful mental match between the picture and all creatures with wings, including lark and blackbirds, but also bats and dragon-flies. Or even with all roughly V-shaped objects, depending on the simplicity of the picture.

But implicit generalization does not even stop here. After some time, the schematic picture of the eagle may also refer to the word "eagle" instead of the object "eagle", and somewhat later to the sound of the word "eagle", and even later to the sound of the first letter of this word. And we have to realize that all these abstractions (or rather changes in the communication code) probably did not result from meticulously negotiated agreements between the artist and the observer. On the contrary, they most likely occurred largely unnoticed, and it would be interesting to know how much confusion was caused during the process.

Apart from implicit generalizations, and other highly confusing meaning-transformers, there is a second process going on that complicates the relation between pictures and the real world. The pictures themselves also seem to evolve according to their own, hidden laws, of which "changing aesthetics" and "artistic innovation" are merely the least mysterious ones. As a result, the implicitly generalized eagle has not only evolved into an "A", but also an A, an A, an A, an A, and an A and to many hundred more distributions of dark on a light background.

Over the last 4000 years, the process of creating and transforming pictures and endowing them with evolving meaning, either concrete or abstract or a mixture of the two, has been a process of gradual evolution interspersed, every now and then, with a quantum leap (the introduction of phonetic alphabets, the invention of perspective, the usage of schematic drawings, the printing process, photography, impressionism, expressionism, abstract painting, ...). Each time, undoubtedly, there was some confusion after each jump, but the time lapse before the next one mostly allowed sufficient habituation to the new communication codes. Until the last couple of decades of the second millennium AD, when computers came along and everything started evolving in accordance with MOORE's law.[4]

In particular, the developments in computer graphics have caused a tremendous increase in the number of available options for visualizing both concrete and abstract information. But the focus of this work has been predominantly on the picture-making process (to be more precise: on the process of algorithmically imitating the physics of photography), and the ties

---

[4] The amount of computing power available per dollar's worth of hardware doubles every eighteen months.

between the pictures and their underlying semantics, as well as alternative strategies for picture generation, have been largely ignored. One lesson to be learned from our small thought experiments on the history of semiotics, outlined above, is that confusion is to be expected if the relation between pictures and their meaning is left unspecified, and new communication codes are introduced before the previous ones have been established.

Visual Representation and Meaning

As we mentioned in the introduction, the new research field of computational visualistics attempts to fill in some of the blank areas that have been left open by mainstream computer graphics research. The central theme in most of the research in computational visualistics has to do with the relation between the visual representation of images and their meaning. This relation is really two-directional:

1. The (visual) contents of an image should be such that this meaning is optimally communicated: the meaning dictates (part of) the pictorial contents;
2. Given the contents of an image, additional (non-graphical) communication modes can be used to support conveyance of its meaning: the pictorial contents dictate non-graphical attributes.

In the first category, there is a rich tradition, dating back to the pre-computer era, where non-photorealistic imaging techniques have been used. In fact, our short excursion to the origin of the Western alphabet is an example. Other examples are simplified drawings, or drawings in which deliberate alterations with respect to the depicted object(s) have been introduced. These drawings are often used in the context of teaching or instruction. The alterations may range from subtle modifications (e.g., local adjustments to the line style, size, or amount of detail), to completely symbolic renderings (organization charts, graphs). Halfway between these extremes we find geographic maps, architectural drawings and sketches, and so on. In many cases, the designer of these types of images is not, in an algorithmic sense, aware of the types of alterations he or she applies. Therefore, in order to program computers to render these types of images, one first has to carefully analyze and formalize the process of non-photorealistic picture-making. It has to be fully understood what choices a human artist would make when choosing levels of detail, line styles, hatching, and so on, as a function of the structure and meaning of the object or scene to depict. Next, there is the more technical challenge of formalizing these choices, and translating them into suitable algorithms.

With respect to the second category, we observe that in some cases even a photorealistic picture on its own is not sufficient to convey the intended meaning. An example would be where the picture is meant to be understood by a visually handicapped person; another example would be a situation in which non-graphical references to the objects in the picture are required (e.g., from an associated text). In both cases, a non-pictorial annotation is required, either in the form of a full non-graphical representation (e.g., a 1-D graph that is translated to a varying sound over time, or a tactile map), or in the form of well-placed textual labels or symbolic icons. In many applications we are confronted with the challenge of automating the process of non-graphical annotation, based on a formal representation of the picture's contents.

The two research fields above can be seen to enhance, extend, and build on traditional techniques in image making. Although this is nowadays much too laborious for large volume production, a human artist could in principle generate many of the visual effects discussed above. There are further research fields, however, where computer graphics have introduced drastically new paradigms in non-photorealistic image production. These are techniques such as selective zooming (enlarging those portions of an image of a 3-D model that are of current interest); manipulating the perspective of such images; (non-photorealistic) animation; synthetic holograms, and others. These are all techniques that only have become available over the last few years.

Perspectives

This book discusses in depth many of the research fields outlined above. It is an anthology of some of the results that have been obtained in Computational Visualistics in the University of Magdeburg over the last two years. Apart from the direct relevance of the methods and techniques, described in the sequel, much of the merit of this work lies in the dawning awareness that effective visual communication critically relies on both the pictorial and the semantic aspects of the communicated picture.

It is my sincere wish that this awareness will continue to inspire fruitful and groundbreaking research.

Eindhoven, The Netherlands, August 1998   *Kees van Overveld*

Preface

This book is about abstraction, or, in simple terms, how to change things in pictures, how to get away from the inherent precision with which computers display information. The topic evolved out of the observation that practically all pictures which have been made by hand deviate from an objective, exact representation of reality in some way, often even in many facets. By the same token, pictures generated by computers almost always have an aura of correctness about them. We hypothesize that certain areas of application of graphics will only become accessible to computer graphics if we get a firm grip on the topic of "changing things" by computers in pictures.

The Computer Graphics and Interactive Systems Laboratory of the University of Magdeburg has had as its goal for the last four years to discover how to "change things" in computer-generated pictures to the point where the pictures become more useful in areas which up to now have been restricted to hand-made graphics. The goal is not to emulate such hand-made graphics, but to make a contribution with computers to these areas.

This book represents the results of the 19 scientists who have worked together in the Laboratory over the last few years. Practically all the work reported has been published previously in refereed conference proceedings. The more polished versions appearing in this book are structured so as to emphasize the methodology they have in common. Hence certain ideas which appear in various parts of the book are shown to be of wide applicability through the diverse areas of application.

The work was carried out within the Faculty of Computer Science of the University of Magdeburg. The Faculty specializes in combining knowledge engineering and image science. This specialization is manifested in the Faculty's degree programs in the area which has been termed *Computational Visualistics* – the study of how pictures are created, stored, transmitted, and analyzed by computers as well as perceived, understood, and processed by computer users. To this end, considerable thought is given in the book to the relationship between language and pictures. The ultimate goal is to make pictures a more flexible medium of presentation of information, and even to give pictures some of the degrees of freedom which language enjoys.

The authors wish to thank those who funded their research. In particular, funds from the University of Magdeburg, the State of Saxony-Anhalt, the German Research Foundation (DFG), and the European Union under the programs "Technology for Disabled and Elderly People" (TIDE) as well as "Human Capital and Mobility" (HCM) contributed to make this research possible.

Quite a number of persons collaborated to turn the original manuscript into a publishable book. The finishing touches on the book were painstakingly applied by Stefan Schlechtweg, who paid particular attention to the layout and the uniformity of the bibliography, and Bert Schönwälder, who worked on the index, the final corrections, and the layout. They were assisted by Ronny Schulz and Birger Schmidt, who prepared the figures. The expertise provided by the Institute's clerical and administrative staff (Petra Specht, Sylvia Zabel, and Petra Janka) proved once again to be invaluable. Ian Pitt and Sylvia Zabel patiently proofread the manuscript. At Springer-Verlag, the copy-editing was carried out by J. Andrew Ross, while Peter Strasser produced and Dr. Hans Wössner published the book. Many thanks to all these persons for their diligent support of our work.

Magdeburg, Germany, August 1998 *Thomas Strothotte*

Contents

I Introduction ... 1

1 New Challenges for Computer Visualization ... 3
1.1 Non-Computer Visualizations ... 4
    1.1.1 Examples ... 4
    1.1.2 Features ... 8
    1.1.3 Observation ... 8
1.2 Computer Visualization: Exploring Complex Information Spaces ... 9
    1.2.1 Information Spaces ... 9
    1.2.2 Requirements for Dialog Systems ... 11
1.3 Abstraction in Interactive Computer Visualization ... 13
    1.3.1 Abstraction ... 13
    1.3.2 Abstraction in the Exploration of Complex Information Spaces ... 14
1.4 Research Topics ... 15

2 Exploration of Complex Information Spaces ... 19
Bernhard Preim

2.1 Orientation in Complex Information Spaces ... 21
2.2 Fisheye Views: A Step Towards Abstraction ... 23
2.3 Applications of Fisheye Views ... 25
    2.3.1 Filtered Views on Source Code ... 25
    2.3.2 Distorting Views of Graphs and Maps ... 26
    2.3.3 Multiple Foci ... 28
    2.3.4 Fisheye Views of Hypertext Structures ... 28
    2.3.5 Fisheye Views for Supervisory Control Systems ... 29
    2.3.6 Zooming Windows ... 29
2.4 Comprehensible Fisheye Views ... 30
2.5 Fisheye Views for 3D Data ... 33
    2.5.1 Implicit 3D Fisheye Views ... 33
    2.5.2 Explicit 3D Fisheye Views ... 36
2.6 Nonlinear Magnification ... 37
2.7 Comparing Visualizations of Information Spaces ... 39
2.8 Abstraction in Computer Graphics ... 40
2.9 Abstraction in User Interfaces ... 42
2.10 Summary ... 43

3 Enrichment and Reuse of Geometric Models 45
Bernhard Preim and Axel Hoppe

- 3.1 Requirement Analysis 46
  - 3.1.1 Basic Terms 47
  - 3.1.2 Information Visualization 49
  - 3.1.3 Interaction Facilities to Explore and Enrich Geometric Models 50
- 3.2 Related Work 50
  - 3.2.1 Integration of Geometry and Structure View 51
  - 3.2.2 Visualization and Interaction in Hierarchical Structures . . 51
  - 3.2.3 Observations in Graphics Editors 52
- 3.3 An Approach to Reuse and Enrich Models 53
  - 3.3.1 Design of an Enrichment Tool 54
  - 3.3.2 Modification of the Object Structure 55
  - 3.3.3 Navigating in the Structure View 55
  - 3.3.4 Navigating in the Geometry View 57
  - 3.3.5 Tight Coupling of Structure View and Geometry View . . . 59
  - 3.3.6 Implementation 60
- 3.4 Concluding Remarks 61

II Controlling Detail 63

4 Rendering Line Drawings for Illustrative Purposes 65
Stefan Schlechtweg and Andreas Raab

- 4.1 Related Work 67
- 4.2 An Analytic Rendering Pipeline 69
- 4.3 Hidden Line Elimination 71
  - 4.3.1 Method I: Quad Tree Based Algorithm 72
  - 4.3.2 Method II: Scan-Line Based Algorithm 76
- 4.4 Drawing the Lines – Shading 78
  - 4.4.1 Line Selection and Chaining 79
  - 4.4.2 Special Line Drawing Techniques 80
- 4.5 Illustrating with Lines 84
  - 4.5.1 Drawing the Contour 84
  - 4.5.2 Shading Techniques 85
- 4.6 Applications and Open Problems 88

5 Rendering Line Drawings of Curved Surfaces 91
Frank Godenschweger and Hubert Wagener

- 5.1 Generation of Meshes 92
  - 5.1.1 Conventional Line Drawings of Freeform Surfaces Versus Evenly Spread Meshes 92
  - 5.1.2 Mathematical Background 94

5.2	Analytic Freeform Surface Rendering Pipeline		96
	5.2.1	Outline Generation	97
	5.2.2	Texture Generation	98
5.3	How to Add Shadow		99
5.4	Examples		101
5.5	Conclusions and Future Work		102

6 Pixel-Oriented Rendering of Line Drawings — 105
Oliver Deussen

6.1	Previous Work		106
6.2	A Pixel-Oriented Graphics Pipeline		107
	6.2.1	Basic G-Buffers	107
	6.2.2	G-Buffer Operators	108
	6.2.3	Half-Toning Using Short Hatching Lines	112
	6.2.4	Generating Long Hatching Lines by Intersections	114
	6.2.5	Half-Toning Using Long Hatching Lines	115
	6.2.6	Computer Generated Copper Plates	117
6.3	Concluding Remarks		118

7 Measuring and Highlighting in Graphics — 121
Axel Hoppe and Kathrin Lüdicke

7.1	Related Work	124
7.2	Approaches and Techniques in Paintings	124
7.3	Theoretical Background	127
7.4	Measuring Color Contrasts	128
7.5	Animation Analysis	129
7.6	Color Discontinuity	131
7.7	Discontinuity in Motion	131
7.8	Emphasizing Objects	132
7.9	Results	135

III Adaptive Zooming and Distorting Graphics — 137

8 Distortions and Displacements in 2D — 139
Rainer Michel and Jörg Hamel

8.1	Methods for Distortions		140
8.2	Distortions Along Linear Features		141
8.3	The Focus Line Distortion		142
	8.3.1	Defining the Shape of the Distortion	143
	8.3.2	Defining the Amount of Distortion	146
8.4	The Interactive Focus Line		148
8.5	Concluding Remarks		149

9 Zooming in 1, 2, and 3 Dimensions ... 151
Andreas Raab and Michael Rüger

- 9.1 Fisheye Zoom Technique ... 152
  - 9.1.1 The Continuous Zoom Approach ... 152
  - 9.1.2 Dimension Independent Zoom ... 154
- 9.2 Visual Constraints ... 157
  - 9.2.1 Recognition Constraints ... 157
  - 9.2.2 Shape Constraints ... 158
  - 9.2.3 Transition Constraints ... 159
  - 9.2.4 Connectivity Constraints ... 159
- 9.3 Conclusions ... 160

10 Zoom Navigation ... 161
Michael Rüger, Bernhard Preim, and Alf Ritter

- 10.1 Zoom Navigation ... 162
  - 10.1.1 Degree of Interest ... 163
  - 10.1.2 Representation ... 164
- 10.2 Aspect of Interest ... 164
- 10.3 The Pluggable Zoom ... 166
- 10.4 The ZOOMNAVIGATOR ... 168
- 10.5 The ZOOMILLUSTRATOR ... 169
  - 10.5.1 API, DOI, and AOI in the ZOOMILLUSTRATOR ... 171
  - 10.5.2 Selection Using the AOI ... 173
- 10.6 Conclusion and Future Work ... 174

IV Textual Methods of Abstraction ... 175

11 From Graphics to Pure Text ... 177
Ian Pitt

- 11.1 Giving Blind People Access to Graphics ... 177
  - 11.1.1 Blind People's Understanding of Graphical Concepts ... 178
  - 11.1.2 Text Versus Tactile Graphics ... 182
- 11.2 Graphics Versus Text ... 184
  - 11.2.1 Fundamental Differences Between Graphics and Text ... 184
  - 11.2.2 What to Translate, What to Ignore ... 186
- 11.3 Translating Graphics to Text – Technical Issues ... 187
- 11.4 Presenting the Text ... 190
- 11.5 Conclusions ... 195

12 Figure Captions in Visual Interfaces 197
Bernhard Preim and Rainer Michel
12.1 Figure Captions in Print Media 198
    12.1.1 Figure Captions in Anatomical Atlases 199
    12.1.2 Figure Captions and Legends for Maps 200
    12.1.3 Generalized Structure of Figure Captions 202
12.2 Related Work 203
12.3 Dynamic Figure Captions 203
    12.3.1 Layout Considerations 204
    12.3.2 Adaptable Figure Captions 204
    12.3.3 Updating Figure Captions 205
12.4 Interactive Figure Captions 206
12.5 Integration of Figure Captions in Interactive Systems 208
    12.5.1 Template-Based Generation 208
    12.5.2 An Architecture for Figure Captions in Visual Interfaces . 209
    12.5.3 Basic Scheme 210
    12.5.4 Representation of Events 212
12.6 Concluding Remarks 212

13 Interactive 3D Illustrations with Images and Text 215
Bernhard Preim
13.1 Related Work 217
    13.1.1 Generating Illustrated Documents 217
    13.1.2 Interactive Anatomical Illustrations 218
    13.1.3 Fisheye Techniques to Explore 3D Models
            and Related Text 218
    13.1.4 3D Fisheye Zoom 219
13.2 Consistency of Rendered Images and Their Textual Labels 219
13.3 Architecture 220
13.4 Zoom Techniques for Illustration Purposes 222
    13.4.1 Zoom Techniques for Navigation in Textual Information . 224
    13.4.2 Zoom Techniques for the Exploration of a 3D Model . . . 226
    13.4.3 Adaptive Graphical Zoom 226
    13.4.4 Enhancing Navigation in Textual Information 227
13.5 Interactive Handling of Images and Text 230
    13.5.1 Managing Consistency when Geometric
            Transformations Occur 231
    13.5.2 Implementation Issues 233
13.6 Figure Captions for Anatomical Illustrations 234
    13.6.1 Important Parameters of Visualizations 235
    13.6.2 Examples 237
13.7 Concluding Remarks 239

V Abstraction in Time 241

14 Animating Non-photorealistic Computer Graphics 243
Maic Masuch and Frank Godenschweger

14.1 A Brief Introduction 243
    14.1.1 Traditional Animation 244
    14.1.2 Computer Animation 246
    14.1.3 Principles of Animation 246
14.2 Non-photorealistic Computer Animation 248
    14.2.1 Why Use Non-photorealistic Computer Animation? . . . 248
    14.2.2 Problems Using Existing Concepts 249
    14.2.3 Rendering Non-photorealistic Computer Animation . . . 250
14.3 Animating Paintings 250
14.4 Animating Line Drawings 252
    14.4.1 Animating Polygonal Models 252
    14.4.2 Animating Curved Surfaces 254
    14.4.3 Animating Line Styles 255
14.5 Future Work 256

15 Interaction Facilities and High-Level Support for Animation Design 259
Ralf Helbing and Bernhard Preim

15.1 Related Work 260
15.2 Creating Animations from High-Level Specifications 263
15.3 Theoretical Foundations 263
15.4 Animation for Educational Purposes 266
    15.4.1 Design of Animation Techniques 266
    15.4.2 Data Structures 267
    15.4.3 Script Language 268
    15.4.4 Architecture 269
    15.4.5 Implementation and Examples 269
15.5 Film Techniques in Technical Animation 271
    15.5.1 Design of Animation Techniques for Technical Animation 273
    15.5.2 Creating Animation Sequences 274
15.6 Concluding Remarks 276

VI Abstractions in Interactive Systems 279

16 Zoom Navigation in User Interfaces 281
Michael Rüger, Kornelia Ullrich, and Ian Pitt

16.1 Prior and Related Work 282
16.2 The Zoom Navigator 283
16.3 Zooming Windows 286

16.4	User Study	288
	16.4.1 General Setting	288
	16.4.2 Hypotheses	288
	16.4.3 Variables	289
	16.4.4 Subjects	289
	16.4.5 Overall Experiment Structure	289
	16.4.6 Experiment Tasks	290
	16.4.7 Collection of Data	290
	16.4.8 Results	291
	16.4.9 Interview	292
16.5	Conclusion and Future Work	293

17 Interactive Medical Illustrations   295
Stefan Schlechtweg and Hubert Wagener

17.1	Interactive Medical Illustration	296
17.2	A Text-Driven Illustration System	298
	17.2.1 The Information Space	299
	17.2.2 Coupling of Graphics and Text	302
	17.2.3 Interaction Support	303
17.3	Comparison to Other Approaches	305
	17.3.1 The Zoom Illustrator	306
	17.3.2 VoxelMan	307
	17.3.3 Other Graphics-Driven Systems	308
	17.3.4 Knowledge-Based Systems	308
17.4	The Road Ahead	309

18 Rendering Gestural Expressions   313
Frank Godenschweger and Hubert Wagener

18.1	The Problem of Visualizing Human Bodies	314
18.2	Drawing Optimization for Gestures	315
	18.2.1 Representing the Hand and Its Movement	315
	18.2.2 Temporal Control	316
18.3	Animation of Gestures for the Manual Alphabet	317
	18.3.1 Interactive Dialogs for Library Maintenance	317
	18.3.2 Building Gesture Sequences	318
18.4	Generating Line Drawings of Freeform Surfaces	319
	18.4.1 The Rendering Process	319
	18.4.2 Demonstration of Drawing Styles	321
18.5	Conclusions and Future Work	322

19 Animation Design for Simulation   325
Ralf Helbing

19.1	Using Simulation to Create Animation Models	326
19.2	Problems in Generating Animations	328
19.3	Plugins for Visualization Modeling	329

19.4 Trace Conversion in a Plugin Based Framework 330
19.5 Future Work 334

VII Abstraction for Specialized Output 337

20 Tactile Maps for Blind People 339
Rainer Michel

20.1 Customized Maps 341
20.2 Map Creation 342
    20.2.1 Data Sources 342
    20.2.2 Map Layout 344
20.3 Symbol Displacement 345
    20.3.1 Overview 345
    20.3.2 Requirements 345
    20.3.3 Detection and Analysis of Conflicts 347
    20.3.4 Displacement 350
20.4 Communicating the Map Fidelity 351
20.5 Concluding Remarks 354

21 Synthetic Holography 359
Alf Ritter and Hubert Wagener

21.1 Holography as a 3D Visualization Technique 359
    21.1.1 Optical Holography 359
    21.1.2 Synthetic Holography 361
    21.1.3 3D Display Techniques to Provide Depth Cues 361
21.2 Methods of Synthetic Holography 363
21.3 Where Holography and Common Computer Graphics Meet . . . 365
    21.3.1 Holograms of Objects Composed of Line Segments 365
    21.3.2 Implementation 368
    21.3.3 A New Approach to Holographic Imaging of Lines 369
    21.3.4 Results 373
21.4 Future Work 376

VIII Epilog 377

22 Abstraction Versus Realism: Not the Real Question 379
Jörg R. J. Schirra and Martin Scholz

22.1 The Naïve Opposition of Abstraction and Realism 379
22.2 Three Examples of Functional Pictures 380
22.3 Several Kinds of Realism 384
22.4 Images as Signs: Considerations from Communication Theory . . 388
22.5 Abstraction in Realism 392
22.6 Realism in Abstraction 397
22.7 Abstraction *and* Realism: Conclusions 399

23 Integrating Spatial and Nonspatial Data 403
23.1 Pictures, Lies, and Abstract Data Types 403
23.2 Spatial and Nonspatial Data 406
23.3 Continuity and Discontinuity in Abstraction 407
        23.3.1 Continuity 408
        23.3.2 Discontinuity 408
        23.3.3 A Comparison Between Image and Language Generation 411
23.4 Conveying Allowable Operations to Viewers of Images 412
        23.4.1 Graphical Comprehension Cues 412
        23.4.2 Linguistic Comprehension Cues 414
        23.4.3 Comparison 415
23.5 The Bottom Line 416

Copyrights 419

Bibliography 421

Index of Names 443

Subject Index 449

Contributors 455

Part I

Introduction

This part sets the stage for the study of the process of abstraction by surveying the current situation in visualization and interaction.

In Chap. 1, Thomas STROTHOTTE observes that computational visualization has yet to have an effect upon a variety of areas of application in which the manual design of images dominates. He shows that a fundamental difference between the images in these areas of application and computer-generated images lies in the fact that many aspects of hand-drawn images do not actually correspond to a correct geometric model of the objects being portrayed. Indeed, computational visualization is generally viewed as the process by which a model is rendered; instead, he suggests that the process of computational visualization can be viewed as an exploration of what he calls a complex information space. The key to the visualization is learning to cope with the differences between straightforward renditions and ones which are modified so as to achieve a particular effect on the viewer. He proposes a definition of abstraction and sets the design and implementation of methods and tools for application as a medium-range research goal. In essence, all the topics addressed in this book chip away at various aspects of the overall problem.

Complex information spaces and their exploration have been studied by a variety of other authors in recent years. Chapter 2, by Bernhard PREIM, surveys the major work in this area, concentrating in particular on fisheye visualization techniques. These techniques have been applied widely in the literature and are an effective way of distorting an image so as to have more screen space for important items, while less important items use less screen space. The chapter concludes with a discussion of the notion of abstraction in the context of the literature surveyed.

It becomes evident that geometric models alone cannot lead to the kinds of visualizations needed to make a contribution to the wider applicability of computational visualizations. Hence Bernhard PREIM and Axel HOPPE address in Chap. 3 the question how geometric models can be enriched to include more information. They survey existing graphical editors for geometric models and then turn to the design and implementation of a new tool for structuring and enriching geometric models. While such a tool is the prerequisite for preparing geometric models for abstraction in the visualization process, the editor itself draws on some of the methods and tools designed later on in the book.

Chapter 1

New Challenges for Computer Visualization

Practically all images which meet the human eye today can, in principle, be classified as computer graphics. Some images are produced from raw numeric, symbolic or geometric data obtained from application programs. Most diagrams are produced with spreadsheets or drawing programs. Many photographs are scanned and postprocessed to improve the quality of the colors; such graphics are tuned in a highly interactive process involving users who are experts at such tasks.

To analyze the utility of images, it is useful to differentiate between graphics where a user has expended a great deal of effort only in the design of a single, specific image, and those where the main effort has gone into describing, and perhaps even designing, the object being portrayed, while the visualization has been created more or less automatically. Indeed, the latter are most interesting from the point of view of the customization for which the current trend in net-based computing calls. What is required are methods and tools for flexibly creating images which suit the current information needs of end-users.

We shall use the term *computer visualization* for the process of generating images by computer algorithms based primarily on a description of the geometry of the objects to be portrayed. Further, we refer to such descriptions as *geometric models*. The emphasis of this book is on areas of application which have so far eluded the widespread use of computer visualization in this sense. Our aim is to learn more about the nature and composition of such visualization with the goal of making visualizations in these applications more accessible to customization by end-users. In insisting on customization, we go beyond the process of rendering ("going from a three-dimensional object to a two-dimensional shaded projection on a view-surface" [Wat93]) by considering the effect of sources of information, other than the purely geometric model, and by going beyond shaded projections.

Throughout the book we shall deal continuously with user interaction. The term "(end-)user" sometimes refers to the person ultimately in need of information, such as a medical student wanting to look up the answer to a specific question in anatomy, or an engineer consulting technical documentation so as to find a bug in a production line. The term "user" may also denote the person providing or organizing information so that the aforementioned (end-)user will be able to find the information being sought. Finally, the term "user" often also refers to the toolsmith, i.e., the computer scientist who devises the software tools others work with. The context of each occurrence of the term "user" determines which of these users is being referred to. In any case, the activities of the various different kinds of users are at the center of our attention throughout the book.

1.1 Non-Computer Visualizations

In a wide variety of application areas, pictures are routinely used which are, in fact, not based on computer visualization in the sense defined above. We shall examine a number of examples of such pictures and study where the problems might lie which have hindered computer visualization.

1.1.1 Examples

Example 1: Medical Illustrations
Despite an immense research effort in medical imagery in recent years, there is still a wide range of examples of images used by medical students and in reference materials which were devised with traditional methods. Figure 1.1 shows an example of a drawing taken from a book on surgery. Notice the fine detail in places where it is needed for the task at hand; other parts of the image which are not particularly relevant are shown with less detail, or are even left blank. Some images are in fact relatively old and are so well done that they have been used in many textbooks for decades. Despite the advent of newer drawing techniques, clearly no one has been able to surpass some of these old drawings in quality. Drawing is often used not only by illustrators to record observations, but also as a vehicle to make observations. Indeed, artists often look down upon photography, which they say does not further their process of seeing objects and their qualities [KE93].

The technology does not yet exist to render images like that of Fig. 1.1 from geometric models. There are a number of key reasons for this inability to produce such images:

- *Missing motivation within the research community.*
  The focus of practically all research in computer graphics has been on

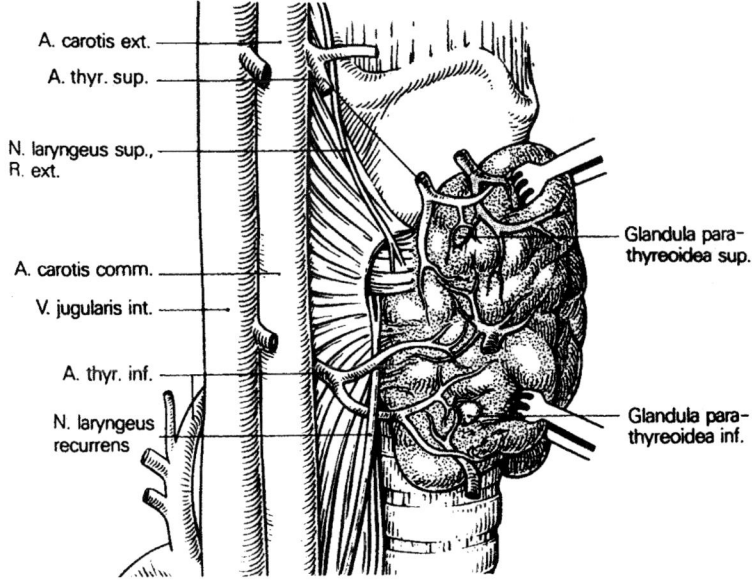

Figure 1.1: Example of a drawing taken from a textbook on surgery [VKPW82]

so-called *photorealism*. Sophisticated methods to produce images in other styles, such as line drawings, are only just emerging.

- *Context-sensitivity.*
  Visualization software has generally been designed to run independently of the specific application. While this clearly has its advantages, the approach fails when specific needs of an application have to be addressed, because the software typically cannot be sufficiently parameterized. In the example, details in the image have been selected and even emphasized to fit the context of its use. Often such images are not even drawn to scale, but show important parts somewhat larger so that the appropriate level of detail can be attained.

Example 2: Architectural Sketches in an Early Design Phase

Architects designing buildings generally begin their work by drawing simple sketches. Indeed, this process of drawing is one which serves not only to communicate their ideas to others, but also to develop further these ideas. Examples of such sketches are shown in Fig. 1.2.

After carrying out an initial design with "pencil and paper", most architects move to a computer to continue their work with a computer-aided design system. Since most such systems only have software for rendering shaded images or wire frames which are both often deemed inappropriate (see [SKS95]), architects are known to place tracing paper over their ren-

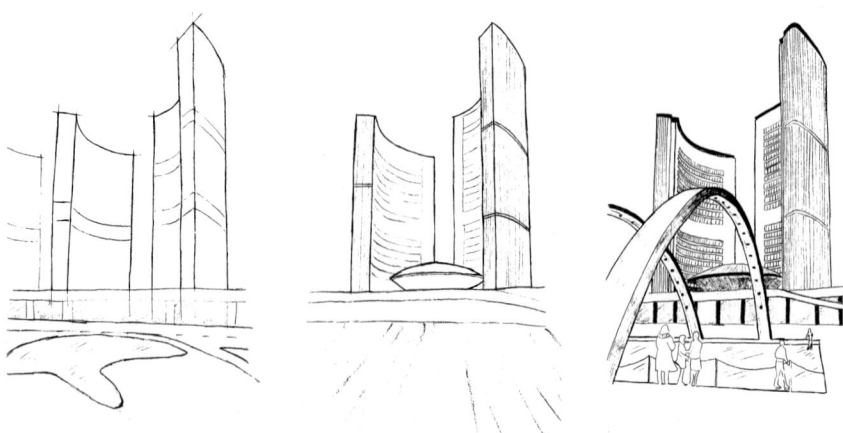

Figure 1.2: Examples of architectural sketches in an early design phase

dered computer output and to trace over the image by hand. This tracing is then used in discussions with clients. This latter situation shows that the process of computer visualization is inadequate for certain situations in which architects need to carry out their work, and hand-drawn images are preferred. This has a number of reasons:

- In an early design phase, an architect's ideas are but vague. No tools exist for enabling an architect to model such vague geometric data. Such modeling must be quick to carry out and should have some positive side effects over and above those gained with the "pencil-and-paper" approach.
- Tools to support computer visualization are lacking in their ability to produce vague images. Facilities are needed to encode visual cues into images which reflect the degree of completeness of the underlying model.
- Computer output tends to lack the esthetic appeal of hand-drawn images. More effort should be expended along the lines of WINKENBACH and SALESIN [WS94], STROTHOTTE et al. [SPR+94], and SCHUMANN et al. [SSRL96] on producing more interesting images as the result of computer visualization.

Example 3: Specialized Maps
Despite the advent of geographic information systems, maps devised for special purposes are still commonly produced with a great deal of manual manipulation. An extreme example is the subway map of Berlin shown in Fig. 1.3. Needless to say, the layout of the map does not reflect the details of the topography of the actual subway, as the lines are not really as straight, the angles not the same as in the figure, and the distances distorted so that the map fits the space available and appears esthetically pleasing. Despite, or

perhaps because of, these changes with respect to the real topography, users of the subway system are able to use these maps for their intended purpose, which is to convey which train(s) to take for how long in order to get from station A to station B.

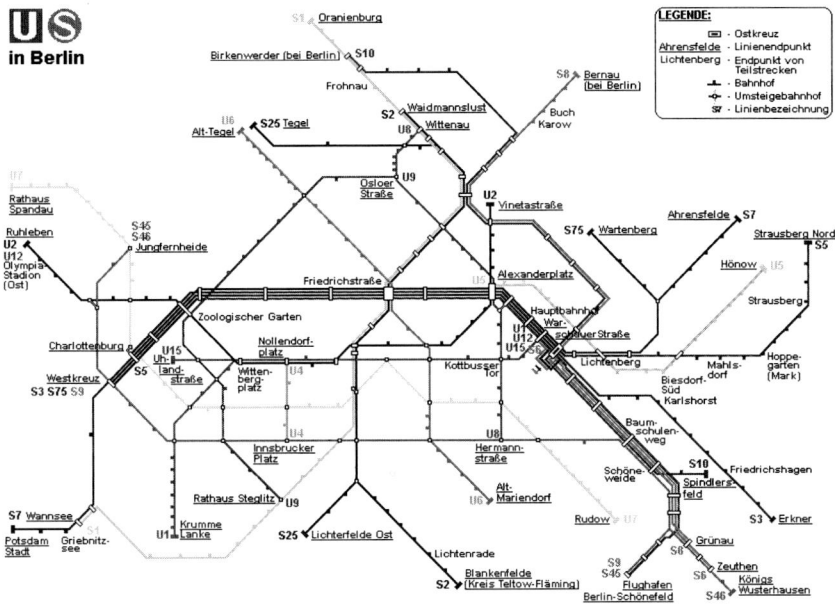

Figure 1.3: Subway system in Berlin

Despite the popular opinion that maps are precise and "tell the truth," cartographers have a whole range of techniques for enhancing maps so that their "message" can be ascertained by their users. In particular, small maps of large areas force cartographers to carry out a process of *generalization* to remove detail and make room for features and landmarks deemed important. Thus, for example, on maps of cities, the downtown portion is sometimes drawn in a different scale because more detail must typically be shown [MS97, HG94a]. The scale is adapted even more when designers, instead of cartographers, create maps for very specific purposes, and whose major claim to fame is their esthetic appeal rather than their correctness.

The techniques which cartographers have developed are not included in their full generality in software for generating maps. It is still a creative process when a cartographer combines the methods available to achieve a good map. This process has eluded automation thus far.

1.1.2 Features

The examples shown in the previous section have a number of features in common:

1. *Creativity.*
   Designing the visualization is a creative process involving a series of decisions by a "visualization expert", be this, for example, a medical illustrator, a photographer, or an industrial designer. While there may be certain guidelines or heuristics which such persons follow, these only form the basis of their work; the work of such experts is highly sophisticated.
2. *Informative nature of the images.*
   The goal of the visualization is *to inform* (or, as FOLEY et al. [FvDFH90] put it, *to convey information to*) a group of end-users ("readers"). This means that the communicative nature of the image is known to the person devising the visualization. Moreover, the images are designed mostly to be presented in unison with surrounding text. Both the images as well as the text focus on certain aspects which are considered to be of importance by the person producing the visualization.
3. *Correctness and completeness.*
   The visualization strives neither for completeness nor for correctness of all aspects and details of the information which could possibly be encoded in the image. Instead, certain aspects which are irrelevant for the end-user's application may be missing, or may even be misleading (recall in particular the map of the subway).

The task of the person devising a visualization, i.e., the person using the tools which computer scientists have developed to aid the process of computer visualization, can be construed as one of search and selection. He or she

- must find out what information is available which can be presented to the user, and
- must then select which pieces of information ought actually be encoded in the image.

The latter process of selection is complicated by the fact that methods and tools are required for emphasizing or deemphasizing certain pieces of information in an image; hence the importance of each piece must be assessed in the context in which the visualization is to be used.

1.1.3 Observation

It must be apparent by now that the usual procedure for producing visualization by computer is fundamentally different from that for producing visualization in the areas of application mentioned above which, indeed, have eluded computerization. In computer visualization, the emphasis has traditionally been on encoding as much information as possible (and necessary) in the geometric model, upon which standard, application-independent rendering tools produce the visualization without any particular creative input. Indeed, the creativity is invested in constructing the geometric model (this modeling is also carried out with application-independent modeling software). By contrast, producing images of the type shown in Sect. 1.1.1 involves a creative process of observation of the object to be visualized, taking into consideration the context in which the information will be used. The product of this process of observation is a visualization. This visualization is delicate in the sense that every detail encoded in it is important and many details are interrelated. On the other hand, unimportant details may be left out or otherwise changed so as to deemphasize them.

We hypothesize that in order to tackle successfully areas of application such as we surveyed above, computer visualization must be construed as a process of *observation* of an information space available to the end-user in need of information. The user best able to assess the information needs to be addressed by the image must search for relevant details among all available information, and must carry out a prioritized selection. It is this process of observation to which we refer as computer visualization.

1.2 Computer Visualization Requires Exploring Complex Information Spaces

The information available about any given scene or situation to be visualized is typically abundant and highly complex, even contradictory. While the models used in computer graphics have up to now focused primarily on the geometry of objects, other areas of computer science have concentrated on models which typically lead to output in the form of text, like words or even whole sentences, numbers, or formatted tables with textual entries. However, the combination of models used for rendering in combination with models yielding text-based output have received little attention in the graphics community.

1.2.1 Information Spaces

We shall refer to such data as that defining the shape and physical appearance of objects as a *geometric model*. Furthermore, we shall define data not directly influencing the appearance of the objects as a *symbolic model*. Together we say that these models form an *information space*. (Later on in Chap. 3 we will refine these terms somewhat more, but these definitions suffice for this introductory discussion.) In the following some examples of these concepts are shown.

Example I

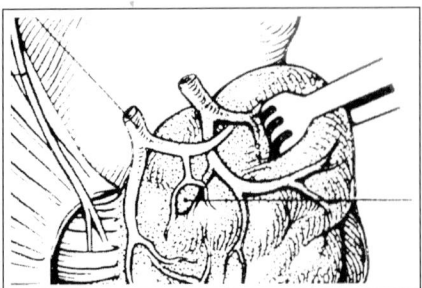

Geometric model:

- shape of parts, represented as polygons or voxels
- surface texture

Symbolic model:

- names of organs and parts
- hierarchy of parts
- function of parts

Example II

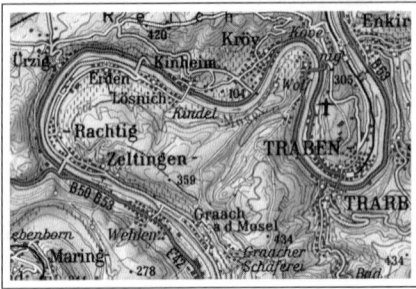

Geometric model:

- altitude at points
- polygons representing roads and rivers

Symbolic model:

- classification of roads
- classifications of cities (political, population)

Example III

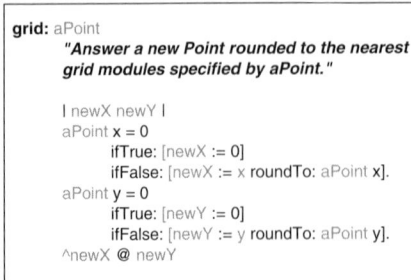

Geometric model:

- fonts
- size and position of window
- shading gray scale and colors

Symbolic model:

- type of window
- syntactic components
- Smalltalk code

It is important to realize that the structure of the information space has a marked effect on the process of its exploration by users, and on the process of computer visualization. Users in search of answers to specific questions need to be able to navigate efficiently in the information space. Furthermore, how this space is structured influences what graphical features can be encoded in the images resulting from the computer visualization.

It is instructive to examine the relationship between the process of exploring an information space and the traditional rendering process. A number of points yield interesting insights:

- *Information hiding*
  Although photorealistic renderers attempt to encode every detail of the geometric model in the picture, they are not successful, of course, as hidden surfaces have to be removed. In an analogous manner, computer visualization in connection with the exploration of complex information spaces also has to hide information. This hiding of information pertains both to the symbolic model as well as the geometric model. Clearly, only a small amount of the symbolic model available can actually have an effect on the visualization; however, as we saw in Examples I to III, not all information in the geometric model need be encoded in the resultant image, either.

- *Visualization of hierarchical structures*
  Rendered images generally do not reflect the object hierarchy of the underlying model, even if it is present. Furthermore, such hierarchies in geometric models generally have only been used to aid users organize and interact with models. For example, even in drawing programs, where objects can be grouped together, the hierarchy can be inspected by the user on the screen, but cannot be printed out (see STROTHOTTE and STROTHOTTE [SS97]). By contrast, we will see that the hierarchy of the objects will play an essential role in algorithms for producing computer visualization, particularly to emphasize the overall shape of individual objects.

The portions of the geometric and symbolic models which are to be visualized must influence one another in a way conventional rendering has not taken into account to date. For example, features which are to be labeled in a visualization should also be visible; such labeling may imply modifying the geometric model or the camera position. Indeed, labeling may in fact entail other changes to the underlying models so as to satisfy other constraints.

It is important to note that the process of observation in an information space must be carried out via an appropriate user interface. Since the product of this process is to be an image, interaction must be possible via such images. This means that data structures must be present which link features of the resultant images with objects and their attributes in the information space and information pertaining to decisions made in the process of visualization. Such data structures must be abundantly supplied to provide flexible interaction methods, but have generally been neglected because the images have been used primarily to look at on the part of users, rather than to support sophisticated interaction (STROTHOTTE and STROTHOTTE [SS97]).

1.2.2 Requirements for Dialog Systems

We now have a situation in which the symbolic part of the information space as well as information gained from the interaction with an end-user seeking information must influence the computer visualization. One of the key issues here is that it must be possible to produce compact presentations of complex data. Table 1.1 shows examples of contractions which are commonplace in symbolic models. Such contractions are generally used for a variety of specific reasons:

Table 1.1: Examples of extracts of symbolic models and the contractions

Extract of Symbolic Model	Contracted Form
List of numbers $5, 20, 10, 2$	Average and standard deviation: 9 ± 3
Ranges on the scale $1 \cdots 3, 4 \cdots 7, 8 \cdots 10$	Fuzzy variables: low, medium, high
Segment of the color spectrum	Name of a color: red

- *The details may not be known.*
  It may be that a more detailed complete symbolic model may not be available so that only the contracted form can be presented to a user. The fact that the composition of a piece of information is not available may in fact not be of relevance to the user.
- *The details may not be calculable.*
  In some cases, a user's query may be too imprecise so that the details may in fact not be calculatable. For example, if the user simply specifies "red" as the color of an object, the system has no way of knowing which of the wavelengths in the range 600 to 770 nm are actually meant. Hence a "red car" may in fact not be the right red color.
- *The details may not be important.*
  A contracted form of the symbolic model may be sufficient for the information needs at hand of the user. Often a user will not even want to get all details.
- *The presentation space or time may not be sufficient to warrant giving the details.*
  In some situations, it may be necessary to give a contracted form as output because there is not enough screen space available to present the complete results. Furthermore, if the context is one in which the user's time is at a premium, it may be more appropriate to give a contracted form so as to save reading time.

Hence there is a whole host of reasons why information extracted from symbolic models may be contracted in a presentation to a user. In fact, precisely the same may be necessary on the geometric side. Similar reasons for wanting to provide a contracted form apply; however, very little is known about algorithms to calculate contractions of information extracted from geometric models. Indeed, we have now arrived at one of the key problems which must be addressed to further the cause of computer visualization.

1.3 Abstraction in Interactive Computer Visualization

The last section called for a greater flexibility in the algorithmic treatment of geometric models than has previously been available. That is a tall order in its own right, but we see it in fact as a challenging opportunity to excel with respect to the new application areas for computer visualization. Although many methods and tools exist for managing symbolic models with respect to tuning the presentation to the specific needs in a particular situation at hand, we contend that there exists a major deficit with respect to geometric models. Indeed, most systems which generate images from geometric models do not modify in a substantial way the models of individual objects "on the fly", but rather stick to the pre-defined models of individual parts and instead concentrate on their composition and on camera settings and movements. In particular, there is an enormous potential in computer animation in making changes to geometric models over time so as to provide users with insights into the structure of the underlying models.

However, much more flexibility is required on the graphical side than is demonstrated by software currently available commercially or in research labs. In particular, what is required is a methodology for emphasizing certain graphical features, as well as for deemphasizing other geometric information. Even though some features described in the geometric model may be visible from the vantage point in question, others may still have to be removed. Rather than just performing hidden surface removal, some surfaces which are classified as being "hidden" in a rendering process may in fact be classified as "visible" in the process of computer visualization, as an obscuring surface can be made to be transparent. By the same token, not all objects which would, in principle, be visible ought to be shown, so that in a process of *selective visible surface removal* must be carried out. A less extreme case of the latter phenomenon is that certain information may be left partially visible. This process must be carried out in a systematic way; in short, what we need is a process of abstraction in computer visualization.

1.3.1 Abstraction

The term abstraction as it relates to the topic of this book is defined in dictionaries in basically two different ways. For example, the Pons dictionary [Pon94] refers to abstraction as "a general idea rather than one relating to a particular object, person or situation". By contrast, the German verb *abstrahieren* is defined in the Langenscheidt dictionary [Lan90] as "die wesentlichen Züge ableiten", or "to derive the essential features". The word abstraction (in its basic form, abstract) stems from the Latin *abstrahere*, meaning "to withdraw". Hence from the etymology of the term, the focus of the term is on removing (irrelevant or unnecessary) detail.

Viewing these definitions in the context of the goals defined at the outset of this chapter, a process of abstraction has something to do with leaving out information, i.e., removing certain graphical detail. Moreover, the process of abstraction has a well-defined purpose, i.e., to separate out important features from less important ones, and to make this choice evident for the viewer. However, leaving out some detail does not happen in isolation, but is also related to emphasizing other details or features. Indeed, in practical situations there may in fact be a continuum between encoding a feature and not encoding it. A graphical feature may even be artificially overemphasized (for example by directing a spotlight at it) in an effort to make clear what the "essential features" are without having to deemphasize or even remove entirely less essential features.

1.3.2 Abstraction in the Exploration of Complex Information Spaces

We define *abstraction* in a computer visualization as

> *a process by which an extract of an information space is refined so as to reflect the importance of the features of the underlying model for the dialog context and visualization goal at hand.*

This process of abstraction is carried out by the computer. However, an end-user exploring an information space influences the process of abstraction more or less directly by his or her conduct within the dialog initializing the process of computer visualization.

The decision as to what is important, and what is not, is generally computed from the data collected during the interaction which has taken place between the user and the system. This fact may seem obvious; nonetheless it is often overlooked in the literature, where images are often rendered without taking into account an end-user's situation. Most papers on rendering in the literature in fact do not at all consider interactive input from end-users.

The need for carrying out the process of abstraction may be any one of those discussed for symbolic models in Sect. 1.2.2. The process of abstraction is carried out in situations in which the context simply does not call for all details of the underlying geometric model to be encoded in the visualization. However, it is also necessary when the screen space prohibits the inclusion of detail (which would no longer be discernible anyway because of finite pixel size) or prohibits the use of many colors. Providing less detail can also reduce the cognitive load on the end-user [SSRL96].

For our purposes we view the following features of the process of abstraction as needing attention in tools for supporting computer visualization:

- *Gradually removing detail and adjusting the rendering style.*
  Details can be removed on a gradual scale by any one of or a combination of several techniques.

- *Adjusting the size, shape and orientation of parts of a model in combination with their level of detail and their style.*
  As we saw in the examples of Sect. 1.1.1, not only the level of detail is adjusted in applications which have thus far eluded computer visualization, but also the size, shape, and orientation of parts. WEIDENMANN [Wei89] refers to this process as *didactification*. While adjusting the level of detail is algorithmically challenging, even greater challenges are posed by adjusting the size, shape, and orientation of individual objects while still achieving smooth transitions between other parts of the visualization. Note that to adjust the size may also mean to make parts of an image smaller, particularly so as to deemphasize a part, but also to make room for other, more important parts.
- *Bringing text and graphics into unison with one another.*
  It is absolutely essential that computer visualization present the extracts of geometric and symbolic models in harmony with one another. This may require adjusting the geometric model or the symbolic model over and above the extract of the information space to make things "fit".

A number of studies have been carried out in which goals were set that are related to the ones outlined here. FURNAS [Fur86] described a process of abstraction analogous to the above for tree structures as well as program text. NOIK [Noi93] applied the three operations

- filtering (leaving out detail)
- distorting (enlarge important parts, reduce in size less important parts)
- adorn (emphasize important parts through presentation variables like color, font, and line style)

to hypertext presentations. SARKAR and BROWN [SB94] have done work on the two-dimensional layout of maps.

1.4 Research Topics

The research goals set in this chapter represent an ambitious research program which must be broken down in order that progress can be made on individual problems. The following organization of the topics to be addressed also corresponds to the structure of the chapters of this book into parts.

Abstraction in computer visualization raises the fundamental problems concerned with the style of visualization being strived for. As a method for achieving abstraction, it is particularly instructive to look at the emerging area of non-photorealistic rendering, as well as the combination of photorealistic images with non-photorealistic parts. This kind of rendering provides a wide range of freedoms of expression which are lacking even in state-of-the-art photorealistic rendering methods. However, it turns out that abstraction itself requires certain symbolic models; less detail in a computer visualization does not automatically mean that the underlying models may be less detailed, but, as we hypothesize, requires even richer models. These topics will be addressed in the following chapters of Part I.

Part II looks at algorithms and data structures for rendering visualization and controlling detail. In particular, rendering of line drawings provides the opportunity to emphasize shapes while leaving some surfaces blank, or at least without full detail. For this reason, indeed, line drawings offer the possibility to carry out abstraction in an unobtrusive manner. Moreover, lines form the complement to surfaces for expressing the shape of objects. Nonetheless, photorealistic images also provide the opportunity for abstraction by adding graphical features so as to emphasize certain pieces of information.

One of the more difficult tasks in the process of abstraction is to adjust the size of individual objects within what is to become a harmonious computer visualization. In Part III, the technique of fisheye zooming is highlighted from the point of view of abstraction. In particular, it is shown how this can be used as a paradigm for navigating in information spaces, and how the paradigm can be applied uniformly in one, two, and three-dimensional models. A particular problem of distortions in two-dimensional computer visualization is also examined in detail.

Given such a basis for abstraction at the geometric end of information spaces, Part IV turns to the navigation in symbolic models and the integration of text into computer visualization associated with this navigation. We begin with the extreme case of wanting to replace visualizations entirely by text. This is of value in some user interfaces for blind people and raises some interesting fundamental problems. Next, the question is examined how a small amount of additional information can be provided about an image to describe the process of abstraction in the form of figure captions. Finally, methods and tools are developed for integrating text directly into images in the form of annotations.

While snapshots or individual computer visualizations are of central interest, animation is ultimately of even greater importance and is studied in Part V. Rather fundamental questions quickly arise with respect to frame-to-frame coherence under the influence of abstraction in each frame. Furthermore, abstraction is also influenced to a strong extent by the choice of camera positions and camera paths which must be brought into unison with the kinds of images to be shown.

Up to this point in the book methods and tools have formed the focus. Part VI now turns to a collection of application areas. These deal with applications in which the visualizations are shown on normal computer screens. These applications are navigation in graphical user interfaces, medical illustrations, facial and gestural expressions, and technical documentation. Each application area uses a selection of the techniques developed in the first five parts. A rich selection of examples serves to demonstrate the viability of the concepts presented.

In Part VII we turn to specialized output, where, albeit for different reasons, abstraction also plays an important role. In synthetic holography, the computational effort to produce holograms must be reduced. Since the amount of processing necessary to produce a hologram is related to the level of detail in the resultant image, abstraction is an attractive technique. Furthermore, current technology enables the synthetic production of only small holograms (on the order of a few cubic centimeters in size), which also imposes restrictions in the amount of detail that can realistically be encoded in an image. Finally, tactile output for blind people also imposes severe restrictions as to the level of detail to be encoded in a graphic. Here it is important to reduce the amount of information to be displayed and simplify its form.

The concluding Part VIII discusses the results of our investigations in retrospect. First, fundamental issues related to the need for realism with respect to abstraction are examined. Then, problems related to mixing spatial and nonspatial data in visualizations are treated as a fundamental issue in abstraction.

Chapter 2

Presentation Techniques for Exploring Complex Information Spaces

Providing intuitive orientation aids and navigation techniques is essential to enable the exploration of information spaces. By *complex* information spaces we refer to information spaces which are not only large but also heterogenous in their structure. Complex information spaces are characterized, for example, by information which relates to different modalities (e.g., tables, graphics, and videos) and which may differ in their dimension.

Due to the increasing amount of data with which we have to cope, the exploration of complex information spaces is gaining in importance. Information exploration deals with interacting with data in order to extract meaningful information. Information exploration has several aspects:

- interaction facilities to browse in an information space and to search for information,
- information visualizations, which depict graphically an information space or search results, and
- analysis techniques to ease the interpretation of the data returned as result of search requests.

Information retrieval is concerned with how to get information with certain characteristics, for example the use of search engines to look for something on the Web is an information retrieval task. In general, information retrieval relies on a more or less concrete notion of what is being looked for.

Information visualization deals with how to depict an extract of an information space, how to visually communicate important features of data. Visualization techniques are particularly important for browsing through data to get new and unexpected insights about relations, that is, when one cannot specify exactly what one is looking for. However, even when a specific query can be formulated the results may be so complex (so many matching records) that an appropriate visualization may help to detect clusters and other important relationships. In these cases, visualization is a kind of data compression.

Finally, *data mining* is the discipline concerned with extracting information from the bulk of data that often results from queries to databases. Data mining includes techniques to look for characteristic patterns in data.

Information exploration is part of basic textbooks on human–computer interaction (see for example SHNEIDERMAN [Shn92]). Keyword search facilities, query languages, and queries which can be specified by example are important aspects in this field. In particular, dynamic queries are very effective. These queries are specified with sliders to define intervals of interesting attributes. As a result of the initiation of dynamic queries, a visualization is generated in which the regions corresponding to the specified query are highlighted. With dynamic queries, search facilities and visualization of results are closely integrated.

In this chapter we do not describe search facilities and query mechanisms but concentrate on the visualization aspect, on *presentation techniques*. These presentation techniques include emphasizing techniques to highlight data values or regions the user is interested in.

This chapter relates techniques for exploring complex information spaces to the concept of abstraction in graphical views. It turns out that views integrating portions at different levels of detail are a key concept for providing intuitive orientation marks during the exploration of complex information spaces. Many studies have shown that the traditional pan-and-zoom techniques alone are insufficient (see [HCMM89] and [SZB$^+$93]) with respect to these questions. An uniform zoom is forced to provide *either* local detail in sufficient resolution at the cost of neglecting the general context *or* an overview sacrificing the user's interest in special local details.

This chapter is organized as follows. In Sect. 2.1, the human ability to cope with large information spaces is analyzed. Based on this analysis, the need to integrate several levels of detail is derived. The general framework of fisheye views for human–computer interaction is described in Sect. 2.2. Included in this section is a classification of fisheye views. In Sect. 2.3, a variety of applications of this framework is presented, which show how powerful a technique fisheye views are. As fisheye views may distort a given layout, the question arises as to which manipulations are acceptable with respect to the user's comprehension. A discussion of this question is included in Sect. 2.4.

The generation of 3D views is attractive because 3D visualizations can incorporate visual cues we are accustomed to from our natural orientation, e.g., shadows and perspective foreshortening. 3D fisheye views are described in Sect. 2.5. While fisheye views rely on focus points and impose a magnification as a side effect, nonlinear magnification systems directly specify the desired magnification for parts of an information space. The basic ideas behind nonlinear magnification systems are explained in Sect. 2.6. Other

– more traditional – mechanisms, like bookmarks and interaction histories, have also turned out to be useful for user orientation. These mechanisms are described in Sect. 2.7.

In Sect. 2.8, the concepts for abstraction in 3D graphics and fisheye techniques are related to each other. User interfaces represent complex information spaces on their own. How to find the widget required to initiate the desired action may not be trivial. Therefore, in Sect. 2.9, methods of abstraction are described which ease the task of "exploring the user interface".

2.1 Orientation in Complex Information Spaces

Visual perception is the basis of enabling users to think. To this end, visualizations should support concentration on local details while providing an overview of important aspects of the context. WANDMACHER [Wan93] gives some characteristics of human vision. The resolution at the center of the retina is quite high – about one arcminute under ideal conditions – which enables *foveated vision*. Foveated vision allows us to concentrate on small areas, e.g., when reading. The resolution falls off rapidly outside the central 2 degree region. At 10 degrees eccentricity, the resolution is about 10 arcminutes.

Foveated vision is supplemented by the perception of dominant objects and movements in a larger range of about 30 degrees. This *peripheral vision* gives us a rough orientation and relates local details to the general context. Consequently, an effective visualization should present parts a user wants to concentrate on in detail while other information should be given in a simplified, abstract form.

Motivated by similar observations, FURNAS [Fur86] introduced fisheye views. FURNAS points out that our thinking concentrates on details that concern us immediately. At the same time, we have a rough comprehension of more distant objects or concepts. With increasing distance, our comprehension becomes less clear. For example, our knowledge of our own neighborhood is high, in other parts of our home town we are aware of the main streets, on a greater scale we only know major cities. Finally, on a global scale, we often know only the name of capitals. Our thinking is obviously determined by the *spatial distance* to locations (see GOULD and WHITE [GW86] who deal with mental maps).

Our knowledge of certain areas is not static. Once we move to another town we get to know in a new area, and at the same time our knowledge of other areas disappears slowly. However, no matter where we live in Germany we have an idea of some very important cities, like Berlin with its wall – these remain always known to us. If we talk to another person we can assume a priori that these places are known. These cities are thus *a priori important*.

Besides spatial aspects, other kinds of distances dominate our orientation. Our ability to remember events is clearly influenced by *temporal distance*, and again some key events remain important for us even after decades. Furthermore, the similarity of concepts is also important. Concepts may be directly associated with each other or be very distant in our cognitive model. NOIK [Noi93] coins the notion of *conceptual distance*. In the field of anatomy, for example, all muscles with a similar function, e.g., to stretch the hand, are conceptually related (and often learned together).

Abstraction is the key that enables us to work on different scales. In a geographic context, we use city maps for our orientation in the small, where areas with a high density of symbols (e.g., city centers or public parks) are often drawn on an even smaller scale allowing more detailed representation (see HAKE and GRÜNREICH [HG94a]). Thus regions with outstanding general interest can be emphasized.

Maps of nations, continents, or the world, help in orienting on higher levels. When working on a larger scale, pieces of neighboring information are aggregated and represented in a simplified form. To give an example involving the temporal aspect, consider the news. Only a few news items from a given day find their way into a weekly chronicle, and hardly any can be found in an annual one. Only important events of one level make their way to a higher level – a rigorous *filtering* process can be observed. Moreover, an annual chronicle cannot consist of a sequence of the old reports of individual news items, but each item must be redone in less detail.

The examples given above reveal a unique strategy we use for navigation in complex information spaces. Effective navigation requires a structure of different levels of detail. At any instant in time, only a small subset of the information is perceived in detail. Visualizations fit their goal of providing intuition about data best when they conform to the nature of human perception.

A traditional way to achieve this goal is the use of *insets*, which can be found for example in maps as well as in technical illustrations (see Fig. 2.1 and RIST [Ris95]). Insets are overlays that show an interesting detail, such as a city center, in large magnification and have a referencing link to the magnified area within the view providing the overall context. Unfortunately, rather great effort is required for the cognitive reintegration of multiple views.

Studies in experimental psychology indicate that humans integrate information that is perceived in a single view much more easily, indeed almost automatically.

Static media, for example maps, are dedicated to a certain group of users. However, it is too expensive to individualize them to the interests of a single user. Therefore, only such information is presented in detail as is a priori important for a variety of viewers. With interactive systems, however, it is possible to tailor a visualization to the items the user is actually interested in. From this, the following consequences for the development of interactive systems can be derived:

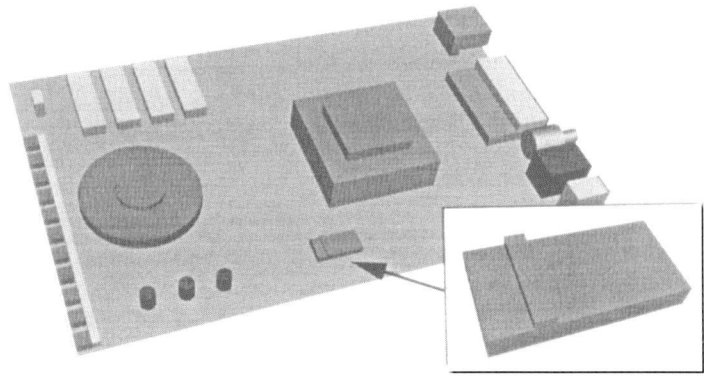

Figure 2.1: A transformator on a modem is magnified with approximate factor 4 as an inset in a technical illustration [Ris95]

- Navigation in complex information spaces requires a careful structuring of the information space. In this process, information must be weighted and prioritized appropriately to enable visualization of an information space on different scales.
- Adaptation of the presentation requires a log of the user's actions in order to determine his or her interest in certain pieces of information.
- A distance function is required which makes it possible to evaluate the user's interest in all pieces of information depending on the user interaction.

With these prerequisites, visualizations can be generated that integrate detail and context within one view. One of the fundamental problems which must be solved is how to handle the transition between areas at different scales within one presentation. Referring to fisheye lenses in photography (wide angle lenses that magnify an image near the lens' focus much more than at its periphery), these views are called *fisheye views*. Fisheye views are characterized by nonlinear transformations with one or more focus points that guide the distortion. Therefore, they are often referred to as "focus+context techniques" (see LAMPING et al. [LRP95]).

2.2 Fisheye Views: A Step Towards Abstraction

Based on his consideration of the human thinking process, FURNAS introduced the framework of generalized fisheye views (recall [Fur86]). To visualize an information space, a *degree of interest*, *DOI* for short, is assigned to each element of the information space. The *DOI* quantifies the current user's interest in that element. The *DOI* is composed of a static component and a dynamic one. The static component is called *a priori importance* or *API*, and characterizes the global importance of the element.

The dynamic component relates the importance of elements to the user's current interest deduced from his or her latest interactions. An element, often referred to as a *node*, is selected as the current focus of interest, called *focus point*, or simply *FP*. An application-specific distance function *dist* that captures the distance between any two elements of the information space is used to measure the degradation of the user's interest in elements when focusing on *FP*. In its simple, additive basic form, the *DOI* of some element x for a given focus *FP* is computed as:

$$DOI_{(x)} = API(x) - dist(x, FP) \qquad (2.1)$$

With this basic equation, the application of fisheye techniques depends on the definition of *API* values as well as of an appropriate distance function. In complex information spaces, the distance function might depend on several factors (e.g., number of inhabitants, importance of traffic connections) which must be weighted carefully. In particular, the distance function may incorporate spatial, conceptual, and temporal aspects.

The *DOI* calculation must be carried out when the user's focus changes. Usually, the *DOI* of all nodes is involved, resulting in a global impact on *FP*. However, as BARTRAM and CALVERT [BC94] point out, in some cases it is useful to restrict the influence of a node to a region or a certain category of nodes. This statement is based on empirical evidence achieved in an extensive usability study. Moreover, a local influence is desirable to achieve an acceptable level of performance of fisheye algorithms. Performance becomes an important question if thousands of nodes are involved.

A number of applications build on and extend the basic concept of generalized fisheye views. A crucial extension is the introduction of several focus points. Several foci have been established in cartography (introduced by KADMON and SHLOMI [KS78]). The incorporation of several foci in interactive systems has been reported by MITTA [Mit90] and elaborated by SARKAR and BROWN [SB92].

Several foci constitute an easy way to classify information a user has interacted with in the near past as more interesting, or to put it the other way, to influence a series of follow-up views by focusing on an object. Thus a certain coherence between successive views can be achieved, facilitating the reorientation of the user and thus the user's interpretation of the visualization.

Up to now, we have been concerned about how to specify a user's interest in different elements of the information space. The second crucial question is which presentation techniques should be provided to emphasize important elements and to deemphasize elements of minor importance.

NOIK [Noi94] presents a taxonomy of fisheye views. He identifies three groups of emphasis techniques:

- *Filtering*
  Nodes with low *DOI* are simply left out. The process of filtering is almost always based on a hierarchical structure imposed on the information space, where entire substructures are left out.
- *Distorting*
  "Classical" fisheye views – similar to the photographic nature of the fisheye – distort a presentation. Size, position, and shape of objects are manipulated in accordance with their *DOI*.
- *Adorning*
  Techniques that emphasize or deemphasize objects by modifying presentation variables like color, line style, fonts, and transparancy are classified as adorning techniques.

It is very common to use a combination of different techniques to emphasize objects, i.e., parts of the information space which are important are displayed with more detail *and* enlarged. A combination of filtering and distortion is often required to adapt the size in the presentation to the density of information to be presented. In addition, important information might be emphasized further by choosing appropriate presentation variables.

Some further terms are crucial for the description of fisheye-based systems. A *normal view* is a presentation without any focus point – usually the initial presentation generated by the system when no information is available as to what is interesting for the user. The position of an element in the normal view is represented by its *normal coordinates* (recall [Noi94]). To ensure that fisheye views are comprehensible it is useful to represent normal coordinates and to record the differences between these coordinates and the actual coordinates. Thus it can be prevented that too-large distortions occur. If large distortions cannot be avoided, additional cues can be provided to guide the user in interpreting the layout.

2.3 Applications of Fisheye Views

In the following we shall discuss some influential applications of fisheye techniques. In most applications, fisheye techniques are employed to visualize abstract and structured data, such as trees or graphs.

2.3.1 Filtered Views on Source Code

FURNAS originally applied filtering fisheye views for navigating in tree structures and in source code texts [Fur86]. In source code navigation the importance of source lines is based on the hierarchical structuring of a (procedural) program. For example, the first and last lines of procedures are especially important. The focus is determined by the current cursor position. The distance function used in this one-dimensional linear sequence of statements is the obvious one based on line numbering. In the community of LISP programmers, folding editors providing such filtered views are extremely popular.

2.3.2 Distorting Views of Graphs and Maps

SARKAR and BROWN apply fisheye techniques to geographic data [SB94], actually to graphs embedded in the plane. The user can place a focus point such that the focused region is enlarged, and simultaneously, other regions are reduced in size. In contrast to the application of FURNAS, several focus points are possible. An essential contribution of this work is the extension of the application area of fisheye framework to domains, where the shape of objects is important for the orientation of the user. Since graphical distortions are interesting as an emphasizing technique in computer graphics we will go into some of the technical details.

As a first example look at the view of large cities within the United States and their connections (see Fig. 2.2). As the distortion is not combined with an appropriate filtering the displacements can produce regions of extreme symbol density.

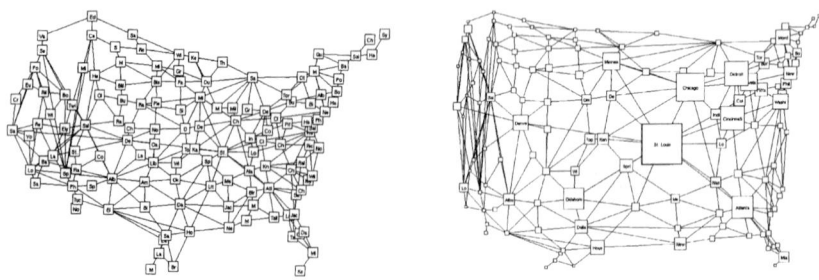

Figure 2.2: Normal view and distorted view of important cities within the continental US [SB94, p. 75]

The resizing imposed by the fisheye algorithm causes displacements and thus a change of shapes. Shapes we are accustomed to are hard to recognize when heavily distorted. Consider for example the outline of the US as in Fig. 2.3. As a consequence, SARKAR and BROWN state the necessity to provide the user with interaction tools for manipulating the parameters of displacement. This is not an easy issue – the challenge is to hide (and thus to abstract) from the underlying mathematical relations and to provide "intuitive" interaction facilities.

SARKAR and BROWN provide a general scheme for graphical fisheye distortions. Starting from the undistorted layout (the normal view), a transformation function specifies the reposition of points. Distorting views should smoothly integrate focus and context. The transformation is based on a

2.3 Applications of Fisheye Views

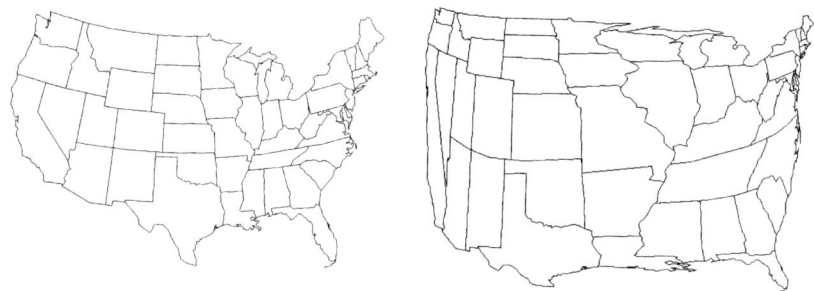

Figure 2.3: Normal view and distorted view of the continental US border [SB94, p. 78]

one-dimensional transformation f_m that is applied either to each cartesian coordinate of a point, resulting in a cartesian or *orthogonal magnification*, or to the radius component of the polar coordinates, giving rise to a polar or *radial magnification* (see Fig. 2.4).

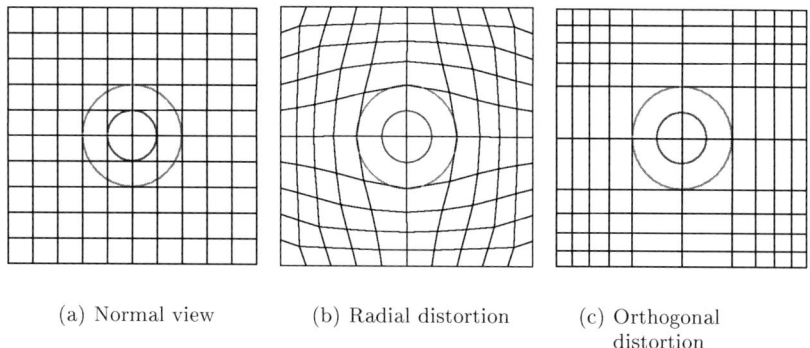

(a) Normal view (b) Radial distortion (c) Orthogonal distortion

Figure 2.4: Radial and orthogonal distortions (courtesy of Rainer MICHEL)

Consider a focus point $FP = (x_{FP}, y_{FP})$. Under orthogonal magnification, the point (x, y) is mapped to $(x_{FP} + f_m(x - x_{FP}), y_{FP} + f_m(y - y_{FP}))$. This way FP remains fixed. Furthermore, vertical and horizontal lines are mapped to vertical and horizontal lines, respectively. To achieve a magnification integrating detail and context, a non-linear transformation f_m is required. The derivative f'_m indicates the local scale factor. If the derivative f'_m is monotonically decreasing the magnification near the focus is larger than in the periphery. Another constraint imposed by most applications is that the image size has to remain fixed. This issue is often referred to as the *screen real estate problem*.

Normalizing the x- and y-coordinates to span the interval $[0, 1]$ and choosing f_m so as to map $[0, 1]$ onto $[0, 1]$ forces the invariance of image sizes.

SARKAR and BROWN suggest using as f_m the parametrized function

$$f_m(x) = \frac{(d+1)x}{dx+1} \quad \text{with derivative} \quad f'_m(x) = \frac{(d+1)}{(dx+1)^2}$$

Thus large values for d result in a high magnification near the focus and high demagnification near the border. The polar magnification can be derived in a similar way. It does preserve angles relative to the focus, but not vertical and horizontal relations.

2.3.3 Multiple Foci

The work of SARKAR and BROWN has been extended in different ways. Several methods for dealing with multiple foci were proposed. Given several foci the transformations can be applied in sequence. Since these transformations are in general non-commutative, this raises the question in what order they should be applied. In an interactive session the sequence is usually derived from the interaction history in a data-driven visualization (e.g., a visualization of search results), an application-specific priority must be assigned to the foci.

Another widely used approach is weighted averaging. Each transformation is applied independently in the original domain. The final transformed point is obtained as a weighted average of these independent transformations. A third possibility consists of assigning to each focus its own domain of influence, and applying the corresponding transformation to this domain exclusively. Another line of extension is the handling of focus areas instead of focus points.

SARKAR et al. [SSTR93] describe an interactive method to deal with multiple convex focal areas. The scaling is uniform within each area. Their approach follows the metaphor of *stretching a rubber sheet* and is based on morphing. The user interactively fixes the boundary of the focus regions in the source layout and in the destination layout. Based on the vectors defined this way, morphing is performed. This method does not guarantee invariant image sizes in a strict sense, and the transformation has no general inverse. Although the visualizations generated this way are similar to fisheye views, they are in fact not in this category, because no *DOI* function is involved.

2.3.4 Fisheye Views of Hypertext Structures

Navigation problems in virtual spaces are especially evident in hypertext systems and cause the feeling of being "lost in hyperspace." NIEVERGELT and WEYDERT argue that the most crucial questions in this context are "Where I am? What can I do? How can I get to ..." [NW80]. Fisheye views enable a better orientation in emphasizing the current viewpoint as focus point (first question). At the same time, the navigation may be improved compared to pan-and-zoom navigation (second and third questions) if changes are animated smoothly.

Hypertext structures are visualized most naturally by graphs. NOIK [Noi93] employs fisheye views to improve navigation in hypertexts. Since in this application the geometric layout of the graph is not restricted to resemble a given shape, distortions are less critical.

The application in the hypertext domain reveals an interesting facet of fisheye algorithms. Usually, fisheye techniques deal with nodes exclusively. These algorithms do not cater for links between nodes. In the hypertext domain it is useful to apply filtering also to links. With this approach, for example, all possible links are displayed for the focus point only while the number of links presented degrades with increasing distance. Some work has been done very recently on distorting the path between two nodes (see Chap. 8).

2.3.5 Fisheye Views for Supervisory Control Systems

The *variable zoom* presented by SCHAFFER et al. [SZB+93] is designed for viewing large hierarchical networks in a real-time application for network supervisory control (see also DILL et al. [DBHH94] and SCHAFFER et al. [SZG+96]).

The interesting point in this project is that information from very different sources and with very different characteristics is handled in an integrated manner. The state of the network can be represented by charts and tables which show, for example, the load in nodes of the system. In addition, videos are employed which monitor parts of the network. Textual information is also available.

The information space is very heterogenous and requires mechanisms to decide *what* should be displayed. In such a complex information space it is not sufficient to derive a *DOI* for each piece of information. Instead, additional considerations are required to decide whether a diagram is more appropriate than a video. The variable zoom is therefore accompanied by reasoning techniques which take into account the state of the network (e.g., broken pipes). This gives rise to the term *intelligent zoom* (see [BOD+94]) emphasizing that a sophisticated mechanism is employed to determine the user's information needs. This project and the lessons learned initiated our interest in fisheye techniques, and it is therefore described in more detail in Chap. 9.

2.3.6 Zooming Windows

On the desktop of our Personal Computer with many windows, the one we need most is usually obscured. Window management is an important application for the development of more sophisticated navigation facilities. BURY et al. [BDD85] performed an analysis which indicates that the overall time to complete a complex task in a multiple-window system is in general longer than in a non-windowed system. However, the actual task completion time (without window management operations) as well as the error rate is reduced considerably in multiple-window systems. In this publication, the portion of time for switching the active window set is 63 percent of the overall task completion time. Even if this percentage appears to be very large, it cannot be denied that the prevailing window managers with independent overlapping windows have a strong influence on user performance. Window management may be time-intensive and distracts users from their actual tasks.

The obvious problem of more effective window management receives only slight attention. BEDERSON and HOLLAND [BH94] argue that the widespread desktop metaphor guides window placement strategies and leads to an underutilization of the new medium. In particular, structural relations which often exist between different windows of one application are neither visualized nor employed for easy navigation. They describe PAD++, an interface with zooming (growing windows at the expense of others) as the basic interaction technique. As an example, a multiple-window directory browser was implemented.

So far, the most extensive work on window management based on zooming has been carried out by KANDOGAN and SHNEIDERMAN [KS96]. They rely on a hierarchical structure of windows and use algorithms for a space-filling layout of the rectangles in which windows are embedded (see [JS91] for the space-filling algorithm). These algorithms automatically arrange as many windows as possible in such a way that no overlapping occurs. Figure 2.5 shows a layout with windows arranged automatically. On the base of the hierarchical structure of the windows, efficient multi-window operations can be performed, e.g., stacks of windows can be moved and resized in their entirety. Furthermore, the windows are *elastic* – they can grow at the expense of others to a certain extent.

This technique has been applied to several domains where typically many windows arise: programming environments for object-oriented systems, CAD applications, and geographic information systems. All these systems are characterized by underlying hierarchies, e.g., OO systems operate on class hierarchies and CAD systems operate on part-of hierarchies.

To conclude, window management can benefit from fisheye views. However, improvements in window placement require substantial structural information about the relationships between windows.

2.4 Comprehensible Fisheye Views

Distorting fisheye views as well as other nonlinear transformations distort an underlying layout to a certain extent. This raises the question as to whether these views can be correctly interpreted and whether they are perceived as

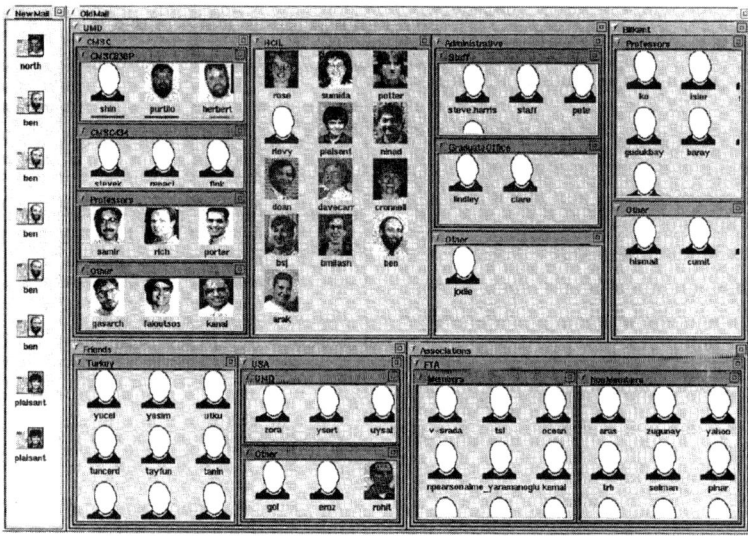

Figure 2.5: Automatically arranged windows [KS96, p. 31]

natural and comprehensible. SARKAR et al. [SSTR93] were the first to discuss this question in detail. They identified the following properties as most crucial for the user's comprehension:

- *Topology.* The topological requirement is that the transformation from undistorted to distorted layout is a homeomorphism; in particular, the inside of a closed continuous curve is mapped to the inside of another closed continuous curve (see EADES et al. [ELMS91] for a more rigorous definition).
- *Sequence in orthogonal directions.* The relative orientation of nodes to each other, the "compass direction", ought to be maintained, e.g., node p is northeast of node q.
- *Membership in clusters.* If nodes are near to each other in the original layout (being perceived as a cluster), they should remain near to each other.

Whether or not these features are maintained has a large influence on the user's orientation. The morphing algorithms by SARKAR et al. do not maintain any of these properties in a strict sense. However, the morphing approach is provided with an easy-to-use interface and can handle multiple polygonal focal areas. The fisheye algorithms described so far maintain these properties. In particular, the sequence in orthogonal directions is preserved if rectangular distortion methods are involved. Radial distortions do not preserve this property in a strict manner. Whether the third property is maintained depends strongly on the definition for cluster membership, but in general fisheye views also do well with respect to this feature.

Besides these properties, some others may be important with respect to the application domain. The most important difference is that the shape of nodes is important in some applications, but not in others. For example, the shapes of geographic regions and countries are familiar to us while abstract visualizations of data, like rectangles and circles, are not as important to maintain. Preserving the basic shape of objects may be even more important than the preservation of the topology. As SARKAR and BROWN point out, radial distortions are superior with respect to shape preservation than rectangular distortions.

As a general rule, it is problematic to distort heavily a layout with which the user is familiar. In particular, known shapes should not be magnified with different ratios in x- and y-directions – the aspect ratio should be maintained if possible. For geographic applications, however, where no empty intervals between the nodes exist, strict maintenance of the aspect ratio is incompatible with a nonlinear magnification.

CARPENDALE et al. [CCF95] support the interpretation of a distorted fisheye view by visualizing the distortion. In their system foci are elevated – resulting in a 3D model. This 3D model is rendered, resulting in light areas for foci and dark areas for parts in the vicinity, thus clearly indicating where a focus point is situated (recall Fig. 2.6). However, with this technique the extent to which a visualization is distorted (compared to the normal view) cannot be extracted. In Chap. 7 an approach for coding the extent of a distortion directly is described.

The comprehensibility of fisheye views also depends on temporal aspects. When a user is confronted with a radically new layout, he or she must *recog-*

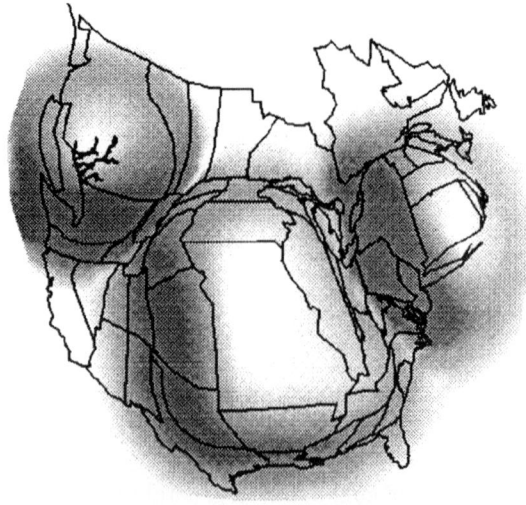

Figure 2.6: The amount of a distortion of the geographic map of North America is visualized [CCF95, p. 224]

nize what has happened. By contrast, when the changes are animated they can simply be *watched*, which imposes less cognitive load (see ROBERTSON et al. in [RMC91]). Almost all papers on fisheye techniques include a description of the efforts to ensure an appropriate frame-rate for an animation which shows the change from an undistorted layout to a distorted one.

2.5 Fisheye Views for 3D Data

The distorting methods discussed so far make no use of 3D graphics. Distorting views integrating detail and context can be obtained by perspective projections of 3D data. NOIK calls these methods *implicit fisheye views*, stressing that a distortion is imposed which is not explicitly stated in an (arbitrary) function but instead results from the perspective projection of 3D data.

By contrast, *explicit 3D fisheye views* distort a 3D model with an appropriate function in a similar way to 1D and 2D techniques. While some work has been done with implicit 3D fisheye views, explicit distortion of 3D views is just beginning to receive attention. First results have been developed by RAAB and RÜGER [RR96] in the context of illustrating 3D models (see Chap. 9). In independent research, another approach was taken by CARPENDALE et al. [CCF96] in the context of 3D data visualization.

2.5.1 Implicit 3D Fisheye Views

Perspective Wall. MACKINLAY et al. [MRC91] suggested the use of perspective projection for integrated detail and context visualizations. The PERSPECTIVE WALL is limited to linearly structured 2D charts, e.g., calendar information arranged on a time-line, alphabetically ordered text, or a sequence of pictures, and supports one focus point (see Fig. 2.7). The focused chart is projected on a center panel, while the neighboring context is displayed on two perspective panels. The trade-off between detail and context can be controlled by manipulating the degree of folding, the width of the center panel, and the angle of view. Changing the focus is accomplished by scrolling.

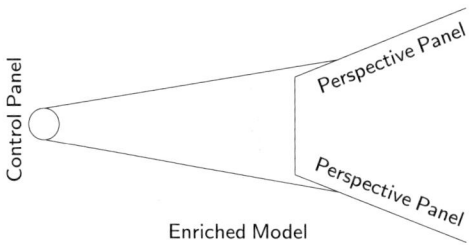

Figure 2.7: Sketch of the PERSPECTIVE WALL

Cone Trees. ROBERTSON et al. [RMC91] developed a tool for displaying large hierarchies as trees. Any node and its children are mapped to a 3D cone yielding a 3D model of the entire tree (see Fig. 2.8). The distortion from a 3D perspective establishes an implicit fisheye view. Choosing a focus node automatically rotates cones to bring the focus to the front of of the display. In addition, a filtering through interactive gardening is provided. Gardening supports three types of operations:

- *pruning:* hides the descendents of a selected node,
- *growing:* restores hidden descendents, and
- *prune others:* prunes the siblings of a selected node.

Thus CONE TREES let users interactively simplify large hierarchies. User studies have shown the efficency of this display technique, especially when the cones are rendered semitransparent and cast shadows (see [ZBM96]).

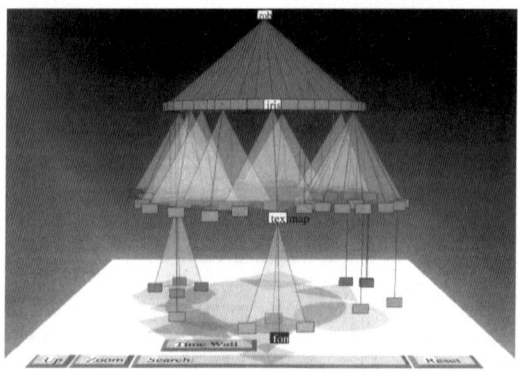

Figure 2.8: Large hierarchies are laid out as 3D CONE TREES supporting our 3D visual cues, like depth and shadows [RMC93, p. 67]

CONE TREES have become popular within recent years. They have been applied, for example, to large websites (see CARD [Car96]). A horizontal variant of CONE TREES, called CAM TREES, is better suited in terms of the legibility of text (see Fig. 2.9). KOIKE and YOSHIHARA [KY93] demonstrate that CONE TREES can be combined with filtering fisheye techniques which are extremely useful for the visualization of large hierarchies. Filtering fisheye techniques are employed, for example, to show the path from a given node to the root node. Moreover, fractal techniques are employed for the tree layout. It is shown that fractal views of hierarchies can effectively use the screen space available.

Document Lens. While CONE TREES and the PERSPECTIVE WALL lend themselves to navigation in structured information spaces (hierarchically or linearly organized) complex information must often be managed without an underlying structure. Again, a smooth integration of focus and context is required. For this purpose the DOCUMENT LENS has been developed at XEROX Parc (see ROBERTSON and MACKINLAY [RM93b]). The DOCUMENT

2.5 Fisheye Views for 3D Data

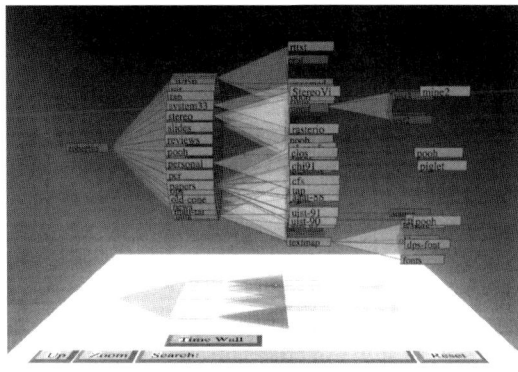

Figure 2.9: CAM TREES –
A horizontal variant of
CONE TREES is better suited
for text legibility [RMC93,
p. 67]

LENS is suitable for laying out the entire contents of a multi page document and for magnifying important places the user is especially interested in. The important places result either from direct user interaction or from a search command executed on the document to locate the occurrences of words.

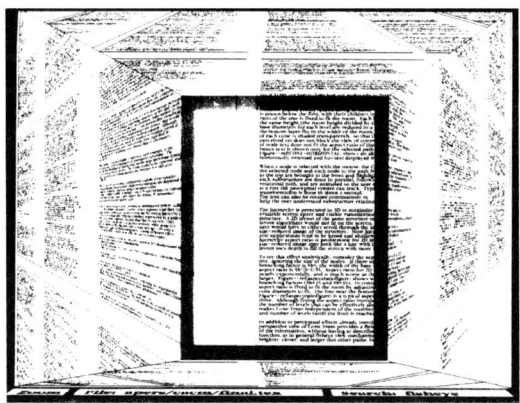

Figure 2.10: Example view of
the document lens ability to
visualize unstructured
text [RM93b, p. 105]

In contrast to traditional magnifying lenses, which necessarily obscure the region in the vicinity of the enlarged area, the DOCUMENT LENS visualizes the context, too. The DOCUMENT LENS is rectangularly shaped as it is used for text display.

Like the PERSPECTIVE WALL and the CONE TREE, the DOCUMENT LENS employs the perspective projection resulting from a projection from 3D to 2D. The entire document is mapped to a pyramid frustum. The lens projects the interesting parts at the top of this frustum so that it appears parallel to the observer, resulting in optimal text legibility (see Fig. 2.10). The user can move the DOCUMENT LENS in the xy-plane as well in the z-direction. Thus the user can control the amount of magnification for the focus as well as the distortion imposed on the context. This freedom, however, has a penalty. If the lens is moved too close to the observer, the text on the sides of the pyramid becomes totally unreadable. Therefore, the content of the DOCUMENT LENS should not occupy too large a region of the overall screen space.

Pliable Surfaces. CARPENDALE et al. (recall [CCF95]) tackle the problem of integrated detail and context visualization of general 2D normal views. They extend the ideas behind the PERSPECTIVE WALL to enable multiple foci. The original layout is mapped to a three-dimensional surface, and subsequently mapped to the screen by perspective projection.

To give at least a rough idea about the working of this technique, we restrict our attention to the simple case of a single focus. Let us assume first that the focus point FP lies in the center of the field of view. Each point p of the 2D normal view is now lifted to a height of

$$h_p = h_{FP}\,{}^{-\frac{s_{FP}}{d_p}} \tag{2.2}$$

where h_{FP} is the interactively chosen height of the focus point, s_f the standard deviation of h_{FP}, and d_p the distance of p from the focus point FP.

This maps the plane of the normal view to a bell-shaped Gaussian surface. A perspective projection for the viewpoint directly above the center of the field of view at height $h_c > h_{FP}$ yields the desired magnification.

It must be noted, however, that the standard deviation of a distribution is not a very intuitive parameter for user interaction as it requires an understanding of the underlying mathematical relation. Off-center focus points require special treatment to avoid part of the lifted normal view leaving the viewing frustum. To deal with several foci, individual Gaussian surfaces are blended by an averaging process.

2.5.2 Explicit 3D Fisheye Views

Although 3D graphics are used to establish implicit fisheye views, the techniques discussed manipulate 2D views. Surprisingly little research has been dedicated to the problem of manipulating 3D scenes. Of course, when visualizing 3D scenes they are usually projected to a 2D display and the techniques for manipulating 2D views can be applied. In many applications, however, this approach is not desirable. For example, consider an interactive application where a series of views from a moving view point is displayed. The application of the 2D techniques for the individual views would result in a lack of coherence. The problems of missing coherence can be avoided by manipulating 3D scenes directly. Moreover, the manipulation of 3D scenes makes it possible to show surfaces which would otherwise be hidden. FAIRCHILD et al. [FPF88] discuss two approaches for 3D data visualization. The *density approach* samples fully around the focus point and less as the distance from the focus increases. The other approach is based on octrees. Octants near the focus are shown at full scale, while more remote ones are displayed at progressivly larger scales.

CARPENDALE et al. [CCF96] discuss the problems of straightforward extensions of 2D methods to 3D. In 3D, for example, it is not enough to scale the important nodes, the foci, because these nodes may be hidden. The most remarkable result of their efforts is a *visual access distortion* which translates all nodes so that the visual access to important nodes is ensured. The visual access distortion explicitly distorts 3D data. The intended domain of application is limited to abstract 3D data, such as 3D graphs.

This transformation is somewhat similar to the use of *cut away views* which are employed in technical illustrations of 3D models (see SELIGMAN and FEINER [SF91a]). Cut away views are constructed by making a hole in an object that appears at the front to clear the view to an important object behind it. Cutting a hole in a frontal object is better than removing it because it often provides the context necessary to understand the detail inside.

As the experiences with CONE TREES reveal, 3D visualizations can be very effective if visual cues like shadows are employed. Shadows, however, complicate the problem of achieving visual access because objects may become completely dark due to their position with respect to the configuration of light sources.

In Chap. 9, a 3D fisheye approach is presented which has been applied successfully for complex 3D scenes, including 3D models from anatomy [RR96].

2.6 Nonlinear Magnification

The concept of fisheye views relies on explict foci and adapts the size and position according to these foci and a distance function. With this approach, the foci can be effectively emphasized. However, the actual magnification which results in a specific node is difficult to predict. In fact, one often takes several zoom steps to achieve the desired size for some nodes of interest. As the size of other nodes is often hard to predict, the amount of information presented is adapted to whatever size remains available.

For this reason, the concept of *magnification grids* has been introduced by KEAHEY and ROBERSTON [KR97]. With this approach, the magnification is no longer a side effect of a distortion but is explicitely visualized and manipulated (see Fig. 2.11). Fisheye views and magnification grids have in common that nonlinear transformations are applied to the original data. The local maxima of the magnification grids correspond to foci in a fisheye view.

Often, several constraints over and above the conservation of the image size are imposed on a visualization. In particular, often certain regions of the data should be excluded from the scaling process. Such constraints are difficult to handle with a fisheye algorithm but can be easily integrated in

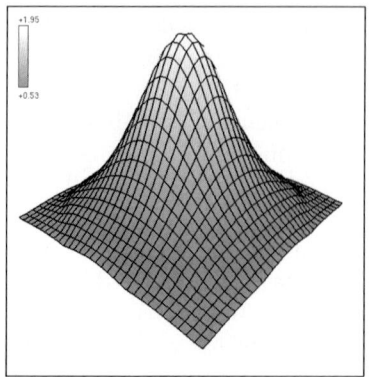 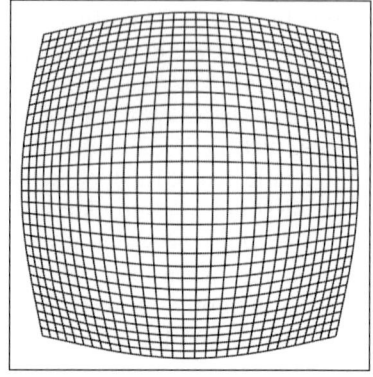

Figure 2.11: A distortion (left) and the corresponding magnification (right) [KR97] (© 1997 IEEE)

the concept of magnification grids. KEAHEY and ROBERSTON show that users can mark arbitrary combinations of nodes and request that these are presented in their original size compared to the average of the other nodes.

Visualizations in Hyperbolic Spaces. Several approaches have been developed to employ the characteristics of hyperbolic spaces for visualization and navigation within large hierarchies. Non-euclidean hyperbolic spaces have some nice features for the visualization of hierarchies. In hyperbolic space, parallel lines diverge and the circumference of a circle grows exponentially with the radius. This is particularly useful for the layout of trees which tend to grow exponentially.

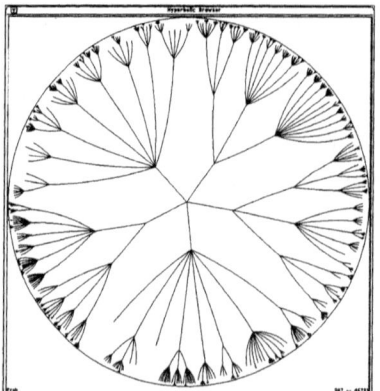 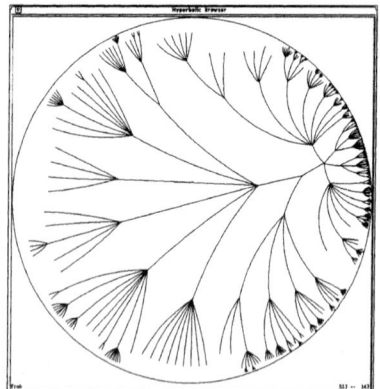

Figure 2.12: Hyperbolic visualizations of a hierarchy. The left image shows the normal view whereas in the right image the focus is shifted to the right – resulting in a detail and context visualization [LRP95, p. 404]

LAMPING and RAO [LR94] (see also [LRP95]) have developed a browser which projects the hierarchy to a hyperbolic plane which is subsequently projected onto a circular region. The nodes themselves are embedded in rectangular areas to ensure optimal legibility of textual information (see Fig. 2.12). These techniques use the screen space much more efficiently than traditional graph drawings of hierarchies, which run into difficulties in displaying a large number of leaf nodes horizontally or vertically.

Originally, the root node of the hierarchy is in the focus. The display space allocated to each node continuously decreases with the distance to the focus. During interactive working the focus can be shifted (either by dragging or by typing the name of the node which becomes the focus). The hyperbolic browser has modest computational requirements compared to CONE TREES and is better suited to give an overview of a large hierarchy.

2.7 Comparing Visualizations of Information Spaces

The smooth integration of detail and context as it can be accomplished with fisheye views is an essential technology, but not the only for navigation within large information spaces.

Current browsers for the World Wide Web include additional navigation aids. Web browsers offer the facility of managing a list of *bookmarks*. These bookmarks can be named by the surfer and can be flexibly organized within folders. Thus, a very personalized view over a large information space can be established. Such a list of bookmarks can even be integrated in the Web and thus allow others to navigate more easily.

Furthermore, the *interaction history* is maintained by the system. With this approach, it is easy to return to any place where one has already been. As an additional navigation aid, a list of URLs explicitly typed in the recent past is maintained to enable the user to get to these places again easily. Note, however, that these navigation facilities rely on URLs and title tags of the Web pages only. These navigation aids are not very useful for remembering images or animations.

Using transparency in user interfaces. Besides geometric transformations, presentation variables play an important role in an appropriate visualization of complex information spaces. In particular, transparency can be used to present more information at some position by rendering a foreground object semi-transparent and thus allowing to look at something behind it. While the use of semi-transparency is established for 3D illustration design (see for example [SF91a]) to communicate depth relations, it can also be used directly in the user interface. HARRISON and VICENTE [HV96] as well as KAMBA et al. [KEH+96] have done experimental studies in the use of transparent menus (see Fig. 2.13). HARRISON and VICENTE deal with semi-transparent menus to manipulate 3D geometric models. Instead of obscuring a large portion of the model on which they operate, the menus are overlaid. Naturally, the legibility of text decreases with a semi-transparent background, but the integration of the commands in a menu with the model outweighs this disadvantage. Furthermore, fonts can be selected which are particularly legible in connection with semi-transparency.

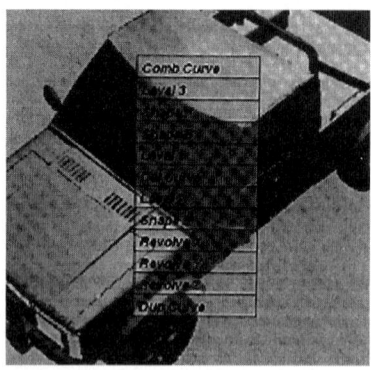

Figure 2.13: Transparent menus to manipulate geometric models [HV96, p. 391]

LIEBERMAN [Lie94] uses semi-transparency to overlay views at different scales of the underlying data, thus integrating detail and context. The approach has been applied to geographic data (an US street map at different scales) as well as to the display of a large file system. However, the combination of three or four layers of data may result in visual clutter. Therefore, it might be useful to reduce the contents of the layers involved and display only the most important nodes and links.

The use of semi-transparency is an interesting approach to integrating detail and context in one view without geometric distortions. Interactive control of transparency values, however, is a must for such systems as it cannot be predicted entirely how different layers interact and whether enough contrasts arise to differentiate between the upper layers.

2.8 Abstraction in Computer Graphics

In the last few years, more and more effort has been spent on reducing the complexity of graphics. Especially for the rendering of complex 3D models, methods have been investigated which reduce the number of polygons to accelerate the rendering process (HECKBERT and GARLAND [HG94b], COHEN et al. [CVM+96], HOPPE [Hop96] and KLEIN et al. [KLS96]). These methods usually operate on the huge geometric models which often result from measured data (e.g., 3D scanners, computer tomography). At its simplest, this reduction process is carried out immediately on the original 3D model and aims at reducing its complexity with only a modest effect on the resulting visualization.

More sophisticated methods of reducing the size of the geometric model are employed if interaction is involved. These methods take into account that from a given position only a part of the 3D model is visible. Even visible parts of the model might be so small in a projection that the number of faces and vertices involved may be considerably reduced without an effect on the resulting image. Although very useful for accelerating image synthesis, these approaches do not correspond to our definition of abstraction (recall Chap. 1). Recently, methods have been developed which deal with reducing the model complexity and simplifying the basic shape of models by taking into account the user's perception. The need for visual abstraction in computer graphics was first mentioned by FEINER [Fei85]. His APEX system is one of the first systems which automatically generates images based on a specification of the communicative intents the visualization should fulfill. Abstraction methods are required to be able to adapt the level of detail to the importance of objects.

KRÜGER and BUTZ [BK96] and [BK97] extended the work of FEINER in different ways. In particular, they investigated which aspects of an image are important to be able to recognize the depicted content and to discriminate similar objects. As the silhouette plays an important role with respect to these questions, 3D models are analyzed as to which polygons contribute to the silhouette of an object from a given direction. In adapting the visual complexity, abstraction methods can thus be used as stylistic means to influence the viewer's visual focus.

Like fisheye techniques, abstraction methods often rely on the hierarchical model structure. If an object is regarded as less important in a specific context, it might be appropriate not to render some of its subobjects (see Fig. 2.14). Since abstraction methods often filter the vertices and polygons, it is often necessary to merge polygons. With this approach, new polygons arise which may not have been part of the original model.

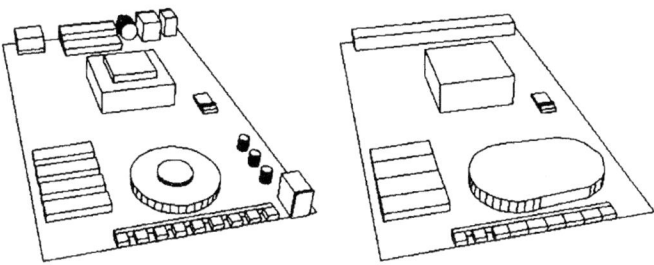

Figure 2.14: Visualizations of a modem platine. Detailed view (left), abstracted view with small objects aggregated, e.g., to cuboids (right) [BK96, p. 248]

As BUTZ and KRÜGER point out in [BK97], abstraction is not limited to geometric aspects. The illumination in a scene has a strong influence on what can be perceived. Important objects may be rendered in full detail and highlighted by an appropriate light source while less relevant objects are exposed to shadows and cannot be looked at in detail.

2.9 Abstraction in User Interfaces

Abstraction techniques are also relevant for the design of user interfaces. As interactive systems become more and more complex, it becomes an ever increasing demand to reduce their complexity, to simplify the user interface by hiding irrelevant widgets. There is no golden rule on how to come up with intuitive and easy-to-use interfaces. However, abstraction techniques play a central role.

Some examples illustrate the point. Abstraction is necessary to avoid a technology-driven terminology, to map commands to the application to meaningful widgets for user interaction (abstraction from the peculiarities of the application). The XEROX STAR pioneered a consistent separation between "normal options" and "advanced options" which are presented only if the user explicitly requires them (see JOHNSON et al. [JRV+89] for a retrospective on the STAR development). With this approach, unnecessary complexity is hidden, especially for beginners and knowledgeable intermediate users. Such designs are not tuned to the current user but instead for the overall user community expected. In the terminology of this chapter "normal options" which are easy to reach represent the a priori important parameters of a class of objects in an interactive system.

Many systems provide a special mode for beginners which actually presents only a subset of the available commands, based on the experience that most of the tasks to be accomplished can be realized with a small subset of the overall available commands.

Some menu-oriented systems provide short and long menus, again for the purpose of not overwhelming casual users or beginners. In fact, all these approaches are abstraction methods which rely on a meaningful structure of the available interaction facilities. Such a structure requires a careful analysis of which commands are of major importance and which ones are activated less often.

Graphical abstraction in user interfaces is important in the design of icons which represent important concepts and tasks in direct-manipulative systems. Meaningful icons are easier to recall (often not easier to leran) than textual commands. Icons are small and simple pictures highlighting the most salient features of the object they represent.

In this context, STROTHOTTE and STROTHOTTE [SS97] provide an in-depth discussion of icon design and use. In particular, they investigate in which aspects icons are related to words and in which aspects they are related to images thus emphasizing that icons lie somewhere in between texts and images.

Finally, consider CAD systems with powerful mechanisms to construct arbitrarily shaped 3D models. For this purpose, they build on a sophisticated mathematics, including Bezier curves and B-splines. The challenge here is to enable a manipulation of shapes which abstracts from the mathematical model of control points, associated weights and approximation functions (see Hsu [HHK92] for suggestions on how to provide easy-to-use tools for shape manipulation). In particular, it should be easy to predict which effect a certain interaction has. Similar considerations are crucial for the parameterization of graphical fisheye views which also rely on mathematical functions.

2.10 Summary

In this chapter, an overview of methods for stretching and distorting spaces for the effective visualization of data has been given. In this context, the need for multi-resolution techniques for navigation in complex information spaces has been demonstrated. Emphasis is put on the interactive manipulation of these visualizations which result in a combination of filtering techniques, geometric distortions, and adaptations of presentation variables.

While a variety of presentation strategies has been mentioned, some important aspects have not even been touched upon. The exploration of complex information spaces can benefit from learning mechanisms which adapt the system's behavior to the habits of the individual information seeker. In general, intelligent presentation systems with application-specific automatic behavior are promising for information exploration.

Most of this chapter has been devoted to fisheye views which are guided by explicit foci. Fisheye views have turned out to be successful with respect to the navigation tasks imposed by large information spaces. The integration of detail and context is particularly useful for editing tasks, because users need a magnified view to be able to edit parts of an information space.

In many cases it is useful to influence the magnification of data explicitly. We have therefore described non-linear magnification which uses magnification grids that can be either explicitly specified or controlled by data values from the application.

Fisheye views as well as visualizations based on magnification grids rely on nonlinear transformations of the underlying data and present the data at multiple scales and/or multiple resolutions.

Although fisheye views have turned out to be superior to traditional pan-and-zoom methods, they have not been incorporated in commercial systems so far. This is at least partly due to a lack of systematic usability studies. Several papers include a description of small usability studies which indicate the potential of fisheye views compared to traditional approaches. However, these usability studies are too small to yield statistically valid results and do not compare different fisheye techniques with one other. Moreover, the measurable usability issues, like ease of learning, ease of use, and task-completion times, should be investigated in more detail.

Fisheye techniques play an important role in several chapters of this book. In Chap. 3, fisheye views are employed for navigation in the structure of complex 3D models as well as for navigation within the 3D models themselves. In Chap. 7, the traditional use of more or less radial focus points is generalized to linear foci. This is particularly useful for distortions of geographic data where properties like the street length have to be preserved. Some fundamental questions concerning fisheye techniques are discussed in Chap. 9, where fisheye views are applied in different dimensions. In particular, modifications of "classical" fisheye views are described which serve the purpose of illustrating complex geometric models.

In Chap. 10, a general scheme is described to cope with heterogenous information spaces. In particular, it is analyzed which aspects of the *API* and *DOI* calculation are generic and can be implemented in a reusable software component. In Chap. 13, we describe the use of fisheye techniques for navigation in the labels and explanations required for understanding complex spatial relations, as can be found for example in medical illustrations. Finally, the evaluation described in Chap. 20 deals with how users cope with fisheye techniques in a complex scenario. The evaluation includes both objective measures of performance and subjective ratings of preference for fisheye techniques compared to traditional zoom techniques.

Contributor of Chap. 2: Bernhard PREIM

Chapter 3

Enrichment and Reuse of Geometric Models

The information encoded in a geometric model is the basis for a "classical" rendering process. The mere geometry, however, is insufficient when the rendered images are *not* the final product. Non-geometric information associated with the objects in the model may be necessary for further operations on the image. Especially structure information is helpful during the modeling process as well as for a flexible reuse of the model. Furthermore, an appropriate structure of the model is indispensable for the interactive handling of models, simply because interaction is only possible at the level of the model's structure.

In the following two examples, rendered images are the starting point for an interactive manipulation or a postprocess. In both cases additional information is needed.

PREIM et al. have developed an illustration system, the ZOOMILLUS-TRATOR (see Chap. 13 and [PRS97]). This system generates interactive illustrations integrating rendered images and textual labels. These illustrations are used for an exploration of the 3D model and its associated textual information (labels and explanations). For explanation purposes, models with considerable detail are necessary.

HOPPE et al. introduce in [HLH96] their tool AKZENT (see also Chap. 7). This system enables the user to emphasize special aspects of objects within a 3D scene. This emphasis can be achieved automatically or interactively controlled, based on additional object information. This information contains specifications about the techniques needed for the emphasizing process.

In both applications, sophisticated geometric models are exploited. Such models are cumbersome to create. Moreover, in some cases special hardware devices, like 3D scanners, are necessary. Therefore, we reuse existing models whenever possible. They are even acquired from commercial providers (e.g., Viewpoint Datalabs offer a large variety of geometric models). The reuse of geometric models, however, requires facilities to adapt the geometry and to enrich it with additional information. For the enrichment it is necessary to locate the related part of the geometric model as well as the corresponding node in the model's structure. The enrichment process requires an understanding of the spatial structure and therefore facilities to explore the geometric model. This, however, requires visualization of both the structure (*structure view*) and the geometric model (*geometry view*).

For a suitable integration of the model and its structure it is necessary that interactions in one view immediately affect the other. A simple example clarifies this: Because selecting an object in a complex 3D model is hard, it is selected in the structure view and subsequently highlighted in the geometry view. In the geometry view, however, it is difficult to locate an object if it is not immediately visible. We deal with this problem and describe a close and bidirectional coupling between these views.

In this chapter we describe the enrichment and reuse of "classical" geometric models. First, we define the basic problems occurring in the enrichment process (Sect. 3.1.1). This leads us to introduce basic terms and to define the required information sets. In Sect. 3.2 we discuss related work. This discussion includes research papers on the integration of structure and geometry view and on the navigation in large hierarchical structures. Furthermore, an analysis of the structuring capabilities of commercially available modeling software is included. In Sect. 3.3 we develop an approach for reusing and enriching geometric models and present our tool, the ZOOMSTRUCTOR. Finally conclusions are given in Sect. 3.4.

3.1 Requirement Analysis

The enrichment process includes the assignment of textual information and an adaptation of the model's appearance. The assignment of text as well as the adaptation of the model's appearance rely on an adequate model structure. This leads to the following tasks which must be carried out in the enrichment process:

- modification of the model's structure,
- classification of objects into categories,
- assignment or reassignment of graphical attributes, and
- assignment of labels and other non-graphical information.

To solve these tasks, a tool is required which allows the exploration of a 3D model and its structure. We distinguish between graphical attributes and non-graphical attributes, which we refer to as contextual information.

3.1.1 Basic Terms

In computer graphics, we often consider a model to be all information which is created during the geometric modeling process. FOLEY et al. define geometric models as a collection of components with well defined geometry and interconnections between components including different application dependent structures. Furthermore, this structure information is regarded as a hierarchy described and represented by a tree [FvDFH90].

As we mentioned above, in selected systems more information is needed. Therefore, we analyze what categories of information are encoded in a model. This is why we have to extend the model definition.

Definition 3.1
A model $\mathcal{M}$ can be regarded as a large information space. This space includes information sets. The elements of these information sets are related to each other. The relations are determined by an object assignment, represented by a set $\mathcal{O}$ of object identification keys. The relations in the model information space are depicted in Fig. 3.1. The information sets included in $\mathcal{M}$ can be classified as follows:

- The set of *geometric information* $\mathcal{G}$ contains the mathematical description of the object's geometries. The elements of $\mathcal{G}$ are well defined geometrical primitives based on the chosen mathematical representation, e.g., polygons or spline patches.
- The set of *graphical information* $\mathcal{R}$ contains all information needed by the rendering system to define the individual appearance of the geometrical objects. This information depends on the renderer and is assigned to the geometrical primitives. Elements of $\mathcal{R}$ are, for instance, surface properties like color, transparency, smoothing.
- Sets of *contextual information* $\mathcal{C}_1, \ldots, \mathcal{C}_n$. All non-geometric information which either enhances the rendering process itself or supports interaction with an image is referred to as contextual information. Contextual information consists of records with a common structure. This structure (attributes and types) is the characteristic feature of a set of contextual information.

    Examples of sets of contextual information are textual labels or attributes for an emphasizing process (like a degree of "importance") – recall the examples discussed in the beginning of this chapter.
- *Structure information* $\mathcal{S}$ describes an order of the objects in the model defined by the user. Thereby we have to distinguish between

    – *Object hierarchies.* An object hierarchy $\mathcal{S}$ can be described as a tree $(\mathcal{O} \cup \mathcal{G}, E)$, in which the leaves are geometric primitives and the inner nodes are object identification keys. E are the edges between all nodes.

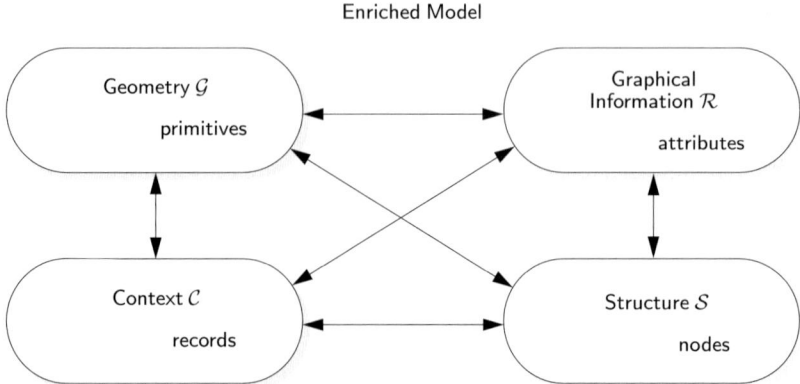

Figure 3.1: An enriched model as an entity of the geometry, its structure, graphical and contextual information

- *Special structures.* For some applications (special animation techniques, enhancement for interactions) it is necessary to define hierarchical structures in a subset of $\mathcal{O} \cup \mathcal{G}$.

A model may contain a variety of structures, but at least the object structure $S = (\mathcal{O} \cup \mathcal{G}, E)$ has to be present.

For the description of the available systems we need two additional definitions:

- *Structure browser*: A structure browser for geometric modeling systems enables the visualization of the model's structure and the navigation therein.
- *Structure editor*: A structure editor is a structure browser which allows one to modify the model's structure. Structure editors can be further differentiated as to whether they facilitate the creation and modification of nodes or whether (only) existing nodes can be cut, copied, or pasted as they are. If the creation and modification of nodes are possible, a large variety of modeling tasks can be accomplished with the structure editor.

An example may clarify this: In the ZOOMILLUSTRATOR which we shall describe in Chap. 13 labels and explanations are assigned to graphical objects to encourage exploration of the textual information behind the model. However, some objects have no labels because everybody knows them (e.g., the eyeball). These objects are displayed for the purpose of orientation but have no contextual information associated with them.

For the interactive handling of the information described above, tools are needed which display the different information sets and provide interaction facilities to manipulate them. This implies that visualization and interaction tasks have to be performed which can be formulated as follows:

- *Visualization tasks:* All information sets must be presented in a suitable and unambiguous graphical representation organized in a *graphical view*. The arrangement of these different views should not hide other information.
- *Interaction tasks:* Graphics editors have to provide navigation facilities to explore the displayed information sets.

  Navigation in the different graphical views must be carried out in a similar manner. An important point is the tight coupling of every user activity in all graphical views to guarantee consistency between these views and the underlying information sets.

Tools which accomplish these tasks are referred to as *graphics editors*. They are described and classified by SCHLEICH in his dissertation [Sch95b].

3.1.2 Information Visualization

For the enrichment of a geometric model, it is important to visualize the geometric model and the related structure (geometry view and structure view). Furthermore, contextual information should be visualized in a context view.

Geometry view: The 3D model should be presented in a viewer which provides basic interaction, as for instance transformations, camera control, and object picking.

Structure view: The structure of a geometric model is basically a hierarchy with *is a* relations between objects and parts thereof. Such a hierarchy can be visualized as a tree with container nodes (nodes with children) and elementary nodes (leaf nodes). Container nodes are characterized by the number of their children, while leaf nodes hold different attributes (depending on their type).

Important layout considerations include the layout of nodes and of lines (connections between nodes). Users should be able to differentiate nodes of different types at a glance. Therefore, the presentation parameters (e.g., shape and color) should be chosen carefully. In the structure view a structure browser or structure editor is presented.

Context view: Because navigation is performed primarily in the geometry and structure view, it is sufficient to display the record which is related to the currently selected object in the geometry/structure view. One record contains several attributes of different types. The attributes of nodes in the structure view and of records in the context view are disjunct. Attributes of structure nodes are elements of the scene description, while the context information is not included in a "classical" geometric model. According to the attribute's type, an appropriate widget is presented for the management of the information. For example, listboxes and radio buttons are provided to select a value from an enumeration, while text widgets are used to specify numbers and character input.

3.1.3 Interaction Facilities to Explore and Enrich Geometric Models

According to the tasks which must be carried out in the enrichment process (recall Sect. 3.1), the following interaction facilities must be provided.

- *Modification of the model's object structure*
  For different applications, a different granularity of the object's structure is required. Hence the modification of an object structure is the first step in the enrichment process. It consists of two subtasks:
  - refinement of an existing structure, and
  - grouping of objects.

  For these tasks it is important to convey to the user carrying the enrichment which elements belong together. Either the system supports the user in coloring parts of the geometry correspondingly, or the user must be offered facilities to color the geometry as he or she likes.
- *Integration of detail and context in the structure view*
  The structure of a complex model may consist of many hundreds of nodes – the view over which is easily lost. Sophisticated navigation facilities are therefore needed to work efficiently with the model's structure.
- *Bidirectional coupling between geometry view and structure view*
  The selection in the geometry view or in the structure view must be propagated to the other view and lead to highlighting of the corresponding part. This bidirectional connection supports the mental integration of a model's graphical appearance and its structure.
- *Management of contextual information in relation to model and structure view*
  When contextual information is updated, it must be clearly recognizable which part of the model and of the object structure it is related to. While it might be obvious that a record of context information is regarded together with the corresponding model part, it is also useful to see the position of the corresponding node in the structure view. Imagine labeling the bones of a foot and seeing that the corresponding node has four siblings. This structural particularity is helpful to identify the object which may be hard to recognize in the geometry view because it is rather small.

In Sect. 3.3 we shall describe how we implemented these interaction facilities and integrated them in an interface.

3.2 Related Work

Our work is inspired by attempts to provide an integrated view of structural and geometric information. It is also related to previous work on navigating in large hierarchical structures. Finally, a look at commercial modeling software is given to relate our concepts to the facilities offered in real systems.

3.2.1 Integration of Geometry and Structure View

Geometric modeling tools are highly developed in terms of the direct manipulative handling of geometric models. Although this is helpful in many situations, the concentration on this kind of interaction is rather onesided and restricted because it neglects the structures which may be behind a model. In the modeling process, objects are grouped together, e.g., because they belong to a common category. Moreover, a *part-of* relation between graphical primitives, elementary objects and high level objects arises.

SCHLEICH and DÜRST point out that this non-geometric information should be visualized as a prerequisite for interactive handling [SD94]. They present an integrated system with different views for geometry, structure information and attributes with changes in one view immediately affecting others. While the work of SCHLEICH deals with consistency between different views, several problems have not been tackled. As it is applied to small models only, the problem of interactive exploration of complex geometric models and of navigating through large amounts of symbolic information is left out. While parts which are selected in one view are emphasized in the other views, this technique is only helpful if the emphasized information is visible and appears large enough.

Our work is also inspired by the survey article from PLAISANT et al. who classify image browsers in [PCS95]. It is pointed out that the integration of detail and context in fisheye views is helpful in this domain. However, they should be applied carefully if information is presented which is not abstract, because the distortions imposed by a fisheye view may lead to problems. We learned from this article that a browser with multiple views should include a window placement strategy. The usual multiple window interface with overlapping windows, the management of which is left to the user, is harmful in terms of usability.

3.2.2 Visualization and Interaction in Hierarchical Structures

FURNAS pioneered the idea of fisheye views to integrate several levels of detail within one view (see [Fur86]), with the level of detail adapted to user interaction, which is formalized in a *degree of interest* (*DOI*) function. This idea has been applied to quite different domains since then. It is natural to apply fisheye techniques for the navigation in hierarchically organized information. In this case, information is presented as a tree with subtrees collapsed or expanded depending on the *DOI* value of the related subtree. FURNAS himself applied fisheye views to the layout of hierarchical information in browsers (see FURNAS, ZACKS in [FZ94]).

LAMPING and RAO present in [LR94] a fisheye version of a structure browser, in which nodes are projected onto hyperbolic space. While this method uses the available space very well, it leads to nonrectangular areas for nodes, which is inappropriate for text display.

With more and more compiling power available in recent years, 3D visualizations of hierarchical structures were introduced (see ROBERTSON et al. in [RMC91]). PLAISANT et al. argue in [PCS95] that this kind of navigation is natural because we are accustomed to turn something around to locate it. ROBERTSON et al. present special trees in which nodes are organized in cones. The foremost nodes are semitransparent, allowing the user to select more distant nodes which are brought forward if selected. Cone trees have been applied in large scale (e.g., parts of the WWW with 20 000 nodes), and allow a better overview of large hierarchies. Although the authors have applied their system to very large data, some questions remain open as to the practical feasibility of this approach, e.g., the handling of the picking.

Although some systems present clever strategies for either the presentation (cone trees, fisheye views) or the integration of structure and geometry (SCHLEICH, DÜRST [SD94]), several problems remain open. Most fundamental is the problem, that the highlighting fails to inform the user if the corresponding part is not visible (which is often the case, especially for small objects), or if it is too small to be recognized.

3.2.3 Observations in Graphics Editors

In the field of computer graphics editors, geometric and structure information is integrated in modeling systems. However, not every kind of non-graphical contextual information can be managed with these systems. Often, even in high end modeling and animation systems such as Autodesk 3D Studio 4.0 (see [Imm95]), structuring of model during the modeling process is not implemented. The user can only define a hierarchical linking for selected animation techniques.

Alias|*wavefront* is an example of a modeling and animation system providing a special window with structure information: the *scene block diagram* (*SBD*) window). The *SBD* appears in an independent window which may cover important information in the underlying view with geometric information (see [Ali94]). Only a detail *or* the global context of the object structure can be displayed at the same time. The *SBD* window's content represents a structure editor although it does not allow one to create nodes. Thus, only limited modeling facilities are possible at the level of the structure.

As to the integration of structure and geometry view, the structure editor GVIEW, belonging to the OPEN INVENTOR package from SGI, is a leading example. This application (see Fig. 3.2) enables the user to browse and

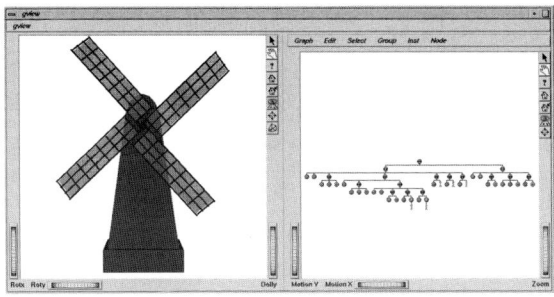

Figure 3.2: The GVIEW editor; left: geometric view, right: structure view

manipulate the structure of an OPEN INVENTOR scene graph (see [SC92]). In contrast to the *SBD* window component, GVIEW makes it possible to create nodes from scratch and can therefore serve for a variety of modeling tasks. The geometry and a structure view are integrated in GVIEW. The structure is visualized as tree with nodes represented by icons. GVIEW also realizes a bidirectional coupling when the user selects an object. In the structure view, the tree is collapsed automatically to include the node selected in the model view. The user, however, has to scroll through the window to see the relevant nodes. For navigation, the usual pan and zoom facilities are provided. Summarizing, we can conclude:

- Tools for structuring models in commercially available systems are provided in rudimentary manner. The navigation facilities of structure browsers are insufficient, however.
- The coupling between structure and geometry view alone is of limited value. An object selected in one view may be selected in another one, but it may not be visible or it may be too small to be recognized. Users have to struggle to find the selected object and perform a variety of navigation operations (i.e., scrolling, rotating).
- Orientation and navigation in large models (and corresponding large structures) is not supported.
- Only graphical information which is directly related to the rendering process (e.g., material description of object surfaces) can be managed. Contextual information, such as special textual information, cannot be managed at all.

The support for visualizing and manipulating geometric information is highly developed; a variety of tools for creating, navigating, and editing in geometric information sets are provided. Support is limited for modeling tasks on a different level than the direct manipulation of the geometry.

3.3 An Approach to Reuse and Enrich Models

This section describes the design and implementation of an enrichment tool which is dedicated to the exploration and enrichment of large models. All kinds of information are integrated in one view according to the requirements outlined above. To prove and integrate our concepts, we developed the ZOOMSTRUCTOR in C++ on SGI workstations. We used OPEN INVENTOR for the implementation of the geometry and structure view to ensure flexibility for future work (see [SC92]).

3.3.1 Design of an Enrichment Tool

As a consequence of the problems with commercial systems, we present structure information, contextual information, and the 3D model in an integrated view (see Fig. 3.3). The user is able to resize the different parts. Other views are automatically adapted in size, so that no overlapping of views can occur. Nodes of the structure are presented as rectangles to display textual information. Because nodes do not differ in shape, different colors are employed to characterize nodes. For this task, the following classification of nodes is employed:

- geometry nodes (nodes representing geometrical information),
- property nodes (nodes representing graphical information), and
- container nodes (nodes with children representing structure information).

Nodes are colored according to the above classification. An extra color is employed as feedback for the selection of a node.

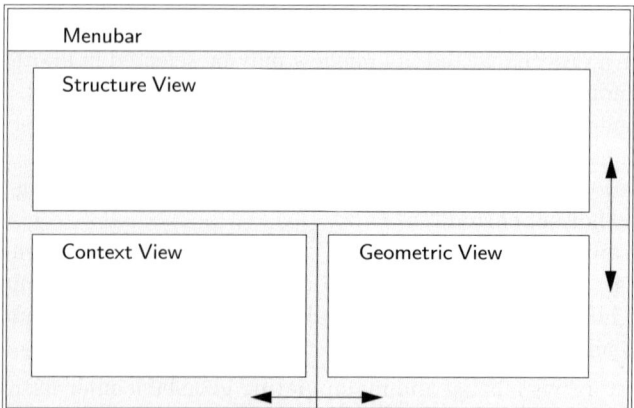

Figure 3.3: Basic layout of the ZOOMSTRUCTOR

One important detail is often neglected in the design of browsers for hierarchical data: The layout of lines. Fig. 3.4 (left) shows the widespread layout with lines directly connecting the center points of nodes and an approach which conveys the structure much better using orthogonal lines only as shown in Fig. 3.4 (right).

Direct connections cause problems when nodes have many children, as shown in Fig. 3.4 (left). Orthogonal lines ensure better recognition, as shown in Fig. 3.4 (right).

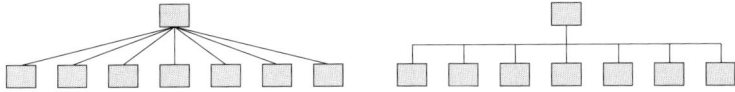

Figure 3.4: Oblique (left) and orthogonal (right) layout of lines in the structure view

3.3.2 Modification of the Object Structure

The modification of the object structure includes the refinement of an existing structure and the grouping of existing nodes. For the refinement, the graphical object to be decomposed is displayed in a separate window. In this view, the object can be handled in the same way as in the geometry view (including rotation and zooming).

In this view, which we refer to as the *refinement view*, single polygons can be selected and grouped to form new objects (parts of the original object to refine, see Fig. 3.5(a)). Here it is important to visualize the membership of nodes. To distinguish the newly generated objects, they are colored differently, whereas the user can modify the colors the system suggested. Note that the differentiation between these objects is updated in the geometry view as shown in Fig. 3.5(b).

This method is cumbersome if complex objects (with hundreds of polygons) are decomposed. The process is supported with a kind of region growing (a polygon selected can be "asked" to select all its neighbor polygons). Despite of this support the refinement is still preliminary. Cutting planes to isolate regions from each other is necessary for more comfortable refinement.

3.3.3 Navigating in the Structure View

The hierarchical structure of a 3D model is presented as a tree. The nodes of the tree are either labeled with a specific name assigned by a user, or with the name of its type. The presentation of textual labels is adapted to whether or not the necessary space is available. The navigation is guided by the type of nodes: The structure consists of group nodes (containers for other nodes) and individual nodes (the leaf node in the tree with a certain set of attributes). The interaction to be performed within a structure is mainly to show more or less detailed information.

The request for more detailed information for an unlabeled node results in its horizontal expansion to accommodate its label. The request for more

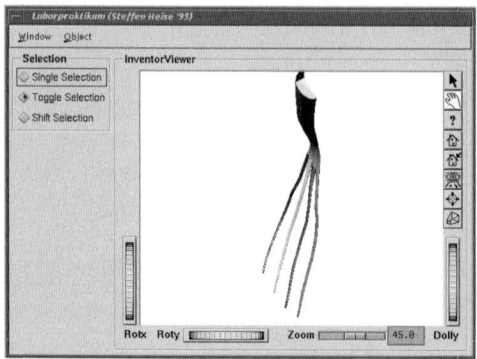 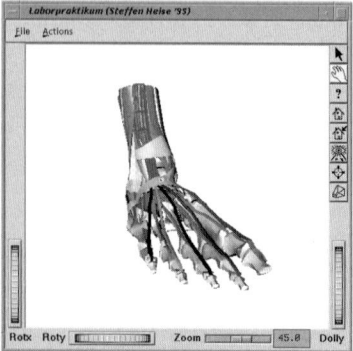

(a) Decomposed object in the refinement view

(b) Updated model view after decomposition

Figure 3.5: Refinement of the object structure (courtesy of Steffen HEISE)

detail for a labeled node is handled differently for group nodes and for individual nodes. Group nodes are expanded horizontally in order to accommodate the labels of their children. Leaf nodes, however, are expanded vertically to display their individual attributes.

All these requests are handled by a fisheye zoom algorithm, more precisely, by a variant of the Variable zoom algorithm (DILL et al. in [DBHH94]), which allows one to continuously scale a rectangular area at the expense of others which are scaled down automatically. Some illustrative images may clarify the effect of the fisheye. An initial view is given in Fig. 3.6. Nodes are embedded in rectangular shapes, the color of which indicates the type of the nodes (e.g., container node or leaf node). The structure view with some labeled nodes is shown. Colored rectangular shapes indicate the children of the nodes.

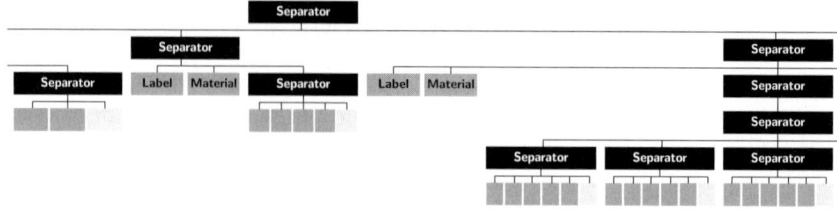

Figure 3.6: A look at the structure view with some nodes labeled

In Fig. 3.7, a container node has been selected. It is scaled up horizontally together with its children until all nodes can accommodate their labels.

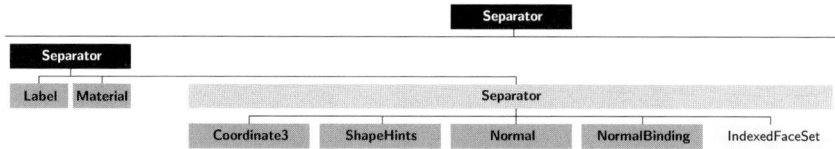

Figure 3.7: Horizontal expansion of a container node to display its children

After one of the child nodes is selected by the user, the child node grows vertically until the names of the attributes can be displayed (see Fig. 3.8).

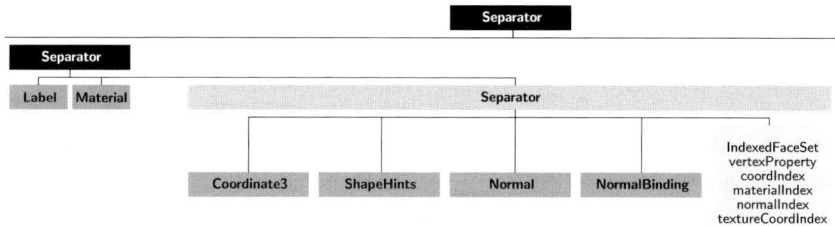

Figure 3.8: Vertical expansion of leaf node to display its attributes

Note that the presentation is automatically adapted to the available space. This means that if the space to display an attribute label is no longer available then it is hidden automatically due to the size request of another node.

3.3.4 Navigating in the Geometry View

In complex models there is typically a large number of objects of very different sizes, leading to the problem of how very small objects can be depicted clearly. It is insufficient to change the viewing direction automatically and to emphasize an object with colors if the projection of this object is too small. In addition, an interactive system for structuring information should support the following tasks directly (cf. RAAB, RÜGER in [RR96]):

- recognizing relationships between objects,
- recognizing the positions of objects in the model, and
- inspecting the shapes of objects in the model.

This is often done by simply scaling the overall model for displaying parts of it or adding separate windows containing objects. However, there are several problems inherent in these approaches. Scaling the model is not always helpful because the context gets lost. Separate windows for the geometry view bring other problems, however, such as difficulties with the user's mental in-

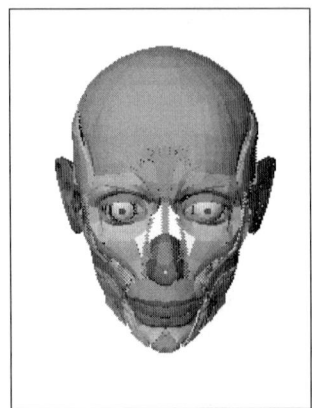 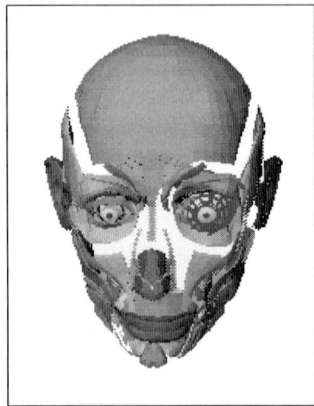

Figure 3.9: One muscle (above the eyes) has been enlarged in the right image by means of a 3D zoom to be explained, while others have been scaled down and moved away

tegration of two or more images in separate windows, and difficulties with navigation in more than one window.

Therefore, a different approach has been used that integrates the fisheye techniques into the graphical part (see Fig. 3.9). Based on twodimensional techniques, the fisheye zoom has been extended to allow navigation in three dimensions (see Chap. 9 and RAAB, RÜGER [RR96]). Here, the regions covered by objects in the model are expressed as 3D bounding boxes facilitating the application of the interval structure independently in each direction (i.e., along the x, y, and z axes) and afterwards the reconstruction of new bounding boxes. The extension includes the handling of overlapping boxes, which is crucial for illustrating 3D models. There are several advantages of this approach for the ZOOMSTRUCTOR:

- *Detail and context:* Objects can be zoomed inside the model's space, enabling the enlarged illustration of small objects in the context of the overall model.
- *Uniform interaction:* Navigation in the structure view and in the geometry view is based on the same techniques and therefore behaves uniformly during interaction.

The latter point is of special importance for the usability. The effort to understand how navigation and interaction is performed decreases. Once a user has understood navigation in the structure view, he or she will probably cope with the graphical interaction. The 3D zoom allows for dual interaction with the structural as well as with the graphical part of the ZOOMSTRUCTOR. The effectiveness of the 3D zoom is partly due to the increased size of small objects. It is also due to the improved visibility and recognizability achieved as the zoom algorithm moves other objects away, which is roughly similar to the effect of an exploded view. Finally, the fact that the object being emphasized as the central point of a movement makes it easy to see which object is involved.

3.3.5 Tight Coupling of Structure View and Geometry View

As in other systems, the ZOOMSTRUCTOR provides a bidirectional coupling between structure and geometry view in adapting the color of the corresponding part in the other view. However, this is insufficient if the part emphasized this way is not included in the displayed information or is simply too small to be recognized. In the case of a complex model, this often occurs. This leads to the question how the visibility and recognizability of the highlighted objects can be achieved. Furthermore, if an object to be highlighted is not visible or not recognizable, the question arises which transformations should occur to ensure the orientation of a user.

Ensuring Visibility. To ensure the visibility of a node in the structure view, it is necessary to represent the position of each node. If a node is outside the visible area, an animated movement scrolls the structure view continuously to center the selected node. To support the user's understanding, we have found it helpful to divide the movement into a horizontal scroll and a subsequent vertical scroll.

The visibility of an object in the geometry view is a more serious problem. While it is possible to find out quickly whether an object is visible or not, it is not as easy to find out which transformation is useful to display an object that is not visible.

To accomplish an automatic transformation, information about visibility from different viewing directions is necessary. This information, however, is not derived online as it is computationally too expensive for an interactive system. Therefore, the model is analyzed in a batch process with regard to the visibility of objects from different viewing angles. This visibility information is used to determine a "good" viewing direction, that is a direction from which an object is visible and as large as possible. If an object should be selected which is not visible, the model is rotated gradually to this "optimal" direction. The rotation takes into account the current viewing direction to minimize the rotation angle. However, a rotation of the whole model forces a user to re-orient himself because all objects have been moved. Some objects even disappear during the rotation. This encouraged us to look for possibilities to reduce the need for rotation.

If an object is not visible, with only one other object in front of it, the occluding object can be rendered translucent so that visibility is achieved without rotation. If several objects hide an object to be highlighted but do not hide each other, then the same strategy can be applied. Only if the object is hidden by some objects occluding each other, the model is rotated. To render a few objects translucent, only a local change of the geometry view is necessary, which we have found is easier for the user's understanding than a global rotation. The ZOOMSTRUCTOR achieves this effect in a small animation, providing a gradual change in the object's translucency value.

Ensuring Recognizability. The graphical zoom – as noted in Sect. 3.3.4 – allows small graphical details to be explained and ensures their recognizability. At first glance it might be not convincing to zoom within the 3D model at all, because the 3D zoom distorts topological relations to a certain extent.

However, adaptive scaling is a common technique for focusing the viewer's attention in static illustrations. We assume that if an adaptive scaling is appropriate in static illustrations, the same ought to be true for interactive illustrations. Instead of confronting a user with a final image, our interactive system carries out a distortion by presenting an animation, i.e., it shows the actual movement from the undistorted to the distorted view. This lets the user know the extent of the distortion. In the final image he or she can see the items of interest better than before the distortion.

The graphical zoom is dedicated to the emphasis of 3D objects which are small in relation to the overall model size. Even these objects are zoomed carefully in order to ensure that the resulting image is not distorted heavily. Figure 3.9 gives an example of an illustration with a muscle enlarged with a 3D zoom. Typical scale factors are between 1 and 2. If such factors are applied to small objects, the overall image is hardly distorted. To prevent heavily distorted views, we do not provide full access to the graphical zoom but invoke it only in a restricted way initiated from the system. It is important that the user can reset the zoom so that all changes to the relative sizes are undone.

3.3.6 Implementation

Our system is implemented using the graphics library OPEN INVENTOR. This object-oriented library is dedicated to the interactive handling of 3D models (e.g., camera control, object transformation). Furthermore, OPEN INVENTOR is useful to realize animated movements which are needed to adapt the presentation gradually. Another important feature of OPEN INVENTOR is the portability to different platforms which is due to the fact that it does not exploit the SGI hardware directly.

In Fig. 3.10, a typical structure view is shown. The structure view as well as the geometry view is realized as a viewing window from OPEN INVENTOR. With this decision, the presentation and interaction in the structure view and in the geometry view (see Fig. 3.11) is unified.

Figure 3.11 presents an integrated view of the context and the geometry view. The context view is composed of standard widgets from OSF MOTIF (recall the mapping of types to widgets discussed in Sect. 3.1.2).

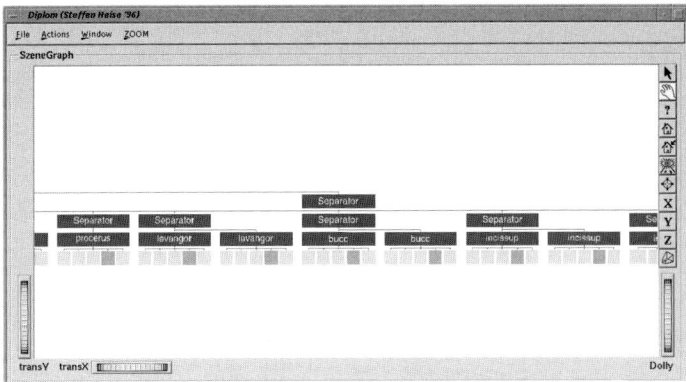

Figure 3.10: ZOOMSTRUCTOR: Structure view

3.4 Concluding Remarks

In this chapter we have developed an integrated approach for the enrichment and reuse of geometric models. Our concepts have been implemented in the ZOOMSTRUCTOR. This system is designed for structuring and for the reuse of geometric models. Our concept integrates a context view, a structure view and a geometry view with a window placement strategy that prevents overlapping windows. In order to explore a geometric model and its structure, we apply fisheye techniques to both structure and geometry view. This enables us to present the structure as well as the model in *one* view instead of a multiple view display with separate overview and detail view. Furthermore, we present relevant objects in detail while maintaining the global context. The application of fisheye techniques in the structure view (2D fisheye) and in the geometry view (3D fisheye) unifies the interaction.

The ZOOMSTRUCTOR has been applied to the enrichment of models for an interactive illustration system, the ZOOMILLUSTRATOR, which will be de-

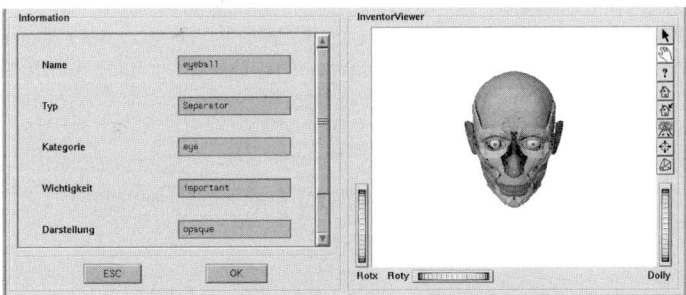

Figure 3.11: ZOOMSTRUCTOR: Context view (left) and geometry view (right)

scribed in Chap. 13. Furthermore it has been tested in context with the AKZENT tool which enhances rendered images (see Chap. 7).

Our structure browser still has scrollbars to support navigation in very large hierarchies. While we have not completely overcome the need for scrolling, we have reduced it considerably and eased navigation.

The connection between structure and geometry views is a tight bidirectional coupling which emphasizes the correspondence between information in both views. This coupling means that information in one view is emphasized in another view. Techniques to emphasize objects include an analysis of visibility and recognizability.

A serious drawback in our system is that the structures displayed are restricted to be purely hierarchical ones. With this restriction, references to geometric objects cannot be displayed, because this kind of multiple inheritance is not purely hierarchical. The system could be improved to handle references using multitrees (introduced by FURNAS, ZACKS in [FZ94]), which are trees with multiple roots.

The ZOOMSTRUCTOR is dedicated to the reuse of geometric models. It assumes that contextual information is submitted from scratch. In many applications the situation is different and related knowledge already exists. This raises the question how the reuse of knowledge can be organized, but that is beyond the scope of this chapter.

Room for improvement exists concerning the management of the context information. The context view can be used to enter search criteria to select information in a database manner. Moreover, consistency checking over and above type checking is necessary to reduce the amount of erroneous data. Furthermore, a user should be supported in assigning contextual information by presenting him or her with an overview about which part of the model has already been enriched with contextual information. While detail and context are integrated in the structure view and in the geometry view, the context view only holds the current record. It would be helpful to have easy access to the records recently processed. A straightforward way to realize this is to provide a history. More elegant, however – and related to the navigation in the geometry and structure view – is it to present the currently processed record together with the most recently processed ones. This can be accomplished using the PERSPECTIVE WALL (cf. ROBERTSON et al. in [RMC91]). The current record is projected to the front wall, while the most recently processed records are projected to the side walls.

Contributors of Chap. 3: Bernhard PREIM and Axel HOPPE

Part II

Controlling Detail

One of the fundamental aspects of abstraction is that the detail to be encoded in an image must be easily controllable and adjustable by end-users who are exploring an information space. This part discusses several fundamental techniques for adjusting the detail during the rendering process. In particular, line drawings are studied extensively (though not exclusively) for visualizing the result of the abstraction process. This is because line drawings emphasize edges of objects and naturally leave blank many areas within a rendition. Between these lines, white spaces dominate in the renditions. This is an opportune way to leave out detail.

The part presents methods which progress from those that yield sparse line drawings (Chap. 4) to progressively more dense line drawings (Chaps. 5 and 6) and enriched shaded images (Chap. 7).

In Chap. 4, Stefan SCHLECHTWEG and Andreas RAAB introduce the reader to the problems involved in rendering line drawings. They discuss an analytic rendering pipeline and show where in the system's architecture the user can influence the underlying algorithms. First, a user can influence algorithms which select the lines to be included in the images, and second, a user can influence the style in which these lines are drawn; these aspects are treated in turn. A particularly interesting aspect of the work is that data which is normally encoded on a surface in a shaded image can now be encoded on lines, for example on the contour of the surface.

Frank GODENSCHWEGER and Hubert WAGENER turn in Chap. 5 to rendering line drawings of free-form surfaces. They discuss methods of converting such free-form surfaces into polygonal meshes. It turns out that when the resultant meshes are converted into line drawings by placing lines along the contours of the patches, some meshes yield good-looking line drawings, while others do not. They introduce the notion of normalized meshes, show how to produce these, and show that they are particularly suited to being converted into line drawings.

Whereas Chaps. 4 and 5 deal with algorithms for producing line drawings directly from geometric representations, in Chap. 6 Oliver DEUSSEN discusses methods of producing line drawings by first rendering shaded images and then carrying out post-processing on these. This yields images which are more dense than with the analytic approach. The method turns out to be more suited for emphasizing the curvature of surfaces than for encoding additional information on the lines.

Finally, in Chap. 7 Axel HOPPE and Kathrin LÜDICKE address algorithms for post-processing rendered images with the goal of encoding additional information within them. They point out that hand-drawn images often use special effects to emphasize selected aspects of objects. Indeed, these effects are simulated in rendered images by setting up a complex and unnatural arrangement of lights. The authors show how some of these effects can be achieved through post-processing of rendered images. Furthermore, they show that their method can be used to encode additional information in rendered images over and above that encoded within a geometric model.

Chapter 4

Rendering Line Drawings for Illustrative Purposes

For many purposes a high-quality photorealistic image is not necessary to communicate intended ideas. "If the ultimate goal of a picture is to convey information", as FOLEY et al. pointed out [FvDFH90] "then a picture that is free of the complications of shadows and reflections may well be more successful than a tour de force of photographic realism." This is especially true for images used for purposes of documentation or as illustrations. Such images are closely related to the text they accompany and utilized to show very specific details of the observed scenario, so a more abstract presentation here often serves the purpose better. A photograph of an engine is of no use for a person in charge of repairing or maintaining it, while a line drawing – possibly a schematic or exploded view – would give the necessary insight to fulfill the task.

In general, high demands are made on images for documentative or illustrative purposes. They have to be of high quality and resolution, it should be possible to transform (scale or rotate) them in order to use them in different places, and they should be clearly recognizable in (almost) any size. Taking this into account, an analytic, vector-oriented image representation is a good choice. Vector images are resolution-independent and can be transformed without creating artefacts or even destroying the visual appearance. It can also be stated that a high quality vector-oriented image needs less storage capacity than a bitmap of comparable size and quality. For future online applications this is very important since the file size is directly proportional to the time spent on network transfer.

Despite all these advantages, bitmapped images are necessary for some purposes. To show surface and material properties exactly, an image that in its appearance closely resembles the real object is needed. Here photorealistic renditions or even photographs are used. They are more suited for depicting very fine details, especially regarding color and texture. However, to be successful, those images have to be provided in a high resolution.

Let us again consider the area of documentation and illustration. We can identify several presentation goals for images which are used here:

- Showing an *illustration* of the scene
  Here lighting and shading is included in the image to enable it to be used for presentations, advertisements, and similar purposes, i.e., to create a "nice" image.
- Showing the overall scene structure and its composition and parts
  This should emphasize the relations between several objects without overburdening the viewer with unnecessary detail.
- Showing the scene from a dedicated point of view
  This means emphasizing different aspects or details and thus focusing on specific parts in the scene.
- Showing the internal geometry of the objects
  This is needed to give a detailed idea of the modeling approach and techniques used. This is a less general goal, however, which will mainly apply to the documentation of geometric models.

To avoid the need to create a new model, images for product documentation should be created directly from the CAD data which are available from the design and construction process. We present a solution to automatically generate images that focus on the presentation goals stated above using such CAD models. The methods presented in this chapter are not restricted to be used within a technical domain. Given any three-dimensional model, they enable us to create illustrations that can be varied in their appearance by using different parameterizations of the presented algorithms. Besides product documentation, medical illustration is a second area of application we have been investigating.

We have chosen to restrict our implementation to polygonal models due to the following considerations:

- Polygonal geometry representations are simple and commonly used in CAD and modeling applications. They are supported by a huge number of systems and thus allow easy data exchange.
- Three-dimensional scanning devices create polygonal models as output. For the intended purpose (documentation and illustration) this is a data source which will be used more frequently in the future.
- Polygonal models of objects from many areas are (commercially) available at different scales and levels of detail (see, for example, [Dat96]).
- Algorithms for the effective handling of polygonal models have been developed over a long period of time and are now standard in computer graphics. These include algorithms for conversion of other representation forms into polygonal models as well as rendering algorithms.

- All other model representation forms can be converted into polygonal models. This allows us to avoid implementing different rendering algorithms for different kinds of models.

Bearing in mind that the final image after the rendering process should be vector-oriented, we use a completely analytic rendering approach. This means that at no point in time will there be an internal representation based on pixels or similar discrete entities. Besides the advantage of accuracy and transformability, analytic rendering offers the possibility to compute and to keep additional information during the rendering process with the same accuracy as the output. This can be used in postprocessing steps which otherwise would require image processing operations at the level of pixels.

This chapter is organized as follows: After a short overview of related work in the area of non-photorealistic rendering (Sect. 4.1), we will develop a new analytic rendering strategy for polygonal models which is particularly suited to the creation of illustrative or documentative images. It will be seen that basically two parts of a traditional rendering pipeline – hidden line elimination and shading – have to be replaced to fulfill the task at hand. Section 4.3 deals largely with hidden line elimination methods. We introduce two particular strategies and discuss their pros and cons. Once the visible lines are computed, the problem of how to finally draw the lines still needs to be solved. We will discuss this topic in Sect. 4.4 and show an easy but effective way to create line drawings which are informative on the one hand and pleasing to the eye on the other. Some techniques for improving the visual quality of the images are shown in Sect. 4.5. Finally, Sect. 4.6 concludes the chapter by explaining the context in which the created illustrations can be used.

4.1 Related Work

The area of non-photorealistic rendering (NPR) has moved into the center of interest in computer graphics research in recent years.

Within the NPR community we can find two directions which seem to be independent of each other. First, there are pixel-based methods for creating more expressive images. Here the work of SAITO and TAKAHASHI [ST90] can be regarded as the basis for many of the approaches used later. SAITO and TAKAHASHI introduced so-called *G-buffers*, data structures which provide a link between the image and the underlying model. A G-buffer stores additional geometric information, for example curvature values, texture coordinates, normal vectors, etc., on a per-pixel basis. Using image processing operations on a G-buffer reveals information about special properties in the image which, in turn, can be used to enhance the image. Here accentuation methods are possible (see Chap. 7 for techniques developed and used in the context of this book) as well as the creation of new kinds of images (see Chap. 6). In [ST90] examples are shown for the superposition of shaded images with line drawings creating "richer", more comprehensible images.

The PIRANESI system as described by SCHOFIELD [Sch94b] can also be regarded as belonging to that group. It works on a so-called *enriched pixel matrix*. This is basically a set of G-buffers storing, for instance, the z-depth or the object-*id* per pixel as well as the (photorealistically rendered) RGB-image. From these input data, a set of *marks* is computed. A mark is a set of pixels which can be described by color, transparency, size, shape, and path characteristics. In general, marks resemble two-dimensional stamp-prints. Those marks are finally placed on the image plane according to information gained from the enriched pixel matrix. Thus, they are aligned and scaled, for instance, according to the current z-depth. PIRANESI is capable of creating images in a wide range of styles at interactive speed.

In contrast to this, the second direction within NPR deals with analytic methods and is basically built upon line creation and drawing techniques. Here especially the work of WINKENBACH et al. is of interest. Their rendering system is based on a binary space partitioning (BSP) approach for hidden line removal. The high quality of the illustrations, however, is mainly determined by the use of so-called *prioritized stroke textures* [WS94], a collection of strokes to produce both texture and tone. The strokes are rendered according to an assigned priority value which determines the drawing order. So for instance strokes contributing to the contour have the highest priority and certain hatching lines the lowest. This ensures that the main idea is properly visualized even with a small number of lines.

A rendering system which can be used for the creation of draft outlines of architectural presentations is presented by STROTHOTTE et al. in [SPR+94]. The renderer here is also BSP-based, but for the creation of hatching lines a pixel-based planar map describing the image for different resolutions is used. The concept for drawing the lines is the basis for our work presented in Sect. 4.4 and consists of two parts. A *model line* is altered based on a *style line* which describes geometric and non-geometric distortions. Even though the method presented in [SPR+94] is limited to straight line segments, interesting results can be achieved.

Not only the positioning of the lines but also the way in which a line is drawn affects the final image. Thus, it is not surprising that there has been a flurry of activity in this area for some time. Many of the researchers here concentrate on painting and drawing simulation. The work of STRASSMANN, for instance, deals with the simulation of brushstrokes to create images resembling the traditional Japanese art *sumi-e* (see [Str86] for some examples). The system devised there is built upon four basic classes of objects: the stroke, the brush, the dip, and the paper. The approach used – moving a tool (the brush) along a path (the stroke) on a surface – is very interesting and will also be applied to our algorithm shown in Sect. 4.4. However, a detailed simulation as presented by STRASSMANN is very time-consuming and thus not appropriate for interactive systems.

In contrast to the pixel-based method of STRASSMANN, a vector-oriented approach is used by HSU, LEE, and WISEMAN. In [HLW93] they introduce

Skeletal Strokes, a technique which is used, for example, in the commercially available drawing program FRACTAL DESIGN EXPRESSION (Fractal Design Corp.) Here also, the general shape of the line to be drawn is defined by a given path. The line is then drawn by transforming a pre-defined picture along that path. The variety of effects gained herewith reaches from very expressive pictures simulating real drawing tools to strange, fantastic images assembled from stretched or distorted cartoon characters.

From this short overview it is evident that two parts of the rendering process are of great importance for line rendering: hidden surface removal and the way a line is drawn. We will examine both aspects in the following sections.

4.2 An Analytic Rendering Pipeline

Rendering, as described by WATT in [Wat93], "... is a general term that describes the overall process of going from a three-dimensional object to a shaded two-dimensional projection on a view surface." This definition – although very general – is appropriate to cover various rendering methods in a simple and understandable way. Interestingly enough, this definition includes *all* rendering methodologies, no matter if the focus is on global illumination simulation or line rendering.

Figure 4.1 shows a rendering pipeline for a photorealistic renderer using a z-buffer for hidden surface elimination as part of the rasterization. We will use this pipeline as a reference and show which parts have to be changed for an analytic line renderer. Obviously, the steps from database traversal to clipping against the view frustum will not change. They basically deal with coordinate transformations and do not alter the structure of the model in any way.

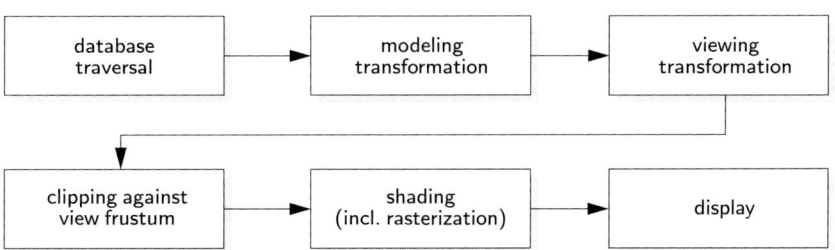

Figure 4.1: A rendering pipeline for photorealistic images (based on [FvDFH90, p. 808])

Compared to the photorealistic rendering approach, where for hidden surface elimination and shading a discretization into pixels has to be performed, an analytic renderer can go on working in object space with the resolution provided in the model. This means that an analytic line renderer will use other hidden surface removal techniques as well as new shading methods based on lines.

The primary task of hidden surface elimination is to remove faces or parts of faces which are not visible from a given viewpoint. This alone is enough for a pixel-based rendering. Within line drawings, a line never exists without its context, and the appearance of a line depends on that context. Thus, for instance, at a point where one line vanishes behind a surface, special attention has to be given to the shape of the line end. Even the contour of the surface screening this line can be drawn differently at this specific point. Hence, it is necessary to have additional information available in such cases. Also, to create line drawings successfully, not all lines should be drawn in the same way. There are special kinds of lines like contour lines or lines showing the internal structure of an object. Those line types have to be determined and the set of lines to be drawn has to be constructed. Finally, especially for technical drawings, "hidden lines" can also be plotted to incorporate more structural information into the image. Here the hidden line elimination process cannot simply discard lines which do not contribute to the visual portion of the image but should keep them for later use, as shown in Fig. 4.2.

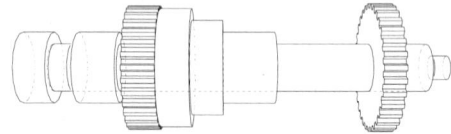

Figure 4.2: Illustration with hidden lines drawn explicitly

We can state that the process of visible line determination is an enormous source of information which can be used for the design of the image. Our investigations in the area of line drawings reveal that the more information is available for the shading process, the more possibilities we have for encoding not only geometric, but also more abstract information in the generated image. In this context, an interesting question is whether this is also true for the generation of other pictorial representations. The work of SAITO and TAKAHASHI [ST90] or SCHOFIELD [LS95] shows that the assertion also holds true for their domains.

For line drawings, there is no process of "shading" in the sense of photorealistic rendering. Instead, lighting information has to be encoded by drawing lines at a certain position and with a certain appearance. There are several techniques, originated in traditional illustration, which can easily be adapted to computer graphics. The change in line width or brightness according to lighting is one example, showing surface structure by hatching is another one. For both, special drawing methods are needed.

The result of a hidden line elimination process is normally a set of line segments characterized by start and end points. For the successful creation of line drawings, simply drawing these segments is not enough. To show the contour of an object, for instance, a curve with changing characteristics will do a much better job than an angular polyline. Thus, curves have to be created from the given line segments, and those curves will be the basis for particular drawing methods.

Putting it all together, the rendering pipeline we use differs from the one shown in Fig. 4.1 in terms of hidden line removal (HLR) and shading. The applied HLR methods work in object space and, instead of shading, a selection of computed lines provides the input for special line drawing techniques.

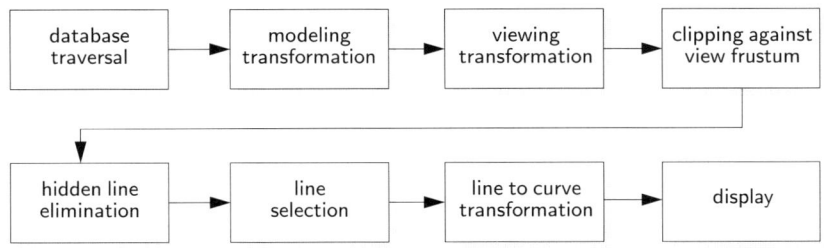

Figure 4.3: A rendering pipeline for line drawings

The following detailed description of our approach focuses on the parts which are different to the reference model. We describe two methods for hidden line elimination, in each of which a different kind of additional information is stored. Thus, the possibilities for "shading" differ and we are able to create variable images by choosing one of the methods.

4.3 Hidden Line Elimination

The task of hidden line elimination – as was already mentioned above – is one of the most important points when rendering line drawings. Special hidden line removal methods have been studied in computer graphics for a long time. The well known painter's algorithm is fast but cannot handle intersections in its simplest form. Approaches based on BSP (binary space partitioning), such as used by STROTHOTTE et al. [SPR+94] and WINKENBACH et al. [WS94], overcome this problem, but they require rather time-consuming preprocessing of the models. In addition, these algorithms generally focus on interactive applications for pixel-based displays and not on analytic descriptions of the resulting visible lines. The algorithm of SECHREST and GREENBERG [SG81] computes visible regions as well as visible lines, but fails to handle intersections. Despite this major disadvantage, we will show in Sect. 4.3.2 that this algorithm has some features which are of convenient use for illustrative rendering of line drawings.

While the algorithms mentioned before solve the general task of hidden line and hidden surface elimination, we have found that an optimized algorithm solves the task of rendering for documentational purposes more efficiently. Observations we have made while examining images rendered for the use in documentations show that typically all lines displayed in these images are part of the geometric model, either in an explicit representation (such as polygon edges in a polygon mesh) or created through a well defined generation process (such as iso-parametric edges in a free-form surface). One reason is that those images are created with CAD programs which are restricted to that kind of drawing. Indeed, we can say that all lines displayed in the final image are explicitly part of the geometric model. This allows us to avoid the task of actual visible surface detection. In the next section we will describe a quad tree based rendering method stemming from this observation.

Having an algorithm available which performs hidden line elimination as well as visible surface determination offers different possibilities for the rendering of line drawings. Here information can be evaluated on how the determined visible line segments are related to form visible faces. This results in information which is of great value within the "shading" process. An example will illustrate this. Knowing of the position of a contour line with respect to the face it bounds (on the left hand or right hand side) gives a clue for the bending direction of this particular line. Also, for the effect of "haloed lines" (here lines are drawn with a distinct separation from any other line, leaving the gap completely white) the relation of lines to faces is of interest. In Sect. 4.3.2 we present a scan-line based algorithm which computes visible lines as well as visible faces.

The two algorithms offer different data which help to produce different drawings. We show examples throughout this chapter. Generally, the scan-line based algorithm is better for drawings in a somewhat artistic style, whereas the quad tree based approach provides interesting results for more exact, technical drawings. It would be interesting to investigate how a combination of both can be used to provide all required information at once.

4.3.1 Method I: Quad Tree Based Algorithm

The starting point for our investigation is a three-dimensional polygonal model. The modeling transformation as well as the viewing transformation and clipping against the view frustum is performed in the standard way. The only difference is that we keep all computed coordinates in the model for further reference.

The concentration on rendering edges derived directly from the triangle mesh representation simplifies the task of hidden line elimination to a great extent. First of all, general line-polygon clipping (such as done by the WEILER-ATHERTON algorithm [WA77]) is not necessary. All we basically need is to clip each edge with a series of triangles. It also allows us to classify the edges (i.e., the resulting lines in the image) so that we can render them in a special order determined by the significance a line has for the final image.

Our rendering algorithm is divided into three phases. In the setup phase, triangulation is performed, and then the edges to be rendered are determined and sorted according to their importance for the final image. In the clipping

4.3 Hidden Line Elimination

phase, a quad tree for efficient face lookup is created, and the basic clipping of all selected edges is performed. Finally, in the update phase, the intersections between faces are calculated.

Setup Phase. In the setup phase, all non-triangular representations are converted into triangular meshes. Generally, we use an iso-parametric triangulation scheme for this task, since iso-parametric lines typically give a good impression of the shape to be rendered.

After this has been done, the edges are prepared for rendering and then sorted such that the most significant edges are rendered first (see Fig. 4.4). The order of the edges is determined as follows:

1. *Contour edges:* These edges segregate an object from its environment and thus give an impression of the general shape of the object. They are considered to be most significant.
2. *Sharp edges:* Edges representing discontinuities between neighboring faces give a strong indication of the internal structure of the model.
3. *Smooth edges:* These edges (typically perceived as curvature) indicate the internal structure at a finer level than the sharp edges.
4. *Triangulation edges:* Although only temporary, these edges can be presented to show the triangulation of the object. (This is only needed for illustrating and documenting geometric models.)

In addition, the edges in each group are again sorted according to the angle between adjacent faces.

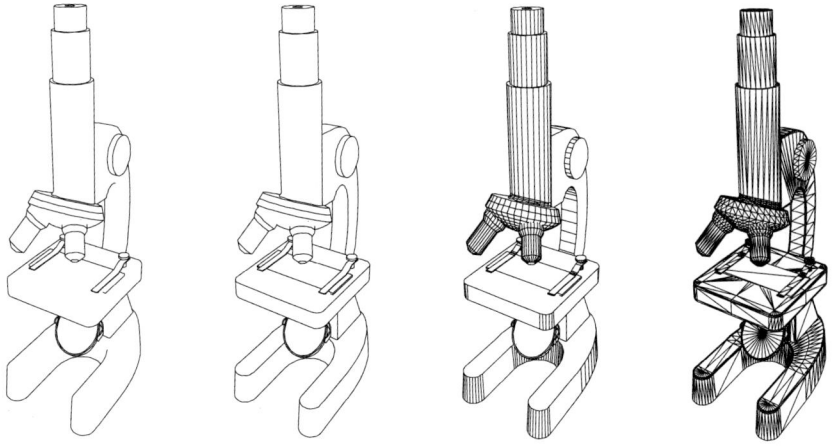

Figure 4.4: Edges displayed after computing the contour, sharp, smooth, and triangulation edges

The order of edges allows us to define certain threshold values for the different line types. So, for instance, a user may define different combinations of the lines (e.g., no triangulation edges, only smooth edges above a certain angle, all sharp edges, etc.). In addition, the threshold values may be automatically defined by the system according to the documentation goal or set by the user interactively.

Clipping Phase. Clipping the edges against a series of faces from the model requires an efficient lookup structure. A quad tree serves this purpose well. However, the creation of the quad tree is somewhat time-consuming and should be done in a way that reflects the complexity of the model. Therefore, we use an adaptive quad tree in which the depth varies according to the number of faces in the model (see Fig. 4.5).

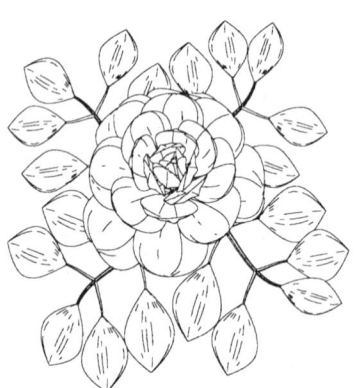 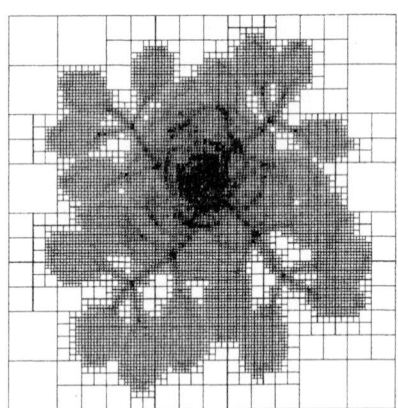

Figure 4.5: The model of a rose (left) and the associated quad tree (right): darker areas in the quad tree indicate a higher number of faces

The clipping consists basically of three parts. After the faces possibly affecting the line to be clipped are selected from the quad tree, each face is clipped with the edge in front-to-back order to efficiently reject completely hidden edges. For each face-edge pair, the following three tests are performed:

- The primitive bounding box test gives information as to whether the edge is affected at all by the given face (if it lies in front of the face we can ignore any further tests), or if we can do non-perspective corrected clipping (if the edge lies behind the face). Note that even though we use a quad tree to reduce the number of faces selected for each clipping operation, the primitive bounding box test can again reject a large number of faces, in particular those which are only touching an area in the quad tree.

- If possible (i.e., if the edge lies behind the face), we perform a non-perspective-corrected clipping operation in 2D. This is generally much faster than a full, perspective-corrected clipping operation. The result of this operation is a hidden interval of the edge which is recorded for later use. In the case that the interval contains the whole edge, the clipping operation can be aborted.
- If necessary (i.e., if the edge intersects the face) an exact perspective-corrected clipping operation is performed. This is more expensive than a simple 2D based clipping operation. We have found that even in models with many intersections the number of perspective-corrected clipping operations is generally far below 5 percent of all clipping operations so that the overall speed is mainly determined by the bounding box test and the 2D clipping. In addition to the hidden interval computed, we also record the intersecting edge and face for the intersection edge calculation performed in the update phase.

Update Phase. It is often convenient or indeed necessary to display intersections between surfaces explicitly as lines in the drawing. To avoid preprocessing we use the information already obtained by previous clipping operations. So, for instance, we already know which edge intersects another face. Obviously, all faces adjacent to this edge generate new intersection edges. We can therefore build well defined face pairs from the already known intersections (Fig. 4.6).

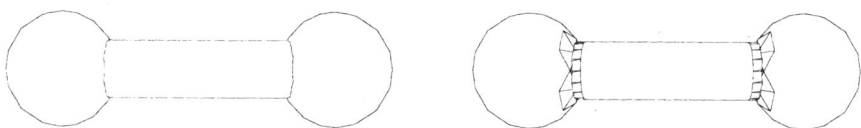

Figure 4.6: Calculated intersections (left) and faces used for exact intersection calculation (right)

Since we only deal with triangular faces, there are exactly two ways in which a penetrating face pair (f_1, f_2) can be defined. Either two edges of the face f_1 intersect the face f_2, or one edge of f_1 intersects f_2 and one edge of f_2 intersects f_1. The information recorded from perspective-corrected clipping can be used to find the appropriate face pairs. However, not all face pairs are necessarily defined, because not all edges of the model may have been clipped yet due to the initial threshold values. For each face pair which still has unknown intersection points, all currently unused edges of both faces are put into the clipping algorithm to resolve these unknown intersections. By doing this, new intersections may be found which have not been recorded before. The new face pairs generated in this process are handled in the same way until there are no more unresolved face pairs. In this way the intersections are updated in an iterative process allowing the calculation of all visible intersections in the model. As can be seen in Fig. 4.6, only necessary edges will be used for the intersection calculation. This, in turn, dramatically reduces the time needed for computation because we do not use every edge from the model.

The complete algorithm as described here provides as output a *sorted* list of lines which are tagged based on the edge classes introduced above. In addition, the lines keep a reference pointer to the model edge from which they were created. For further processing, the output list can be traversed applying several conditions to select particular lines to be drawn. Some examples created with this algorithm can be seen within this section as well as later on.

An interesting property of the quad tree based approach is especially useful for network applications. The algorithm computes the visible lines in a special order (sorted by the visual importance) and, thus, by drawing the lines in this order we go from a rough outline to a more detailed image. The drawing process can be stopped at any time[1] revealing an image which reflects a certain level of detail. This and the streaming capability (it is not necessary to have *all* data to draw the image) offers potential for network based applications such as client/server configurations where the server renders the image and the clients draw it until the desired level of detail is reached.

Although it has the advantage of being a very efficient method, the quad tree based approach has one major drawback. It does not keep any information on how the created lines belong together to form faces. Thus, no information of this kind is available within the "shading" process to evaluate properties that depend on the relationship between several faces.

In the following section we present a second approach, where the process of hidden surface elimination is performed based on a scan-line algorithm developed by SECHREST and GREENBERG in 1981 [SG81]. With this algorithm it is possible to create not only a set of visible lines but also a set of visible faces which are bounded by those lines.

4.3.2 Method II: Scan-Line Based Algorithm

The original algorithm by SECHREST and GREENBERG [SG81] was developed as an elegant and fast way to perform visible line determination in connection with visible surface determination. It works at object resolution and is invoked after the projection of the scene has taken place. Thus, it works in (three-dimensional) screen coordinates. In contrast to other scan-line approaches where the distance between two scan-lines is fixed, an adaptive scheme is used by SECHREST and GREENBERG. The scan-lines are placed at the locations of so-called *events* which occur in the scene. Those events are

---

[1] So-called "anytime" algorithms are popular in the area of artificial intelligence. See for instance [DB88].

vertices defined in the three-dimensional model and crossings of two edges in the picture plane. We will call them *vertex events* or *crossing events*, respectively.

The algorithm is divided into two phases which we will describe in more detail below. Note that the algorithm used is very similar to the original by SECHREST and GREENBERG. It has been extended to suit our needs in such a way that it extensively keeps track of the operation steps performed and assigns additional data to the generated lines as well as to the generated faces. However, it cannot handle intersecting faces. To avoid this, preprocessing of the model is possible in which all intersections are resolved to obtain a non-penetrating model.

Visible Line Determination. For the algorithm to work properly, an order has to be defined over the vertices in the model. We say that a vertex v_1 at (x_1, y_1) lies *before* a vertex v_2 at (x_2, y_2) if $y_1 < y_2$ or, if the y-coordinates are equal, $x_1 < x_2$. The algorithm works on two data structures which are initialized at the beginning:

- An active edge table (AET) containing all edges in the model which are currently of interest. This table is initialized to be empty.
- An entry list containing all minimal vertices sorted by the order defined above.

The algorithm works on the data structures as long as at least one of them contains entries. If both are empty, all visible lines have been determined. The procedure (which is applied repeatedly until the end condition is reached) is as follows:

1. Select the next minimal event (according to the defined order) from the entry list or the AET.
2. Update the AET. At vertex events, remove all edges which end here and add all edges beginning at the current vertex. Determine the visibility of all edges processed. If a visible edge ends, write out the coordinates of the respective line. At crossing events, swap intersecting edges in the AET and determine the visibility for the edge segments. If a visible segment ends, write out the coordinates of the created line.

At crossing events in the second step above, in contrast to the approach taken in the original algorithm of SECHREST and GREENBERG, we generally divide the screening edge into two parts, even though the visibility may not change. We do this to assign a special line type to the resulting segments. At those points, an edge belonging to the silhouette of an object may change in an edge representing a self-occlusion. For determining the silhouette of the object within the drawing process, we will need this information. We can also keep all hidden segments for further reference.

Visible Surface Determination. The visible surface determination is done in parallel with the visible line determination. In general, visible surfaces are polygons bounded by visible lines. For ease of surface reconstruction, additional information has to be preserved in the visible line algorithm from above. On either side of a visible segment, a linked list of output vertices is created in such a way that on the junction of two segments a new vertex is placed in those lists. For polygon reconstruction, closed chains of output vertices are traced.

The differences between our implementation and the original algorithm consists mainly in the preservation of additional data. As already mentioned above, edges – and the resulting visible lines – are marked with a type attribute. The types used are comparable to those introduced in Sect. 4.3.1. An *inner edge* has two visible faces on either side. Here smoothing information from the model is used to determine whether the edge is sharp or smooth. At a *contour edge* a visible polygon and a polygon representing a back face meet. *Silhouette edges* can be regarded as special contour edges building the border of an object to the environment.

If we regard all edges as being directed towards growing y- and x-coordinates (in that order), we can say that faces are to the left or right of a particular edge. This is especially useful when drawing the lines as curves (as will be seen in Sect. 4.4) since here the curvature can always be applied to the correct direction (out of the object). Also the use of "haloed lines" needs a definite statement of the direction inside the object.

In addition to the type information assigned at each edge, we also compute an *edge normal* which is comparable to the *vertex normal* in photorealistic techniques. The edge normal is a vector which is calculated from the arithmetic or geometric mean of the two faces adjoining the edge. For the incorporation of lighting in the drawing, we found that this information is sufficient for simple and fast drawings. More elaborate methods, however, require the exact evaluation of an illumination model. Furthermore, in the context of shading not only the projected coordinates in the view plane are required but also world coordinates. These coordinates are kept aside during the rendering, and at points where new vertices are generated an interpolation is performed to get appropriate coordinate values. This prevents us later on from applying the inverse transformations to gain original coordinates, which is especially tedious for the viewing transformation.

4.4 Drawing the Lines – Shading

With the output of the extended hidden line elimination algorithms as described above we are now in a position to create line drawings which go far beyond the simple wireframe rendition shown in Fig. 4.7(a). Both algorithms examined in the previous section provide a set of visible lines as output. All lines are basically described by their end points, and we require points to be *identical* in terms of the internal representation. Furthermore, we have at least a reference to the original scene object the line belongs to and the type of the line (contour, sharp edge, smooth edge, triangulation edge). All additional information which is available will be used for special drawing techniques. In the following we show how different effects in line drawings can be achieved first by selecting special lines to be drawn, and second by a certain drawing method.

4.4.1 Line Selection and Chaining

The following figures show some simple examples of drawings which can be created just by evaluating the type of the line. As can be seen, the selection of lines in this way makes it easy to create drawings which focus on different aspects. Whereas in Fig. 4.7(c) the construction of the scene can be recognized in great detail, Fig. 4.7(d) focuses more on the subobjects contained in the scene. Another example can be found in Fig. 4.4.

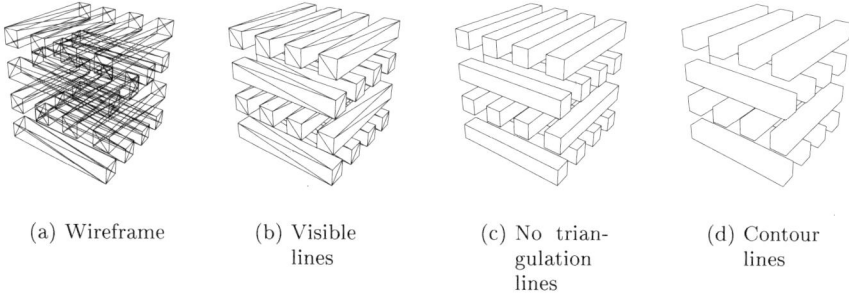

(a) Wireframe   (b) Visible lines   (c) No triangulation lines   (d) Contour lines

Figure 4.7: Several line drawings from the same model where different line types are selected for drawing

Up to this point we have still been working with single line segments which are created during the HLR process. Those line segments stem directly from the model's edges and their number is thus dependent on the model's triangulation. To overcome this problem at least partially, we connect matching line segments to chains which are then drawn either as polylines or interpolated or approximated by spline curves. A prerequisite for this is that shared vertices are indeed identical. In most programming languages this speeds up the execution since there is only the need for pointer comparison instead of comparing somewhat complicated structures element after element.

The algorithm for the creation of line chains is rather simple. We start with a line which we know belongs to the chain and then simply search for continuing segments. The choice of the actual segment to use is done by simple selection mechanisms. For contour lines this might be the angle between the current segment and the candidate line, for other lines some more complicated selection strategies may apply. Those are based on values kept during the rendering process, such as for instance the continuity (smoothness) between adjacent faces in the model. After the chaining process, the drawing is now described by a set of polylines. They can be drawn directly but also regarded as a control polygon for different spline curves. Figure 4.8 shows an example of how this affects the actual appearance of the drawing. Note in the right two images that – since now the drawing is only an approximation of the model and no longer an exact representation – different densities of the triangulations do not affect the final image that much. This is indeed an advantage of our rendering strategy.

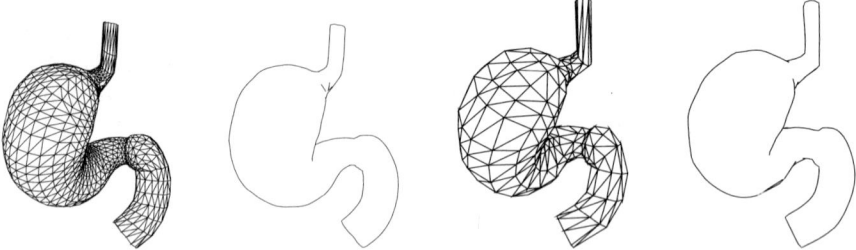

Figure 4.8: Wireframe drawings and line drawings of two differently dense triangulated models: note the effect of a more sparse triangulation (in the right two images) on the line drawing

4.4.2 Special Line Drawing Techniques

All the images shown above are interesting for technical illustration, but they do not include any "shading" information, e.g., lighting and/or material information. For more elaborate images we must first analyze how lighting is depicted within line illustrations before we can find an algorithmic solution. However, we will not carry out a detailed analysis of drawing techniques here. An excellent insight into scientific illustration techniques can be found in [Hod89].

An indication of lighting conditions in line drawings can be achieved by varying the line width or the line brightness. In darker areas, wider or darker lines are drawn, whereas in regions which are lit up, lines are very thin and bright or even not completely drawn. Also, the connection between lines at points where a line vanishes behind a surface has to be drawn carefully to suggest correctly that the line does not just end at the surface's border but instead is continued underneath.

An analysis of traditional pen-and-ink drawings reveals that all lines can be considered as consisting of two parts. The *path* describes the overall course of the line, i.e., its geometry. The final appearance is mainly determined by the way the pen is moved along the drawing surface, the pen angle, the amount of remaining ink, the pressure which is applied to the pen, and other

4.4 Drawing the Lines – Shading

deviations from the exact path (due to surface irregularities or inaccurate hand movement). We refer to all these values collectively as the *style*. The superposition of path and style finally results in the *line* which is then drawn.

The path and the style are both described as parametric curves over the interval [0, 1] by a set of control vertices. Furthermore, an interpolation or approximation method determines the type of curve used. At the moment Bézier curves, Catmull-Rom splines, and polylines (as a special interpolation method) are supported, and more curve types can be added easily in our system.

Since the path mainly describes the line's geometry, all deviations from this are encoded into the style. Thus, the style describes how the given geometry will be perturbed to result in the final line. For easier judgment of the effects which the style has on the line, its definition is based on a straight line. This means that the style basically describes how a straight line would be distorted in terms of geometric and non-geometric attributes (more on this later). This is not a restriction, since the possibilities offered by the superposition method are independent of the underlying curve type. Before we show how path and style are used, it is of utmost importance to note that both are completely independent of each other. It is even possible to use different curve types defined at different scales. This makes it possible for the renderer to deposit data pertaining to physical phenomena in a data structure associated with a path while its interpretation in the form of a line style can be adjusted later to yield the final line.

Besides the geometry, path and style can be attributed with non-geometric information. Those attributes will then be translated into visual properties of the line. So, for instance, different pressure or saturation of a drawing tool can be simulated by mapping them to line width and brightness. Also here, the model can be extended easily to other properties. As for the geometry, the change of attributes is described by polynomial functions. To define them, it is necessary to supply either

- specific attribute values at the curve's control vertices,
- independent attribute values for specific parameters $t \in [0, 1]$ which are then interpolated, or
- an explicit interpolation function defined over the interval $t \in [0, 1]$.

So far we have examined how the path and the style are defined. We shall now describe the mapping of the style onto the path and thus how to compute the final line. A wide variety of methods exists for the geometric superposition of path and style. The simplest approach would be to transform the style so that it matches the scale and orientation of the path and then compute the final line to be the arithmetic or geometric mean of path and style. However, the result is not easy to predict and thus another approach seems to be more promising.

To map the style geometry onto the path we use the line segment from the style's starting point s_s to the end point s_e (see Fig. 4.9).

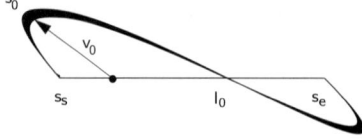

Figure 4.9: Computation of the difference vector v_0

We then compute the point $l_0 = s_s + t(s_e - s_s)$ for a given parameter value $t \in [0, 1]$. Furthermore, we calculate the point s_0 on the style curve for the same parameter value t and the *difference vector* $v_0 = s_0 - l_0$.

This difference vector is then added to the point p_0 which is the position on the given path for the parameter t, and we get the final point p. Fig. 4.10 illustrates how the direction of the vector can be applied to the path:

1. The direction of the difference vector does not change. The angle α of the vector to a horizontal line is kept constant (left). Here $p = p_0 + v_0$.
2. The vector is rotated by an angle β so that α is seen with respect to the tangent vector of the path at p_0 (right). Here we add the rotated vector v_r to p_0.

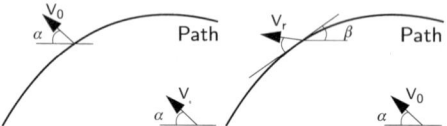

Figure 4.10: Application of the difference vector to the path point: based on a horizontal line (left), rotated to match the path's tangent direction (right)

In both cases, the scale of the difference vector is somewhat problematic. Since the path and the style might be defined in different scales, the length of the vector is not necessarily appropriate. We currently use the ratio between the path length and the style length as the scaling factor. The user can also specify a *style scale factor* that is applied before the mapping.

The mapping of the geometric properties leads to a *skeleton* of the curve which is to be drawn. In contrast to the work of HSU, LEE, and WISEMAN [HLW93], where the *flesh* of this skeleton is computed by transforming an arbitrary picture, we create the flesh from the given pressure and saturation values yielding a hull shape for the line to be drawn. The superposition of the attribute values (in this case pressure and saturation) is simply calculated as the arithmetic mean of the given value for path and style at each position $t \in [0, 1]$. This is directly included in the calculation of the output curve.

From this point on we use a discrete step size Δt. For subsequent parameter values t_i, we compute the position, width, and brightness by combining path and style as described above. For each pair of value sets, a quadrilateral is drawn as output according to Fig. 4.11. The width of those quadrilaterals is determined by the pressure values at t_i. This width is seen either with respect to the normal direction of the path or to a given *pen angle*. Problems arise in regions of high curvature when the step size is relatively small compared to the line width. In this case we may get quadrilaterals with self-intersecting bounds which have to be handled separately.

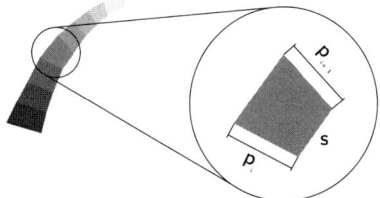

Figure 4.11: For the output the line is drawn as a sequence of polygons. Their size is determined by the pressure values for $t = t_i$ and $t = t_{i+1}$ (p_i and p_{i+1}). The brightness results from the saturation values s_i and s_{i+1}

Figure 4.12 illustrates the effects which can be achieved by applying differently parameterized styles to a simple path (which, in this case, is given directly in 2D).

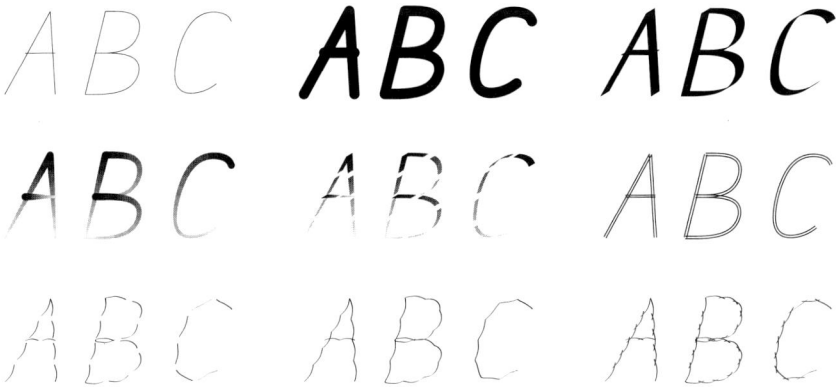

Figure 4.12: Effects of different styles distorting a simple path shown in the first image. Different line widths and pen angles produce lines resembling those drawn in pen and ink. The last three images show how different stroke settings affect the image (courtesy of Lars SCHUMANN)

The line drawing method introduced here is very simple to implement and needs no further supplements from any specific graphics library. Also, the distinction in path and style makes it easy to create different images from one model just by replacing the style applied. Using this drawing method in connection with the line selection mentioned above offers a wide range of possibilities for the design of illustrative drawings. In the following section some of the points which have to be considered are discussed. More examples and possibilities for further development can be found in Sect. 4.6.

4.5 Illustrating with Lines

So far in this chapter, we have developed techniques which can be used to create illustrative drawings. Their application ranges from illustrations which will be incorporated in technical documentations up to medical and other scientific illustrations. In the following, some detailed insight into the area of illustration is given. The main focus here is on using the techniques developed above to fulfill the presentation goals stated at the beginning of this chapter.

Within illustrations, there are several aspects which must be clearly communicated to the viewer. The most important here is the form of the objects shown. Besides that, structural information – how are objects "assembled" from smaller parts and shapes – and texture information are to be depicted. In this section both aspects will be examined. First we show how contour drawings can be enhanced to communicate structure as well as lighting conditions. In addition to this, techniques for showing surface detail and textures are presented.

4.5.1 Drawing the Contour

The most elementary means of depicting form is a simple outline. However, this is often not sufficient to give a clear understanding of what is drawn. So adding structural lines (these are basically the outlines of smaller parts of the subject) or drawing the outline differently will offer some more possibilities.

To distinguish visually several objects in an illustration, it is often useful to draw them differently. Also, it is worth considering differentiating between the actual contour lines of an object and lines depicting internal structures. To achieve this, the concept of drawing the outline can be extended by drawing the outline of different levels of the model's (scene's) whole-part hierarchy. This assumes the model to be extensively structured. Indeed, observations here revealed that to communicate successfully a detailed structure in the image, the underlying model has to be enriched with structural and contextual information (see also Chap. 3).

Within the rendering process, the evaluation of the model's structure leads to attributes which are assigned to the lines to be created. Doing this allows one to process lines which are attributed differently in a special way during the drawing process. The distinction in path and style as introduced earlier helps to fulfill this task. A different style is chosen for the inner lines – preferably a discreet, soft one – than for the contour (a firmer, bolder style). This will emphasize the outline but still make the internal structure recognizable. This applied emphasis can also be based on other criteria, for instance, the (user-supplied) importance of an object or the distance from any given center of interest, for instance the viewpoint (recall the degree-of-interest *DOI* mentioned earlier). Figure 4.13 shows some examples.

Even though line drawings are a limited and limiting medium in terms of the possibilities offered to show attributes other than structural information,

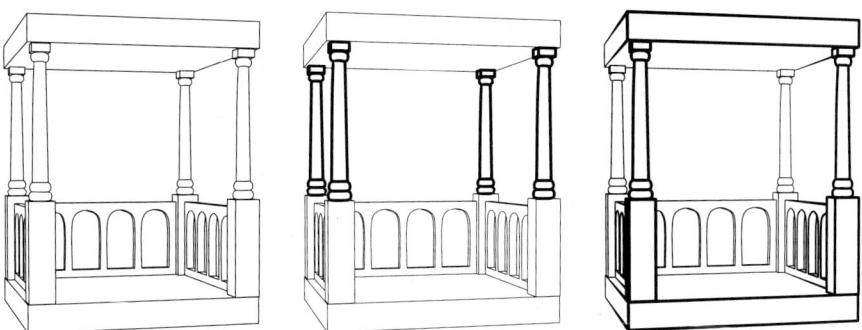

Figure 4.13: The same model without any change (left), emphasized columns (center), and simulated depth-cueing (right) (courtesy of Bert SCHÖNWÄLDER)

there are some methods to depict for instance lighting conditions in a simple contour drawing. The path and style model is particularly well suited for doing this. Let us consider the encoding of light and shadows by different line widths. The actual line width at a certain position is given by the intensity value obtained by evaluating the illumination model, and thus should not be affected by a possibly given drawing style in a way that other lighting situations are suggested. By coding this information as attributes directly to the path we can ensure that they influence the final line in the desired way. In practice, this means that for each path contained in the drawing, we need to compute appropriate attribute values.[2]

Provided there is a link between the edges in the model and the line segments created in the rendering process, the incorporation of lighting is not hard to accomplish. For each path vertex we take the respective model vertex and evaluate the illumination model at this position. (Here already the evaluation of the edge normal for the whole segment suffices, but better results can be achieved with more elaborate methods.) The resulting intensity value is then applied as the pressure attribute at the given path point. This means that when finally drawing the lines, the line width changes in relation to the given lighting situation. Figure 4.14(a) shows the model of a foot rendered without any changes in line width and brightness. By including lighting information we gain the image in Fig. 4.14(b) which nicely illustrates the improvement of visual quality.

4.5.2 Shading Techniques

For many cases the depiction of contour and structure is sufficient; however, the shape of the surface cannot be easily recognized. Texturing and hatching

---

[2] This is not a bad idea anyway, because it gives the path a definite state which is especially useful for animations (cf. Chap. 14).

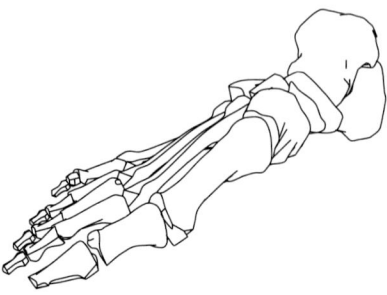 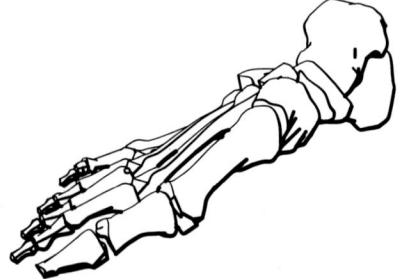

(a) The "plain" drawing without further attributes

(b) Lighting information included and mapped onto the width of the line style (slightly overdone)

Figure 4.14: Two renditions from the same model (courtesy of Bert SCHÖNWÄLDER)

can immensely improve the visual appearance as well as the "comprehensibility" of the image. The algorithms presented above can provide all the information needed to incorporate at least simple texturing. In particular, the scan-line based algorithm keeps track of visible faces and their relations to edges and faces in the model as well as the lines drawn.

In hand-drawn images, hatching with lines is frequently used to show spatial relations and material properties. A great variety of techniques exists here, and they are employed according to the intended purpose and in a differentiated way. In general, the choice of the hatching method to be used and of the parameterization of this method is hard to formalize. In this area the work of SALESIN et al. (cf., e.g., [WS94], [SABS94], or [WS96]) is a valuable approach worth considering.

Besides typical hatching techniques, there are other approaches of how to depict surface structure and texture within line drawings. In the following we will show two examples: *stippling* and *overlay images*.

Stippling. Stippling is very frequently used in the area of scientific illustration. With this drawing technique, form is suggested by gradations of tone. Different tonal values are depicted by groups of dots, where the distance between the dots and the size of the dots depends on the brightness of the specific part of the surface. Figure 4.15 gives an idea of how tonal values are represented with stipples.

Stippling by hand is very time-consuming. It is difficult to achieve the proper scale and spacing of the dots. The distance between two adjacent dots should be larger than the diameter of one dot to make the single dots recognizable even after a reduction of the drawing of 50 percent or more. It is also important in very light areas that the dots appear as being put there on purpose and thus they have to be distributed equally but irregularly. In dark areas where the stipples are close together they may create totally black areas. These areas should be kept to a minimum to stop them dominating the picture.

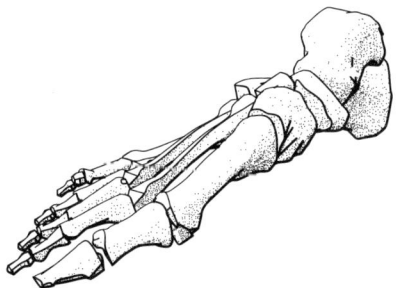

Figure 4.15: With stippling, form is suggested by the placement of dots depending on the lighting conditions (courtesy of Bert SCHÖNWÄLDER)

Implementing stippling as a shading method for computer graphics requires the computation of all visible faces of an object. They, in turn, are then filled with randomly distributed dots where the median distance and size of the dots depends on the calculated intensity value (based on an illumination model). For ease of processing, a heavily triangulated model is assumed so that for each triangle to be filled a single intensity value suffices. However, the choice of the proper distance and size for the dots not only depends on the illumination model but also on the final output device. Different resolutions cause the objects to appear differently.

Overlay Images. Besides drawing techniques that suggest texture with the same means as structure (i.e., using line drawing methods for both), computer graphics enables one to combine totally different rendering methods in one picture. The shaded image of the foot bones in Fig. 4.16(a) is – due to the material information – hardly recognizable on a bright background. A combination of shading and line-based techniques in one image can combine the advantages of both, as shown in Fig. 4.16(b). This was already mentioned by SAITO and TAKAHASHI [ST90], who referred to those techniques as "comprehensible rendering".

In contrast to the work of SAITO and TAKAHASHI, our line drawing techniques are based on an analytic model representation and provide an analytic representation of the drawing. To make sure that the line drawing exactly fits into the shaded image it is of utmost importance that the camera models used are the same, although a slight difference between the images will be tolerated by the viewer since the line drawing is only seen as an approximation of the form of the model.

The method of overlaying a shaded image and a line-based rendition nicely combines the advantages of both techniques. In particular, surface structure and textures can be depicted with photorealistic means, whereas the line drawing enhances the visual properties of the image in terms of object differentiation and figure–ground distinction.

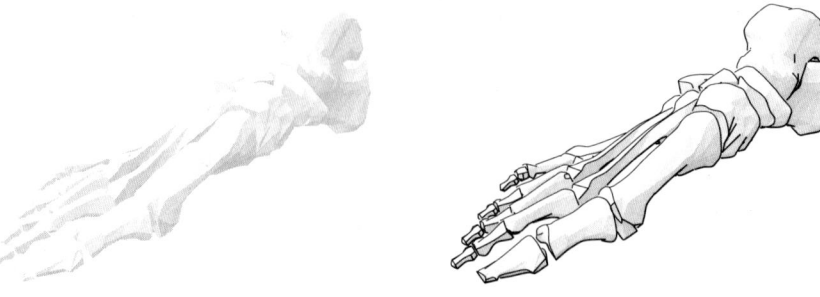

(a) Shaded image of the bones   (b) Image enhanced with line drawing techniques

Figure 4.16: Suggesting texture and surfaces (courtesy of Bert SCHÖNWÄLDER)

4.6 Applications and Open Problems

As can be seen in the technical description and the sample images above, the methods presented bear a high potential with respect to their application. A possible area where our techniques can be used is scientific – or more specifically – medical illustration. According to HODGES [Hod89] this is "... the production of drawings of measured accuracy and other graphic images that help the scientist-author to communicate."

Within this area, the viewer's requirement regarding a good illustration is to get reliable information about form, structure, and sometimes texture of the depicted objects. This means also that all parts of the image may be identified immediately, and hence the context of a specific object is of importance. These requirements lead to the observation that abstraction in medical illustration is crucial. HODGES states: "A medical or surgical illustration that literally copies visual fact would be no more useful than a decent photograph." Photographs, however, are seldomly used in the field of anatomy or surgery. This is due to the uniform colors of different tissues and other parts. HODGES goes even further: "A good medical illustration is neither a photorealist exercise nor an oversimplified diagram. Ironically, the skill is more often in knowing what to leave out than what to put in."

This skill has been developed by medical illustrators over a long period of time. In 1543, the Italian anatomist A. VERSALIUS wrote a book titled *De Humani Corporis Fabrica* which contained woodblock illustrations produced in TITIAN's workshop. This work can be regarded as the foundation of the art[3] and science of medical illustration. From this time on, certain techniques and conventions developed. Nowadays several universities offer courses and degree programs in this area.

---

3 The term "art" is used here to demonstrate that also special artistic skills are required to successfully create medical illustrations.

Nevertheless, even today most of the medical illustrations are drawn by hand. There are almost no tools with which medical drawings can be created, and – even more important – getting accurate models on which such a drawing system can be based is still hard. Moreover, a good illustration also includes an artistic handling of the subject. This is impossible to simulate on the computer. The tools and methods we have presented here can be seen as a first step towards opening up this area for computer graphics. Despite all this, computer generated medical illustration remains an opportunity to excel. In Chaps. 13 and 17 we show how computer graphics can be used to assist a student in learning anatomy, or for medical reference.

A second application area for the line drawing techniques presented here is technical documentation. Here similar demands are made on the images used. However, the models are often easier to handle since the objects observed contain fewer irregularities than anatomical objects. Nevertheless, to succeed in this area, other problems have to be solved, such as the inclusion of hidden lines in the drawings typical for this field. This requires extensions to the hidden surface removal algorithms that are applied.

As can be seen, the presentation goals stated initially can be achieved by using different techniques presented in this chapter, but there are still lots of unexplored paths ahead. Rendering the illustrations for product documentation directly from the 3D CAD data is tempting, but without knowledge of the tools it is as easy to produce "visual noise" as it is to produce "typographic noise" with modern word processing programs. We have presented some tools for rendering documents and illustrations here, and one area of application will be examined in Chap. 17. By all accounts the area of non-photorealistic rendering is moving from a relatively new field in computer graphics, in which it is possible to create new and interesting, "different" pictures, into a workshop for tools for the creation of expressive, expedient images.

Contributors of Chap. 4: Stefan SCHLECHTWEG and Andreas RAAB

Chapter 5

Rendering Line Drawings of Curved Surfaces

Freeform surfaces are very common in the design and modeling of objects, especially when modeling complex objects with curved surfaces. The advantage of working with freeform surfaces is the ability to control the shape of a surface with control points so that the location of the control point influences a well defined part of the curved surface. The greater the complexity of the curve, the greater the number of control points. For a deeper insight into the mathematical matter of freeform surfaces we refer to [Far91, Sei93].

Almost every CAD package handles at least bicubic surface functions for complex 3D object modeling. It is interesting to note that characters in the animation movie *Toy Story* were animated using this kind of surface. Therefore, it is not surprising that advanced modeling software for PCs also includes this feature. For example, the 3D Studio R4 has recently been extended with plugins for both freeform patch modeling and deforming (see [For95]).

There exist some possibilities for polygonal renderers to work with complex models designed using freeform surfaces. The freeform surfaces can, for example, be converted into polygonal representations. Those polygonal representations can be used for rendering line graphics as described in Chap. 4.

One advantage of freeform surfaces is their behavior after applying deformations which are performed by the movements of one or more control points. If the control points are well chosen, smooth transitions of the curvature are achieved during an animation. Imagine, for example, an animation of a head movement in a character where the part moving most is the throat. But the throat remains smooth in every way although the shape changes when the head moves forward and backward. Such deformation behavior is lost if a conversion into a polygonal representation is carried out before the animation is computed.

The use of freeform surfaces is very appropriate for animating line drawings of complex models. Up to now, line drawings of freeform surfaces have been used mainly as previews in modeling and animation design. This is done primarily because of the limitation introduced by processing speed.

We will show that there are also advantages in using this kind of representation for the generation of line drawings or illustrations for the final rendering of scenes. Therefore, this chapter is arranged as follows. A new technique for converting freeform surfaces into a special polygonal mesh as well as its mathematical background are described in Sect. 5.1. This conversion is one step of the analytic rendering pipeline for generating line drawings of curved surfaces which we discuss in Sect. 5.2. The addition of shadow in a scene in order to gain a more realistic illustration is described in Sect. 5.3. Section 5.4 points out the variation of drawing styles with some examples, and Sect. 5.5 concludes the chapter and gives some ideas for further work.

5.1 Generation of Meshes

In this section we introduce a new technique to approximate freeform surfaces with a special mesh from which, ultimately, the line drawing is computed.

Two types of freeform surfaces exist: quadrangle isoparametric freeform surfaces and triangle isoparametric freeform surfaces. The models we use in this chapter are composed of the first type of freeform surfaces (actually tensor product surfaces of cubic B-splines).

The property of the newly generated polygonal mesh from an isoparametric representation is an even spread of the mesh in 3D space. The density of the mesh is adjustable to achieve both rough approximations of the surface and a smooth transition in surface curvature. The influence of the surface parameterization on our mesh is weaker than on isoparametric meshes. We will show by example that, as a consequence, the new mesh tends to support better the impression of curvature.

5.1.1 Conventional Line Drawings of Freeform Surfaces Versus Evenly Spread Meshes

Typically, line drawings of freeform surfaces are strongly dependent on the parameterization of the surface. In the design process, regions of high curvature are modeled using more control vertices. A standard method of generating wireframe representations (of tensor product surfaces) is to compute an isoparametric net with rows and columns placed at the knots of the knot vectors. Wireframes generated in this way may lead to a confusing representation. Figure 5.1 shows such a freeform surface representation generated with Alias|*wavefront*. When viewed from the top (right image), the line drawing fails to indicate the curvature. On the other hand, isoparametric meshes may also suggest curvature that is not there.

5.1 Generation of Meshes 93

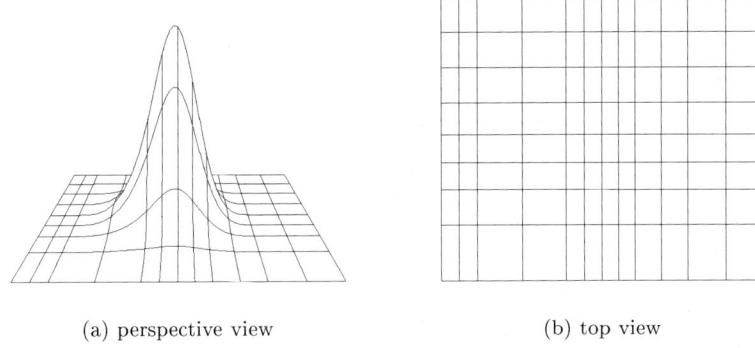

(a) perspective view   (b) top view

Figure 5.1: Appearance of isoparametric wireframes may be misleading for special viewing directions: in the top view no curvature is recognizable

When presenting surfaces with high curvature, e.g., human faces, it would be convenient if the wireframe adequately suggested the curvature of the surface. This would make a direct visualization of the representation more intuitively expressive.

A partial solution is to present wireframes as an evenly spread mesh, where the mesh has the topology of a grid (see Fig. 5.2). The vertices in each row and column are roughly equally distributed in 3D space, and so it should be easier for a viewer to perceive the actual curvature of the surface in a 3D scene. Our implementation shows that this is in fact the case.

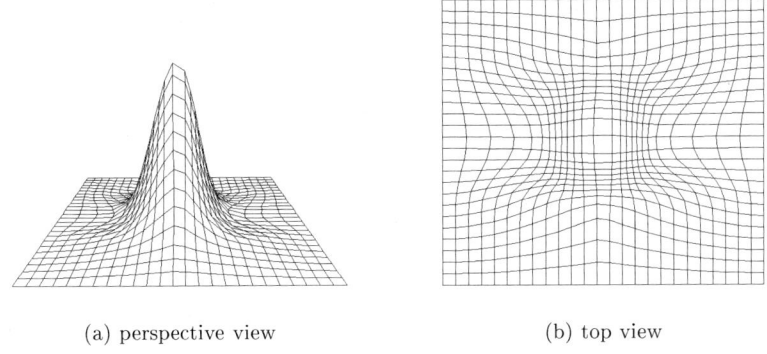

(a) perspective view   (b) top view

Figure 5.2: The evenly spread mesh gives a different presentation style. The top view in this new style reveals the curvature which is hidden in the top view of Fig. 5.1

After the evenly spread mesh is computed, very simple algorithms suffice to produce a "final" line drawing. It is presented by computed contour lines and shadings within its quadrangles. In the lines finally drawn, various parameters for an adequate line style, such as width, brightness, and pressure can be chosen. The technique of applying distinct line styles is described rigorously in Sect. 4.4.2. The shading is performed with cross hatching (created with wobbly lines) and stippling.

5.1.2 Mathematical Background

Assume a NURBS surface

$$S(u,v) = \frac{\sum_i \sum_j C_{ij} W_{ij} N_i^m(u) N_j^n(v)}{\sum_i \sum_j W_{ij} N_i^m(u) N_j^n(v)}$$

with $u,v \in [0,1] \times [0,1]$, where C_{ij} are the control vertices, W_{ij} are the weights, and $N_i^m(u)$ and $N_j^n(v)$ are the basis functions of degree m and n, respectively, for the given knot vectors.

An isoparametric net I for S of size $k \times l$ is a polygonal mesh with vertices

$$V_{ij} = S(\tfrac{i}{k-1}, \tfrac{j}{l-1})$$

with $0 \leq i < k$ and $0 \leq j < l$. The polygonal 3D curve $(V_{0j}, \ldots, V_{(k-1)j})$ is called j-th column of I, and $(V_{i0}, \ldots, V_{i(l-1)})$ is called i-th row.

A fully evenly spread mesh N is a mesh with vertices V_{ij} that lie on the surface S, and adjacent vertices of the same row (and column respectively) are equidistant from one another (in 3D space). Furthermore, vertices on the boundary of the mesh are restricted to lie on the boundary of the surface.

For our purposes, approximately evenly spread meshes suffice, that is we no longer require that adjacent vertices of a fixed row (column) have equal distance, but we require that these distances be only roughly equal.

Up to now, the algorithm approximating an evenly spread mesh of size $n' \times m'$ follows a quite straightforward strategy:

1. An isoparametric net N of some large size $s \times t$ is computed.
2. The polygonal path P_j given by the jth column is considered as an approximation of the isoparametric curve

$$C_j(u) = S(u, \tfrac{j}{t-1}).$$

Thus, the length of P_j approximates the length of $C_j(u)$. The length of P_j, denoted by l_j, is computed.

3. The distance between adjacent vertices in some column K of the intended evenly spread mesh can be estimated as

$$d_j = \frac{l_j}{m'-1},$$

provided that K is placed near $C_j(u)$.

4. An auxiliary net N' is constructed by choosing n' vertices on each curve $C_j(u)$, such that adjacent vertices are a distance of about d_j from one another (the initial net N is used for estimating distances). A net N' of size $s \times m'$ results.

5. The rows of N' approximate curves on S that are equally spaced on S with respect to Euclidean distance in 3D space, but typically not isoparametric in v. The final net I is obtained by placing n' vertices in the neighborhood of each row R_i, where adjacent vertices have a distance of about

$$d_i = \frac{l_i}{n' - 1}$$

with l_i denoting the length of R_i.

The following figures illustrate this process. Figure 5.3 shows an isoparametric wireframe of a freeform surface as it is drawn in Alias|*wavefront*.

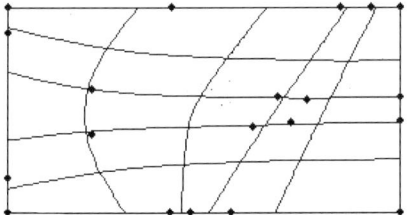

Figure 5.3: An example of a wireframe created with Alias|*wavefront*

Applying the first phase of the mesh conversion yields the mesh N' of Fig. 5.4. A higher number of columns (or rows, respectively) yields a better approximation of this surface. Note that after the first phase is performed, the higher number of rows is already reduced to the requested density in this direction.

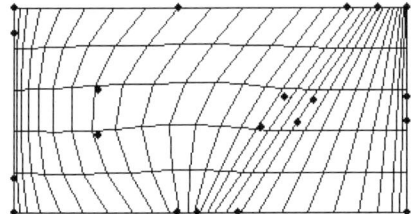

Figure 5.4: The surface of the example of Fig. 5.3 after performing the first step of conversion

The final mesh I obtained from the mesh N' is shown in Fig. 5.5. Note that the higher number of columns is reduced to a lower requested number.

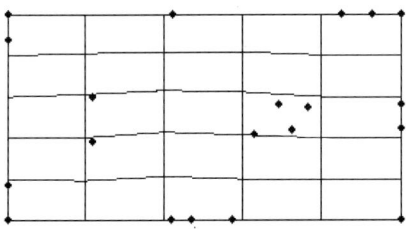

Figure 5.5: The shape of the surface from the example of Fig. 5.3 after the conversion is completed

5.2 Analytic Freeform Surface Rendering Pipeline

In this section we discuss the process of rendering line drawings incorporating the algorithm for converting meshes presented above. A schematic illustration of this process is shown in Fig. 5.6.

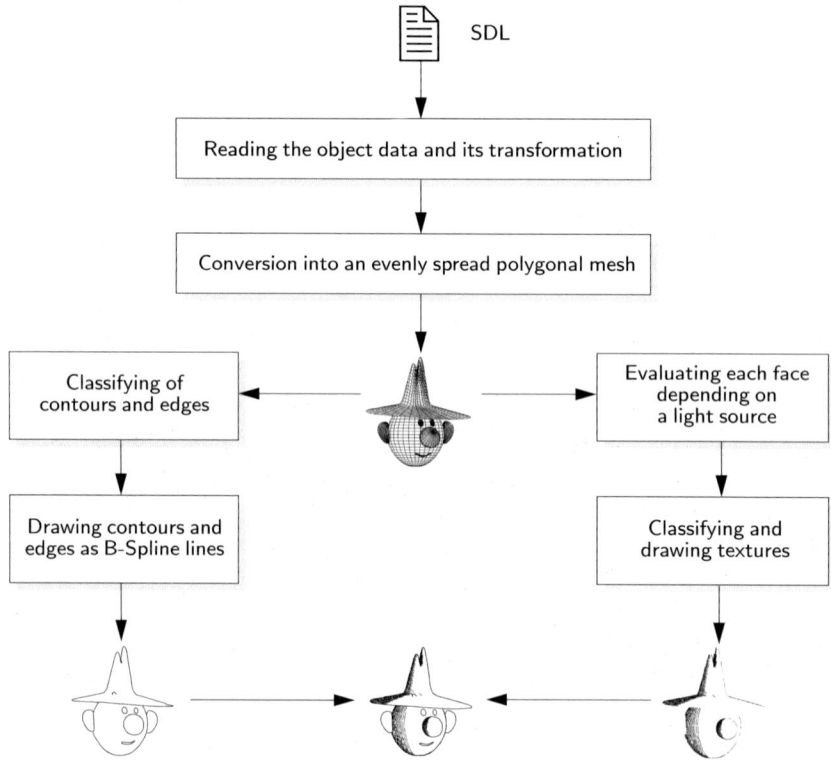

Figure 5.6: The analytic rendering pipeline

The rendering process consists of analytically computing the faces of the evenly spread meshes. Hidden surface removal is achieved by vector-oriented classification of the visible parts of the faces. The actual line drawings consist of outlines and textures.

The following steps of the rendering pipeline are carried out:

1. From a 3D description encoded in the Scene Description Language (SDL), which is exported from Alias|*wavefront*, the objects and their transformations are loaded into the renderer.
2. After the transformations are applied to the objects, the conversions into evenly spread meshes are performed using the algorithm presented in the previous section.

3. From the evenly spread meshes, the following steps are calculated separately:
   a. Classification of contours and inner edges. The inner edges are classified with respect to angles of adjacent faces for controlling the level of detail. The assembled chains of contour lines and inner edges are then approximated by cubic B-splines, which can be drawn in different line styles.
   b. Evaluation of each face depending on the angle between the normal vector of the face and the view vector of the virtual light source. A texturing is applied to those faces which span a higher angle and therefore get a higher value. With this technique, shading is easy to achieve.

In the remaining parts of this section we shall go deeper into the steps of classification of contours and textures. A "Sombrero" is our running example illustrating these steps of calculating line drawings.

5.2.1 Outline Generation

Figure 5.7 (left) shows the Sombrero as an evenly spread mesh. This mesh is used to identify outlines which consist of contour lines and inner structural lines (e.g., where the top of the hat hides some parts of the brim).

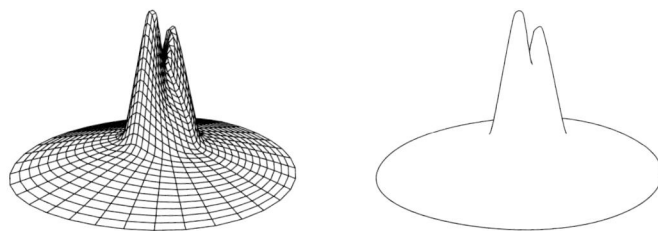

Figure 5.7: The Sombrero as an evenly spread mesh (left), from which outlines are classified and then drawn as B-spline lines (right)

All edges of the evenly spread mesh that possess the following properties are classified as outline edges:

- edges that are shared by a non-backface quadrangle and a backface quadrangle, and
- edges that lie on the boundary, i.e., are not shared by two quadrangles.

The projection of the visible outline edges constitutes the outline in polygonal form which we actually interpolate with B-spline curves. The outlines generated for the Sombrero are shown in Fig. 5.7 (right).

5.2.2 Texture Generation

We aim at a method for the representation of freeform surfaces as line drawings which is fast enough to allow online rendering. Hence, the texturing algorithm we apply is very simple. Each individual quadrangle R is hatched with up to ten wobbly lines depending on the light intensity of R. With an evenly spread mesh, where the edges are equidistant in each row and column, the size of the quadrangles tends to be similar and changes smoothly in 3D space. Therefore, the textures generated with this simple, local method, when applied to this special kind of polygonal mesh, tend to generate homogeneous cross hatching.

In order to achieve a 3D look, we roughly simulate shading using a virtual light source. Hence we evaluate, for each quadrangle of the net, a discrete value depending on the angle between the normal vector of the quadrangle and the vector of the light source.

In the given example we have chosen the range of values from $[0, 10]$. If the angle between the normal vector and the light vector is less than 90 degrees, the quadrangle gets the lowest value 0. If the angle is in $[90°, 180°]$, values ranging from 1 to 10 are assigned to the quadrangle. If the value is greater than 0, a texture is applied.

When using textures for cross hatching, each quadrangle is cross hatched with lines whose density depends on the discrete value φ indicating the intensity of light. If $1 \leq \varphi \leq 5$, the hatching will be performed parallel to the rows only. This value φ then determines the number of hatching lines. If $\varphi > 5$ we switch over to cross hatching. In this case, the number of hatching lines along the rows remains 5 and the number for the hatching lines along the columns is $\varphi - 5$.

When performing texture with stippling, each quadrangle is provided with a number of dots also depending on the discrete value φ. The dots are placed randomly in the quadrangle.

In order to generate textures which resemble handdrawn ones, the hatching lines will be drawn as wobbly lines. Figure 5.8 shows our example, the Sombrero, after texture generation.

In addition, the brightness of the texture lines can be changed in a stepwise fashion according to the illumination. Thereby the effect of grayscale is gained as shown for the Sombrero in Fig. 5.8 (bottom left). The last texture type is stippling to produce a harmonious view, which is shown in Fig. 5.8 (bottom right).

A drawback of this texture procedure is the limited variation in hatching styles. Our approach of generating hatching in a manner that is strictly local to individual quadrangles of the net should be generalized to allow more flexible hatching strategies that can be based, for example, on hierarchical or multiresolution versions of evenly spread meshes.

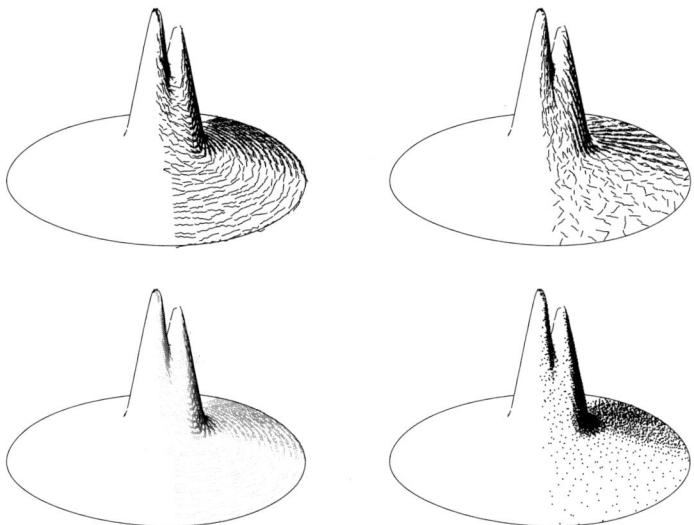

Figure 5.8: The Sombrero with cross hatched vertical (top left) and horizontal (top right) texture lines, with vertical hatched texture and grayscale (bottom left), and with stippling (bottom right) in order to suggest shading

5.3 How to Add Shadow

In this section we discuss the calculation of shadows in an analytic vector-oriented rendering process.

Usually shadows are used in graphics to emphasize a light source and so achieve a more realistic look. In reality, every object produces a shadow if there is light and another surface onto which the shadow can be projected.

With the help of shadows in computer graphics, it is possible to make objects fly or stand on the ground. In Fig. 5.9, two equivalent line drawings are shown, demonstrating the difference in appearance with and without a shadow. The shadow in the left image gives the feeling that the pin is standing on the ground, whereas in the right image the pin is hovering in midair.

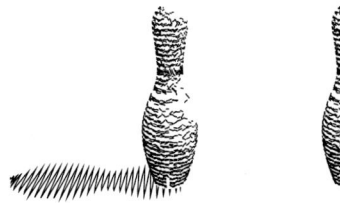

Figure 5.9: A bowling pin rendered with and without a shadow. The shadow "puts" the pin on the floor (left), whereas without shadow the pin seems to hover in midair (right)

The calculation of a shadow is not as simple as it looks. In an analytic rendering process, a projection toward the light source is performed. This means that all objects are transformed in the direction of the light. Then a vector based description of the hidden faces in the direction of the light is used to classify the areas of the shadow. During the classification of the areas lying within the shadow, the following restriction should be considered and omitted:

- backfaces in the view direction, and
- faces which are hidden in the view direction.

The difficulty which occurs during analytic shadow rendering is the localization of the exact area of the shadow. This computing process is very time-consuming if the exact description of the areas within shadows plays an important part.

In our rendering process, the shadow is calculated from the evenly spread mesh. A greater exactness of the calculated shadow on a surface can be achieved with a high density of the evenly spread mesh. If the areas of the shadow are found to have a particular required quality, appropriate drawing types can be used to visualize the shadow. Figure 5.10 demonstrates the schematic flow for adding shadow to a scene.

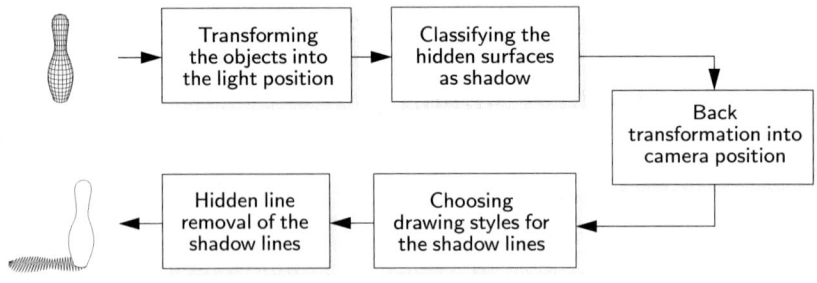

Figure 5.10: The shadow calculation flow

The following steps of the shadow calculation flow are performed:
1. Transformation of all objects toward the light as a temporary view position.
2. Execution of a hidden surfaces classification in which the hidden surfaces define the shadow.
3. Back transformation of all objects into the camera position.
4. Visualization of the defined shadow areas with the appropriate drawing style.
5. Checking of the shadow lines for visibility and removal of the hidden lines.

This last step (5) of the calculation flow is repeated after every change of the camera position, whereas a new shadow classification is performed only when the light position changes or objects are transformed (and deformed as well).

In the next section we show some examples of line drawings. Two animation scenes have been prepared to demonstrate variants of line styles, shadows, and deformations.

5.4 Examples

In order to give an overview of the possibilities which can be achieved with the rendering system introduced here, we will show a scene created with Alias|*wavefront*. More examples using the algorithms presented in this chapter are shown in Chap. 14, where deformation of objects play an important part in creating animations.

Figures 5.11–5.13 show a scene with a perpetually drinking bird to allow a comparison of shadows in illustrations. This popular example, in which the bird cannot stop sipping water from a glass, has been prepared to demonstrate the influence of the mesh density during calculation of the shadow. A light source is located above the bird so that a shadow is projected to the bottom, right underneath the sipping bird. With the shadow added the scene appears more realistic. In Fig. 5.11, a very low density of the bottom mesh is used for the calculation of the shadow. The shadow displays roughly the contour of the objects but the calculation is not so time-consuming.

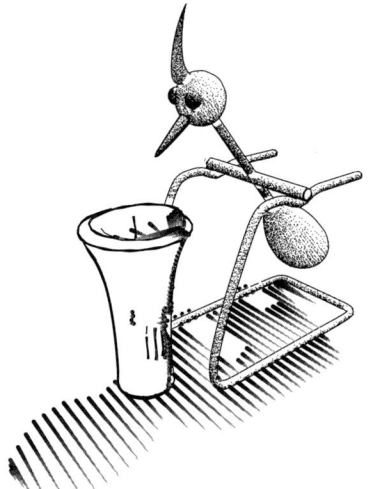

Figure 5.11: The drinking bird scene: low resolution of the projection mesh results in a rougher shadow calculation

The same low density of the bottom mesh for calculation of the shadow is used in Fig. 5.12. The difference in the way the shadow is drawn lies in the direction of the wavy lines which in this case are computed horizontally. Furthermore, different textures are applied to the glass and the support stand, but there is no texture on the bird. This causes a change in the appearance of this scene.

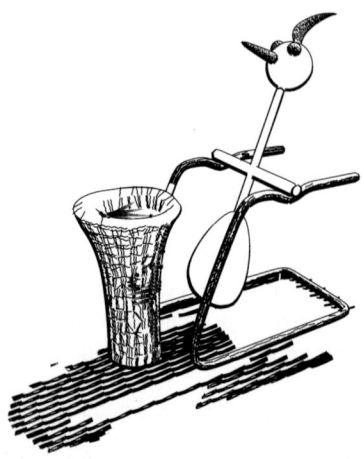

Figure 5.12: The same rough shadow calculation as in Fig. 5.11, but with different textures applied to give a different appearance to the drinking bird

In Fig. 5.13, a very high density of the bottom mesh is used to gain a finer shadow contour of the objects. This results in a more precise projection of the drinking bird and the glass on the bottom. In this case, the mesh is calculated with a grid resolution of 100 × 100. Therefore, the calculation takes a lot of computing time.

5.5 Conclusions and Future Work

We have shown in this chapter a rendering process to present freeform surfaces as line drawings. In order to compute these line drawings, the freeform

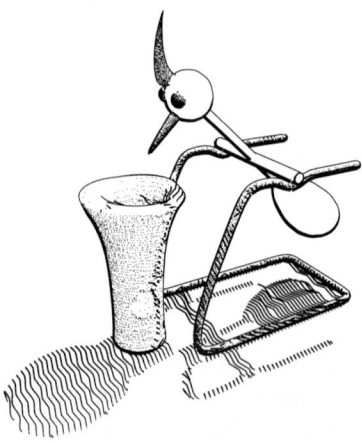

Figure 5.13: When a high density of the projection mesh is chosen, a fine contour of the shadow is calculated. Compare this illustration with Fig. 5.11 and 5.12

surfaces are converted into polygonal meshes. We have found that in evenly spread representations, the curvature of usual models can be recognized more easily. Our studies have also shown that the quality of the representation is quite independent of the viewing direction.

Furthermore, we illustrated a simple and fast hatching and stippling method. If these texturing methods are applied to evenly spread wireframes to generate line drawings, the spatial impression is more satisfactory than applying the same method to isoparametric wireframes.

Unresolved problems are the simulation of different materials, which is still a challenge in the field of line drawing calculation. The drinking bird we introduced in Sect. 5.4 is actually produced from glass, and so transparent areas should be shown.

Another problem are reflections like those produced by chrome or mirrors. Questions arise as to how areas of reflections can be classified in an analytic rendering process and then visualized with appropriate drawing styles.

We discussed the process of adding shadows in order to give a virtual scene a more realistic look. At the moment the shadow is visualized with vertical or horizontal wavy lines. In future work we must include an interaction tool for building distinct shadow drawing styles.

Contributors of Chap. 5: Frank GODENSCHWEGER and Hubert WAGENER

Chapter 6

Pixel-Oriented Rendering of Line Drawings

In Chaps. 4 and 5, several analytical approaches for creating line drawings were introduced. These methods allow the generation of a broad variety of drawing styles, and some applications of scientific and medical illustrations were given.

In the following, a pixel-based method is presented. A set of G-buffers is used for encoding visual and geometric properties of the models. G-buffers store information for each pixel of the image. These buffers are combined with other geometric data to form the line drawing.

In comparison to analytical solutions, a pixel-oriented approach has several advantages and also shortcomings. While working analytically, the results are resolution independent, which is not the case for pixel-oriented methods. An analytic hidden surface removal algorithm may generate more and other information about visible lines and surfaces than can be achieved by a pixel-oriented method. This makes analytic methods more flexible and also more general than pixel-based algorithms.

A pixel-oriented strategy, however, offers the general advantage of easily using graphics hardware which makes algorithms very fast. In addition, the methods are independent of the graphical primitives used to form the models. Everything that can be processed by the hardware can also be used to form the line drawing. Also, the algorithms can be parallelized easily, and in general they are much simpler to implement and to maintain than analytic methods. This makes pixel-based approaches preferentially applicable where results have to be generated quickly and where huge or complex data sets are to be handled.

After discussing previous work and presenting the ingredients of the method, some results are shown. A statue and a bust of Beethoven are used for this purpose. The models have been chosen because of their slightly curved but complex geometry, which is also the case with most of the medical models shown in this book so far. In the last section some suggestions on combining analytic and pixel-based methods are given.

6.1 Previous Work

Pixel-based algorithms for solving visibility problems have a long tradition in computer graphics. CATMUL [Cat74] presented the idea of using a z-buffer, an array storing the color and depth for each pixel of the image. This buffer is used to compute visible parts of the given geometric data by comparing depth values of the surface pixels with the values already stored in the z-buffer. The amount of memory needed by this method can be reduced by using a scan line method which works only with one line of the z-buffer (cf. [Mye75]). ROSSIGNAC refined this method for Constructive Solid Geometry [RR86]; other work was done on processing of data stored in Binary Space Partitioning Trees. Hardware implementations, as described by BOOTH, FORSEY, and PAETH (cf. [BFP86]), of z-buffers can be found in nearly all graphics hardware.

SAITO and TAKAHASHI [ST90] applied image processing to the z-buffer and introduced other pixel buffers (they called them G-buffers) to enhance images in the case that the underlying geometry is given. Their work is stated to be one of the roots of non-photorealistic imaging.

Though extended in some ways, the real breakthrough for non-photorealistic imaging and especially for the use of line drawings took place in more recent years, motivated by the work of LANSDOWN and SCHOFIELD [LS95], STROTHOTTE et al. [SPR$^+$94, SSRL96] and WINKENBACH, SALISBURY and SALESIN (cf. [SALS96, WS96, SWHS97]).

While SCHOFIELD mostly used pixel-based methods for non-photorealistic rendering (he invented G-buffers independently of SAITO and TAKAHASHI), STROTHOTTE et al. focused on generating line directions that are drawn by applying different line styles.

It was the idea of WINKENBACH et al. to use prioritized stroke textures for generating hatching lines. These textures are placed on the surface of objects to form the line drawing. Extensions like resolution dependent textures and orientable textures are given.

LEISTER [Lei94] introduced a special kind of ray tracing in combination with image processing operators for generating line drawings. His method can be seen as an application of volume texturing in order to visualize objects with an outlook similar to copper plates.

The method presented here is an extension of the work of SAITO and TAKAHASHI. Additional G-buffers and cross sectional information are used to form the typical outline of hatched line drawings. Half-toning on the basis of the hatching lines is used to approximate the intensities of a given image.

6.2 A Pixel-Oriented Graphics Pipeline

A pixel-based method for achieving line drawings is quite different from analytic approaches. First, some basic G-buffers are calculated. Image operators are applied to the basic buffers in order to generate additional buffers representing necessary information for the drawing process like structural lines or vector fields.

In the next subsection the set of G-buffers and corresponding image operators is presented, and some extensions to standard image operators are given. In Sect. 6.2.3, a half-toning scheme for short hatching lines is introduced. Their placement is controlled by an error diffusion algorithm.

The generation of long hatching lines (as needed especially for generating medical illustrations) is shown in Sect. 6.2.4. In this case the half-toning must control not the placement but the appearance of the lines; this is described in Sect. 6.2.5. Some results show the usability of the approach.

6.2.1 Basic G-Buffers

A set of buffers forms the basis of all subsequent operations (see Fig. 6.1). Each of them can be calculated efficiently by using standard graphics hardware. For simplification the domain of each pixel is assumed to be the set of integers.

The first G-buffer is the image itself. It is represented as the pixel array I with values describing the light intensity for every point of the image. For the purpose of creating black and white line drawings, a gray-scale map suffices.

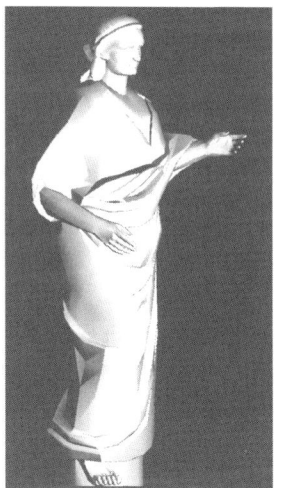
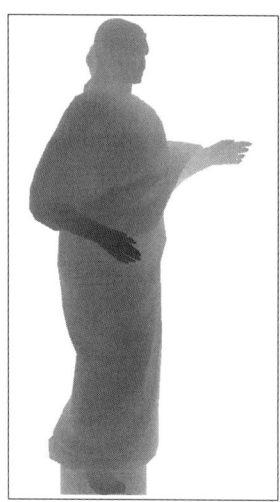
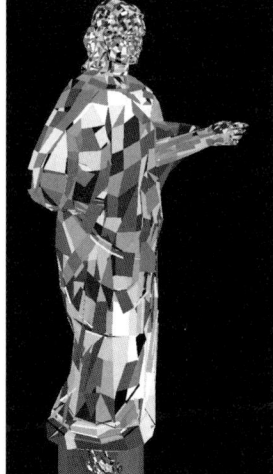

Figure 6.1: Basic G-buffers: image intensity (left), depth values (center), and primitive index (right)

The second G-buffer (Z) is called the depth buffer or z-buffer. The values determine the distance of the model to the viewing plane for each pixel. Later, some image operators will be applied to this buffer in order to generate other buffers.

Another useful buffer is the id-buffer, refered to as ID. The value (color or gray-scale value) of every pixel encodes the index of the visible geometric primitive at this point. For instance, this buffer can also be used for computing efficiently a high quality representation of the image I, as the hidden surface problem is already solved if an id-buffer is present.

The last basic G-buffer (N) stores normal vectors of the geometry. For each pixel the corresponding normal vector of the visible geometry is stored (if it is defined). Usually one needs three images to store the values, the pixels of each image storing one coordinate.

Table 6.1: Basic G-buffers

Description	Symbol	Domain
Image	I	$\mathbb{I}$
Depth values	Z	$\mathbb{I}$
id-buffer	ID	$\mathbb{I}$
Normal vectors	N	$\mathbb{R}^3$

It should be pointed out that numerical accuracy is often crucial for obtaining good results. Therefore, intermediate G-buffers might be stored by using floating point numbers or long integers.

6.2.2 G-Buffer Operators

In the following the set of image operators is shown. These operators are applied to the basic G-buffers to compute other G-buffers necessary for generating the line drawing. A functional notation is used for the operators. For example, the bitwise "and" of two images I_1, I_2 is denoted as "$And(I_1, I_2)$".

Tables 6.2 and 6.3 list the image operators used for generating the line drawings. Most of them are known from standard image analysis literature (e.g., [RK82]). The implementation of the others can be found below.

Difference Operators. Calculating the value of first and second order differences from a pixel image is a classical operation in image analysis. In [ST90] the SOBEL operator (cf. [RK82]) is used. In the following, $G_{i,k}$ denotes the value of the pixel in line i and row k of G-buffer G.

$$d1(G_{i,k}) = \frac{1}{8} \begin{pmatrix} |G_{i-1,k-1} + 2G_{i,k-1} + G_{i+1,k-1} \\ -G_{i-1,k+1} - 2G_{i,k+1} - G_{i+1,k+1}| \\ +|G_{i+1,k-1} + 2G_{i+1,k} + G_{i+1,k+1} \\ -G_{i-1,k-1} - 2G_{i-1,k} - G_{i-1,k+1}| \end{pmatrix}$$

The purpose of this operator is to detect discontinuities in the basic G-buffers. These discontinuities can be used to form structural lines. Therefore the operator is normalized; k_{d1} denotes the threshold, $d1_{min}$ and $d1_{max}$ the minimal and maximal differences.

$$Diff1(G_{i,k}) = \begin{cases} \dfrac{d1_{min} - d1(G_{i,k})}{d1_{max} - d1_{min}}, & \text{if } d1_{max} - d1_{min} > k_{d1} \\[2ex] \dfrac{d1_{min} - d1(G_{i,k})}{k_{d1}}, & \text{if } d1_{max} - d1_{min} \leq k_{d1} \end{cases}$$

To detect discontinuities of second order, the following operator is used by SAITO and TAKAHASHI. It is also normalized to allow the generation of uniform lines:

$$d2(G_{i,k}) = \frac{1}{3} \begin{pmatrix} 8G_{i,k} - G_{i-1,k-1} - G_{i-1,k} \\ -G_{i-1,k+1} - G_{i,k-1} - G_{i,k+1} \\ -G_{i+1,k-1} - G_{i+1,k} - G_{i+1,k+1} \end{pmatrix}$$

Table 6.2: Unary G-buffer operators

Description	Symbol	Domain
Bitwise operators	$Set()$	$\mathbb{I} \to \mathbb{I}$
	$Unset()$	$\mathbb{I} \to \mathbb{I}$
	$Round()$	$\mathbb{R} \to \mathbb{I}$
Value of first order difference	$Diff1()$	$\mathbb{I}^2 \to \mathbb{R}$
Value of second order difference	$Diff2()$	$\mathbb{I}^2 \to \mathbb{R}$
Direction of pixels with same value	$Iso()$	$\mathbb{I}^2 \to \mathbb{R}^2$
Integer conversion of direction vector (angle)	$A^{-1}()$	$\mathbb{R}^2 \to \mathbb{I}$
Retrieval of direction vector from integer value	$A()$	$\mathbb{I} \to \mathbb{R}^2$

Table 6.3: Binary G-buffer operators

Description	Symbol	Domain
Bitwise operations	$And()$	$\mathbb{I} \times \mathbb{I} \to \mathbb{I}$
	$Or()$	$\mathbb{I} \times \mathbb{I} \to \mathbb{I}$
Pixel-wise arithmetic operations	$Add()$	$\mathbb{I} \times \mathbb{I} \to \mathbb{I}$
	$Sub()$	$\mathbb{I} \times \mathbb{I} \to \mathbb{I}$
	$Max()$	$\mathbb{I} \times \mathbb{I} \to \mathbb{I}$
	$Min()$	$\mathbb{I} \times \mathbb{I} \to \mathbb{I}$
	$Mul()$	$\mathbb{I} \times \mathbb{I} \to \mathbb{I}$
	$Div()$	$\mathbb{I} \times \mathbb{I} \to \mathbb{I}$
Multiplication with scalar value	$Smult()$	$\mathbb{I} \times \mathbb{R} \to \mathbb{R}$
Threshold operation	$Tresh()$	$\mathbb{I} \times \mathbb{I} \to \mathbb{I}$

$$\text{Diff2}(G_{i,k}) = \begin{cases} d2(G_{i,k}), & \text{if } d1_{max} \le k_{d2} \\ \dfrac{d2(G_{i,k})}{(d1_{max}/k_{d2})^2}, & \text{if } d1_{max} > k_{d2} \end{cases}$$

Although these operators allow to extract discontinuities in a desirable way, a second operator for detecting first order differences was designed to generate "lighter" lines which are needed for high-quality pixel–vector conversion (as needed below). The difference operator *Diff1* generates lines, as can be seen in the center part of Fig. 6.2. Vertical and horizontal lines are generated as required, but diagonal lines are too fat. Application of the operator *Diff1a* leads to a better (lighter) result.

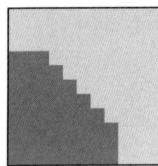
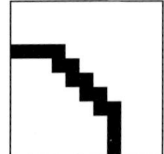
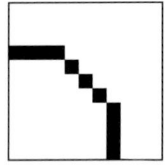

Figure 6.2: Results of difference operators: Original image, after applying *Diff1*, and after applying *Diff1a*

The operator *Diff1a* is also normalized, i.e., it delivers binary values and no information about the level of discontinuity is provided.

The operator has a procedural implementation that works in two steps: First, the image is scanned line by line. If the horizontal differences are above the threshold k_{d1}, the pixel is set. Second, the image is processed row by row. In this step a pixel is set only if either the upper or right neighbor is not set at this time.

```
proc Diff1a()
    for k := 0 to height − 1) do
        Unset(G_{i,0});
        for i := 1 to width − 1) do
            if |G_{i−1,k} − G_{i,k}| > k_{d1}
                then Set(G_{i,k}) else Unset(G_{i,k}) fi
        od
    od
    for i := 1 to (width − 1) do
        for k := 0 to (height − 1) do
            if |G_{i,k+1} − G_{i,k}| > k_{d1} ∧ (G_{i,k+1} = 0 ∨ G_{i−1,k} = 0)
                then begin
                    Set(G_{i,k});
                    if G_{i,k−1} > 0 ∧ G_{i−1,k} > 0 then Unset(G_{i,k}) fi
                end fi
        od
    od
end
```

6.2 A Pixel-Oriented Graphics Pipeline

An application of the difference operators to G-buffers is shown in Fig. 6.3 (center) and 6.3 (right), where structure lines are generated using the image and the z-buffer by application of difference operators. These results can be seen as first sketches of the given statue.

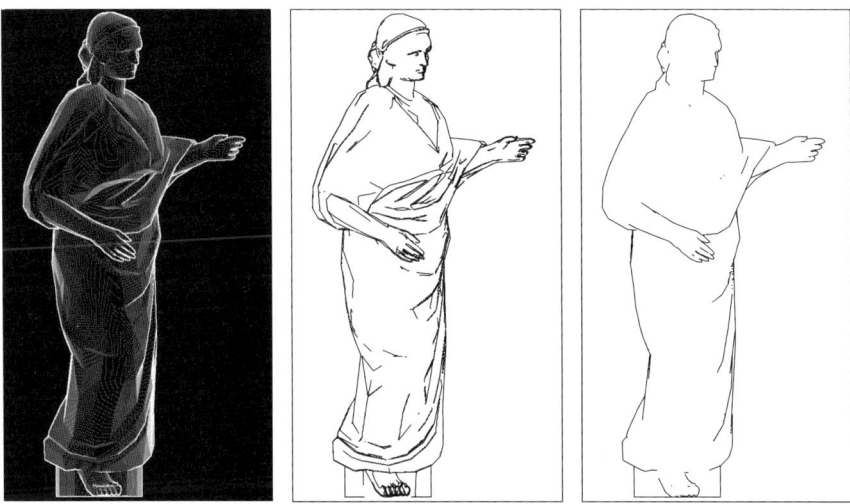

Figure 6.3: Application of difference operators to the image and the z-buffer: $Diff1(I)$, $Tresh(Diff1(I), 30)$, $Tresh(Diff1(Z), 30)$ (from left to right)

The Iso-Operator. During the generation of hatching lines it is sometimes necessary to draw lines along pixels with the same depth value. This is done by using another G-buffer that stores the directions of pixels with the same value (if this direction is unique).

This buffer can be generated by applying the *Iso*-operator to a G-buffer. The *Iso*-operator is defined by the perpendicular vector of the pixel-wise gradient direction:

$$\begin{aligned}
Grad_x(G_{i,k}) &= -G_{i-1,k-1} + G_{i+1,k-1} - G_{i-1,k} \\
&\quad + G_{i+1,k} - G_{i-1,k+1} + G_{i+1,k+1} \\
Grad_y(G_{i,k}) &= -G_{i-1,k-1} + G_{i-1,k+1} - G_{i,k-1} \\
&\quad + G_{i,k+1} - G_{i+1,k-1} + G_{i+1,k+1} \\
Iso(G_{i,k}) &= \bigl(Grad_y(G_{i,k}), -Grad_x(G_{i,k})\bigr)^T
\end{aligned}$$

In Fig. 6.4 the direction of the vectors is visualized. The vectors are stored by their direction angle using the functions $A()$ and $A^{-1}()$. The other operators of Tables 6.2 and 6.3 should be clear to the reader, who is otherwise referred to the standard literature of image analysis.

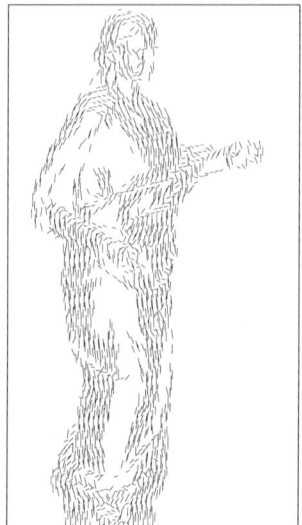 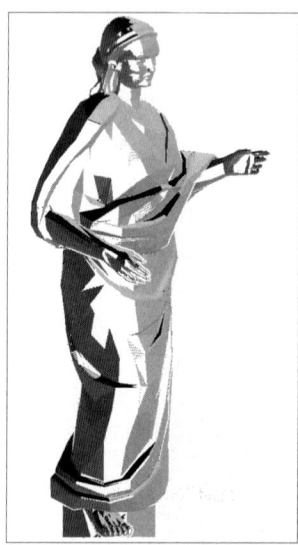

Figure 6.4: Visualization of *Iso* depth vectors and the associated G-buffer

Until now it was shown how G-buffers can be created by using image operators applied to the basic G-buffers. In the next subsection two half-toning schemes working on hatching lines are described. First, short hatching lines are distributed on the image, later the outline of lines is changed according to a given gray-scale value.

6.2.3 Half-Toning Using Short Hatching Lines

The half-toning process is a function which maps an image of gray-scale values to another image composed by the colors black and white. The half-toning process must preserve the integral gray-scale value over each (sufficiently large) part of the picture.

A classic method is the algorithm of FLOYD and STEINBERG [FS76]. The image is processed row by row. For each pixel the error that arises with drawing a black or white pixel is accumulated and added to the next pixel, thus spreading the error over a larger area.

In Fig. 6.5(b) the half-toned image of the given reference (Fig. 6.5(a)) is shown. Points can easily be replaced by short hatching lines, if the error is treated appropriately (cf. Fig. 6.5(c)). If two line directions and smaller lines are used, the result gives a good approximation of the reference image.

Usually, during half-toning no knowledge is assumed about the content of the image to be processed. This is not the case here, as we want to do a special kind of half-toning which leads us to hatched images.

Figure 6.6 shows how information about the model can be used by a half-toning process. Figure 6.6(a) shows the result of half-toning the robe of the

6.2 A Pixel-Oriented Graphics Pipeline

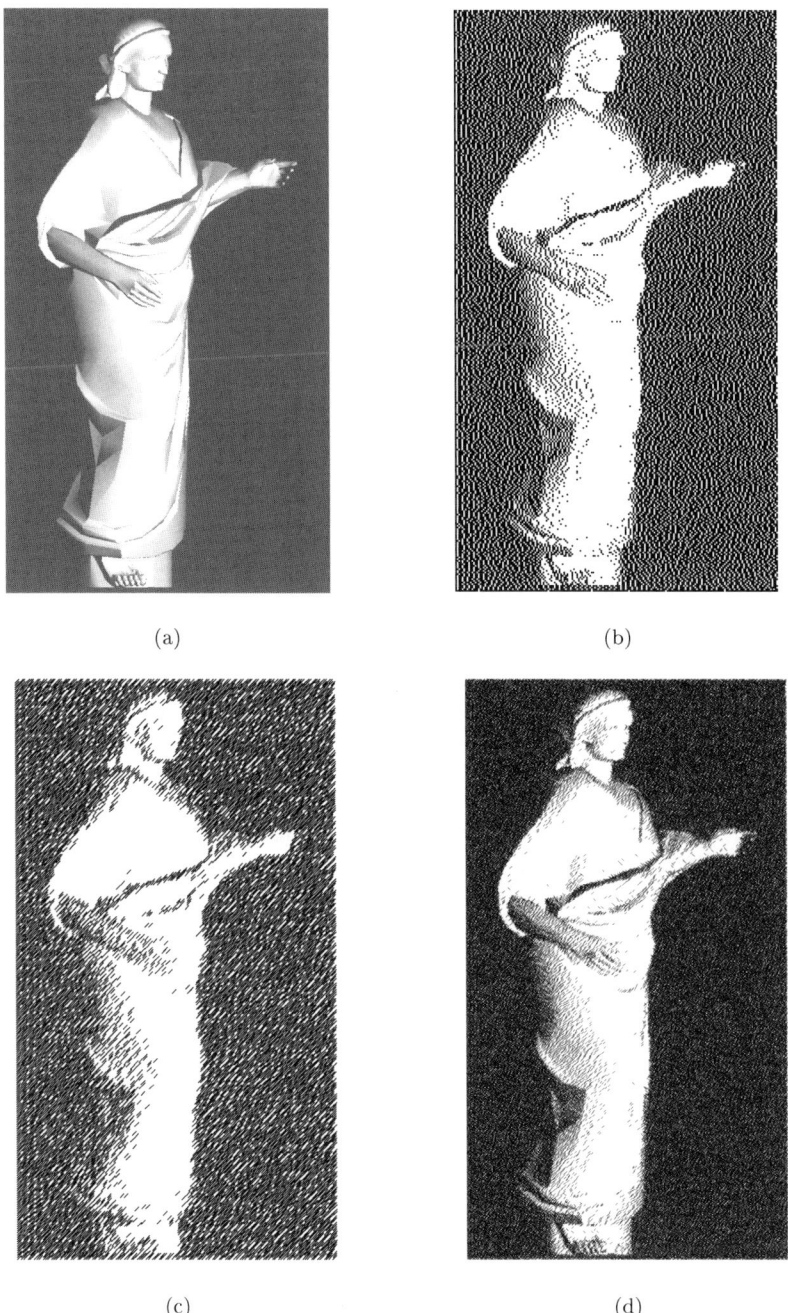

Figure 6.5: A half-toning process with short hatching lines: (a) reference image; (b) application of an error diffusion algorithm using points; (c) the same done by using short lines; (d) two line directions combined, smaller lines used

statue using short hatching lines with a slope of ±45 degrees. In Fig. 6.6(b) the same is done using iso depth values for redirecting the slope of the lines.

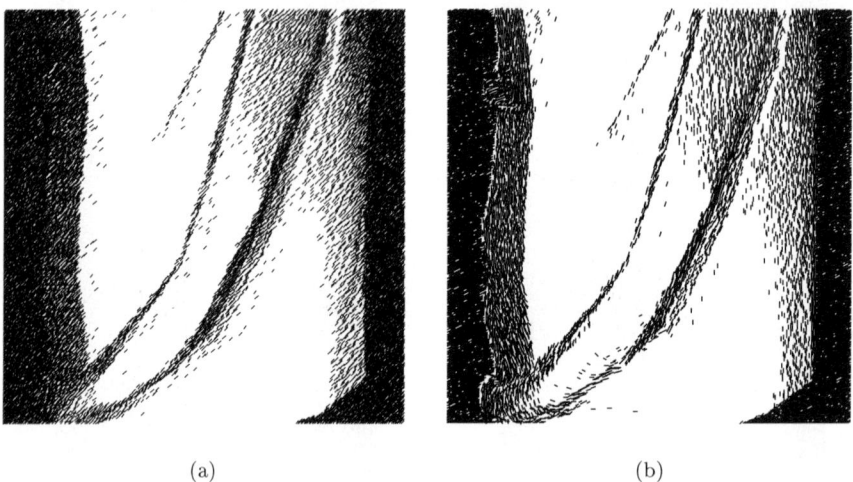

(a) (b)

Figure 6.6: Enhanced half-toning using short lines: (a) half-toning with two static line directions; (b) redirecting the slope of the lines to the direction of *iso* depth values

In the next section the focus is on generating long hatching lines. A half-toning method based on these lines is described below.

6.2.4 Generating Long Hatching Lines by Intersections

In scientific illustrations long hatching lines are widely used. The hatching lines in Fig. 1.1 might be interpreted as intersections between the object and a set of planes.

Such a set of intersecting lines should help in directing subsequent half-toning operators along the surface of the objects. The lines can be created either analytically by intersecting the model with a set of planes, or by a combination of pixel-based operations and image analysis. In both cases the result should be a set of curves in 2D.

Currently the intersections are generated using the latter method (cf. Fig. 6.7). The process has several steps: First, the full model is shaded using flat shading and a dark background. By applying the operator *Diff1a* and performing a pixel-vector conversion, the outline of the model is generated.

Now the same is done by using additional clipping planes (Fig. 6.7(a)). The operator *Diff1a* is applied again and the outline of the model is subtracted. What remains is the pixel representation of the intersecting line (Fig. 6.7(b)). A pixel-vector conversion is carried out to achieve the desired pixel vector. The whole set of vectors can be seen in Fig. 6.7(c).

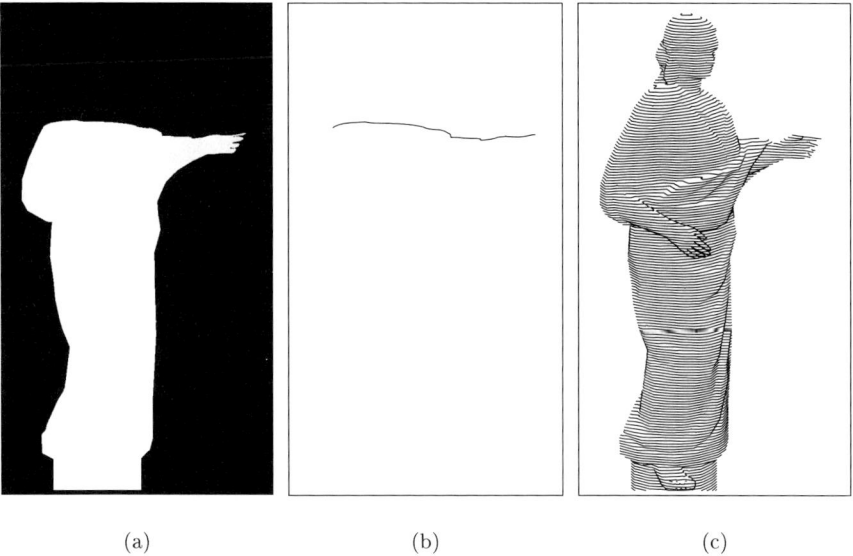

(a) (b) (c)

Figure 6.7: Pixel based generation of intersecting lines: (a) flat shaded image of the model by using an additional clipping plane, (b) resulting vector after subtracting the outline of the full model, (c) the whole set of intersecting lines

6.2.5 Half-Toning Using Long Hatching Lines

The generated lines have to be drawn in an appropriate way. To match the half-toning requirements, each line l_i is responsible for a tube t_i (cf. Fig. 6.8). The outline of the tube lies between the line and its neighbors. Using such tubes results in partitionizing the surface of the object to be hatched.

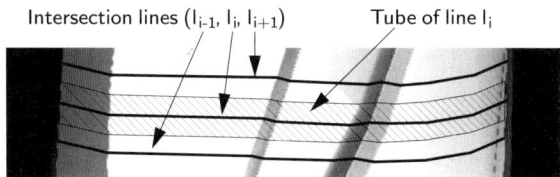

Figure 6.8: For half-toning the appearance of each intersection line l_i is responsible for approximating the gray-scale values belonging to a tube around the line

If the overall intensity of the line l_i equals the intensity of the pixels in t_i, a correct half-toning is achieved. A simple method is to modulate the width of l_i according to the intensities along the line. Doing so supposes that we have uniform intensities in t_i perpendicular to l_i.

In Fig. 6.9, a set of intersection lines is used for half-toning the bones of a foot. The intensities of the image at the top were used for controlling

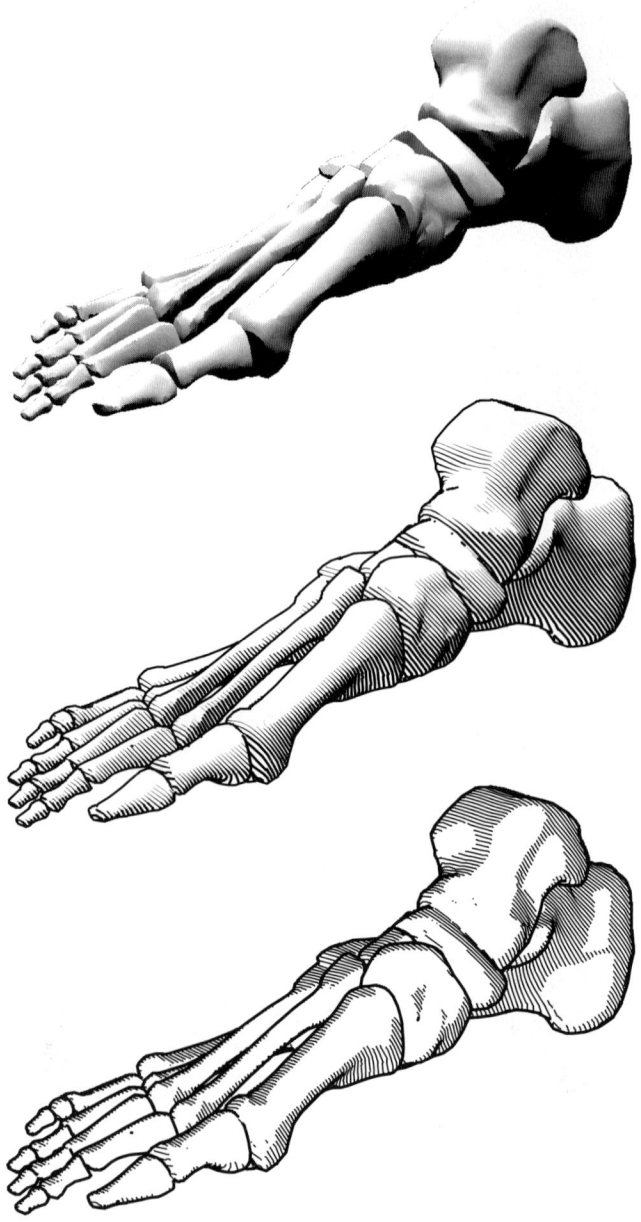

Figure 6.9: Using intersection lines for hatching: A set of intersection planes was used to generate the lines. The intensities of the image at the top were used for controlling the line width of the picture in the middle. At the bottom a style similar to Fig. 1.1 was approximated

the line width of the picture in the middle by using the above method. At the bottom a style similar to Fig. 1.1 was approximated. Here, a uniform line width was chosen, and the line was drawn for those places where the intensities of the picture belong to a given interval.

6.2.6 Computer Generated Copper Plates

As mentioned in the introduction to this chapter, LEISTER used a modified ray tracing algorithm in combination with black and white volume textures to simulate the generation of copper plates. This approach is quite similar to explicitly generating intersections, as was done above. If the volume texture consists of parallel planes, the ray tracing algorithm tests for each pixel if one of these planes is present at the point where the ray hits the surface of the visible object.

The advantage of explicitly generating intersections is that these intersections can be postprocessed later by applying a half-toning method that generates the hatching lines individually. In Fig. 6.11 a copper plate is simulated. Several parts of the model were processed separately and later combined by using z-buffers. The size of the generated dots was chosen according to the intensity of the model's image I.

Artists use several tricks while developing copper plates. It is too simple to assume one can achieve a computer generated copper plate by just intersecting the model with a set of parallel planes. Real copper plates are made by using non-parallel planes or even other objects. Sometimes several planes are overlaid as can be seen in the face of the nun in Fig. 6.10 (left). In Fig. 6.10 (right) different styles are used for the light and the dark parts of the face.

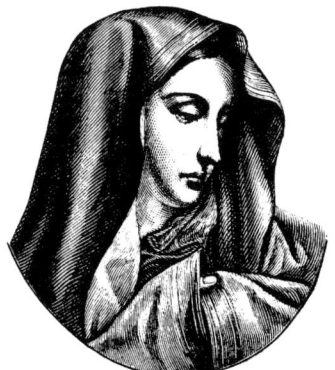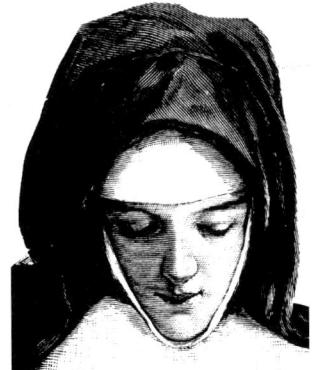

Figure 6.10: Two copper plates of nuns demonstrate the usage of different styles within the same image [Gra90]

The same was done for the computer generated copper plate of Fig. 6.11. The face was drawn by using two sets of intersecting planes and the rest was

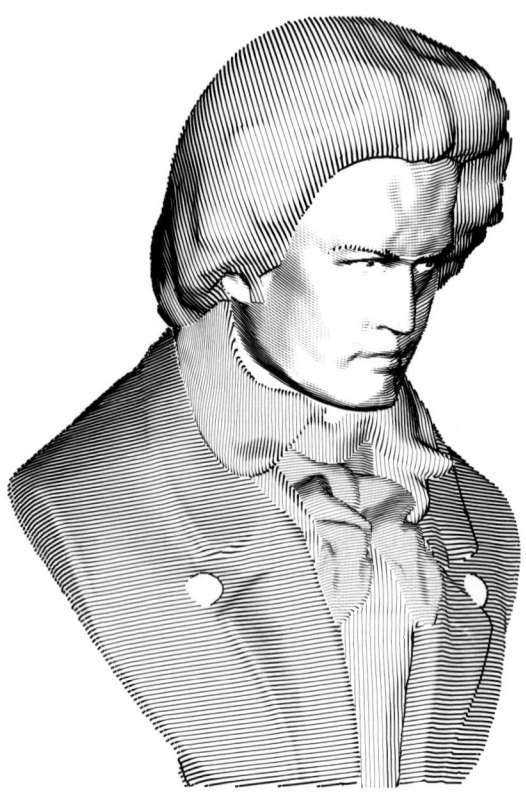

Figure 6.11: A computer generated copper plate showing a bust of Beethoven. The face was drawn using two sets of intersecting planes, the rest using one set

generated using one set. The main difficulty was to direct the orientation of the intersection planes in an appropriate way.

6.3 Concluding Remarks

In this chapter a pixel-based rendering pipeline was given. The pipeline consists of three steps. First, basic G-buffers have to be generated. By application of image operators additional buffers are created in a second step. One may also create intersection information, if appropriate. In the last step a half-toning process is applied to the data which maps the intensities of the image buffer I to the size, direction, and style of the generated lines.

For high quality images sometimes a high resolution of intermediate G-buffers is needed. Therefore, it can be useful to partition the buffers (OpenGL works with images of at most $2\,000 \times 2\,000$ pixels).

Analytical and pixel-oriented methods can be combined in many different ways. On one hand the analytical generation of intersections can be used to get 3D results, on the other hand their pixel-based generation can be mapped into 3D by using back projection (parts of the intersections may be missing if not visible). The results are now usable in an analytic approach.

G-buffers can be used in places where it is sufficient to store information at discrete points. Every analytic approach involves the creation of the image for a pre-defined view. At this point, pre-computed G-buffers may introduce additional information like vector fields (e.g., iso-values) or depth information.

Pixel-oriented methods may also be used to obtain some kind of image-based control on the number of and distance between hatching lines. The avoidance of Moiré patterns is an important problem during the generation of line drawings. It depends on the resolution of the output devices how closely curves can be placed together without obtaining a Moiré pattern. If a line drawing is to be rendered for a specific output device with given resolution, G-buffers may allow efficient calculation of the pixel distance from line to line.

The generation of intersecting lines may now be an iterative process: A new intersection is generated, the maximal and minimal pixel distances to their neighbors is measured and the intersection plane is moved if the distances do not match pre-defined criteria. Such methods were proposed by SAITO and TAKAHASHI in [ST90] and also by TURK and BANKS [TB96] for generating stream lines. Their application to line drawings is future work.

The fast generation and rendering of pixel-based hatching lines can be used for displaying and interacting with complex environments like botanical scenes. Based on our work on modeling and rendering realistic plants and plant ecosystems [DL97, DHL+98], the techniques presented in this chapter will be applied to those scenes in order to provide interaction with objects that otherwise require the display of tens of millions of polygons.

Contributor of Chap. 6: Oliver DEUSSEN

Chapter 7

Measuring and Highlighting in Graphics

In 3D graphics modeling systems, the properties of the surfaces of objects are defined by a special material editor module. In most cases the values of a surface material (for instance color values, effects like shininess, textures) are defined separately on a sample object. Typically, this work is done *outside* the visual context of the scene. To see the material in the context of the whole scene, the image must be rendered.

If we look at photorealistic computer graphics, we can observe several problems concerning

- the discernibility of the dimensions,
- the relationships between the objects in the scene, and
- the figure–ground distinction.

These problems are part of the representation of three dimensions, to reach the impression of "space" on a flat surface (discussed in detail in [Woo83]). These problems are based on the transformation of a 3D scene into a 2D image plane and the physically based model of illumination and object surface shading in photorealistic computer graphics.

The experienced user can reduce the appearance of such problems in changing the properties of the object surfaces and in adding local light sources. We assume that detailed information about the relation between the color contrasts of different objects can support the user in the process of defining the material properties. It can help in understanding the mechanisms of different effects of color contrasts in the scene on a viewer.

Figure 7.1 may illustrate these observations: A part of a rendered image showing the model of a nutcracker can be seen. This model was created with commercially available rendering software. On the left in Fig. 7.1(a), only one spotlight source and the ambient light are defined. A side position for the

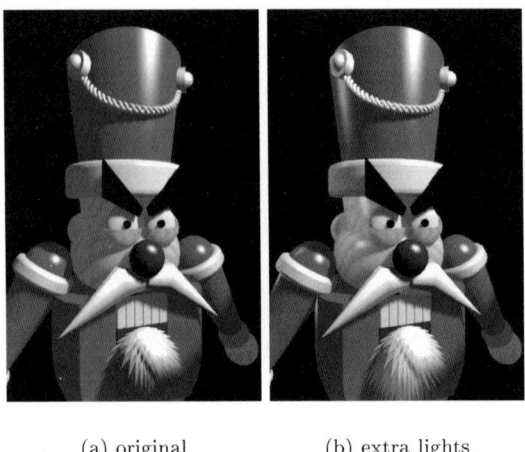

(a) original   (b) extra lights

Figure 7.1: Detail of a nutcracker

spotlight was chosen to make the model appear sculpted – details should be well recognizable. This scene – objects, ambient light, and one light source – corresponds to a physical model of illumination. We notice that some details, especially those in shadowed areas, appear flat or they are hardly recognizable (e.g., the right ear). The experienced user remedies this by defining local point light sources. In Fig. 7.1(b), nine different local light sources are defined to emphasize the object contours (e.g., the right ear), to make the shape and dimensions of objects more comprehensible (e.g., the right side of the head, the right eye) or to let objects appear more interesting, more solid (e.g., the hat). An assessment of color contrasts is only possible in a rudimentary way: some commercial 3D animation software provides special functions for checking the saturation of colors in order to avoid unwanted color effects after encoding the animation on video tape. A change of contrasts is possible in a post-production process, but can only be applied to the whole image.

For the explanation of animation problems we assume a typical hardware solution for digital animation production. For the rendering a workstation pool is used. The video encoding workstation is at a different location. Problems concerning the color information appear during and after the postprocessing of animation. Sometimes, when depicting the encoded animation on video, unwanted effects like a colored "flash" or discontinuities in motion can be observed. These effects can be attributed to errors which happened in the post-production process and may have the following causes:

- *Distributed modeling.* The animation was developed on different modeling and rendering platforms. The modelers approximate the same mathematical description in different ways – this leads to a different appearance of the same scenario.

- *Distributed rendering.* This may cause synchronization problems between different computers. Here errors in the handling of different versions may occur.
- *No evaluation.* The size of an animation is so enormous that the frames cannot be checked as a computer video for verifying the motion flow and for detecting artifacts.
- *File transfer.* During the file transfer, which may be necessary when the rendering and the video encoding workstations are on different locations, files can get lost or duplicated because of hardware errors or user mistakes.

Our work was inspired by postprocessing problems in an animation project: "The BUGA tower Magdeburg 1999" – an architectural presentation for the German Horticulture Exposition BUGA. A scene of this animation is shown in Fig. 7.2. The animation consists of about 6 000 frames, modeled and rendered with Alias|*wavefront* and Autodesk 3D Studio. To ensure a similar appearance of any parts, all atmospheric effects (fog, etc.) were inserted in postprocessing. Because of the image size the frames were stored at different locations. For video encoding, all data was transferred to a digital film editing workstation. After the very time-consuming video encoding we discovered artifacts with the following effects on the viewer:

- color discontinuities, perceptible as quantitative color jumps, and
- discontinuities in motion, perceptible as breaks in the motion flow.

The exact position of an artifact was hard to find on video tape. The number of the corresponding frame in the animation could not be found. A software tool for an automatic analysis of quality (detection of possible artifacts from postprocessing) and consistency (are all needed images available in the right version and right order?) *before* the final video encoding is carried out can obviously save valuable time.

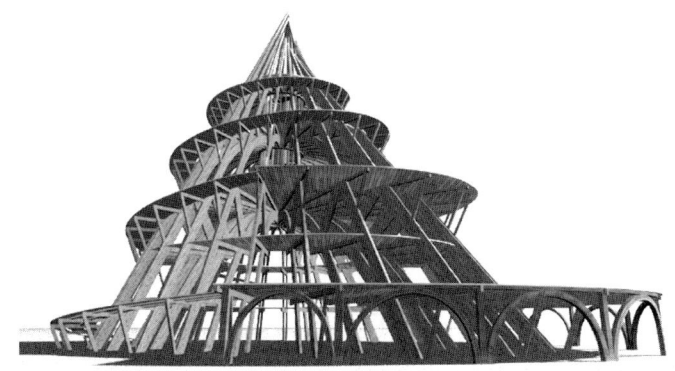

Figure 7.2: Animation shot from "The BUGA tower Magdeburg 1999"

7.1 Related Work

In the literature, one can find several approaches to "enhance" photorealistic images or to use techniques based on examples in paintings.

A first approach to apply methods for an emphasis of objects in rendered images is introduced by SAITO and TAKAHASHI. In [ST90] they develop techniques to enhance edges and contours in photorealistic images. Image processing operations are applied to produce an emphasis of objects in the resulting image. These methods are applied in a more technically oriented way, not paying attention to colors or contrasts and their effects in the process of emphasis.

In [LS95], LANSDOWN and SCHOFIELD presented their extended painting system PIRANESI. This system enables the user to recreate a rendered image in many different styles applying techniques used in paintings or drawings. Techniques for an explicit emphasis of objects or parts of objects are not implemented.

An approach for applying techniques from drawings in art to non-photorealistic images, specifically in computer generated line drawings, is introduced in [SP95]. SCHLECHTWEG and PREIM present a sketch rendering system which makes it possible to control the degree of detail in which an object is depicted with lines. The presented techniques are limited to line based rendering systems.

Also in the literature, many approaches have been discussed dealing with colors during post-production processes. In their blue screen matting system SMITH and BLINN [SB96] discuss problems of separating background and foreground objects and their colors for mixing images. SHONEMAN et al. reproduce light source parameters taken from analysed colors a designer painted on surfaces in the scene [SDS+93].

Many approaches deal with animation analyses based on the geometric model, such as HUGHES et al. [HDLM96]. These approaches consider no animation design after the rendering. BRUDERLIN et al. use signal processing methods for a motion control system [BW95]. Many solutions in multimedia systems or image processing science deal with video film analyzes. AKUTSU et al. [AT94] present a tool for estimating motion, in particular camera movements in videos. ARMAN et al. [ADHC94] present a system for rapidly viewing video sequences based on the extraction of the typical characteristics of a sequence. These methods cannot be used for an exact object observation over a sequence because of the classical motion detection problems in image processing [GW93, Jäh97].

7.2 Approaches and Techniques in Paintings

Designers or artists include color in their considerations: A clearly perceptible difference by the comparison of two color effects is called *color contrast* (refer to [Itt70]). Color contrasts can be classified according to their effects on a viewer. In the literature, we find several similar approaches for classifying color contrasts, based on different models to describe color relations.

ITTEN [Itt70] constructs a 12-segmented color circle and arranges the colors beginning from the center and introducing three orders: The primary colors yellow, red and blue (first order colors), the mixed colors orange, green, and violet (second order colors), and the neighboring colors yellow-orange, red-orange, red-violet, etc. (third order colors). Colors fixing the maximum contrast are called *poles*. Based on this color model, ITTEN distinguishes between seven color contrasts. This classification is listed in Table 7.1.

Table 7.1: Classification of color contrasts (according to ITTEN [Itt70])

Contrast	Description
Color by color	perceived as "colorful" described by three colors minimum, far away from each other in color circle; poles are red, blue, yellow
Bright vs. dark	described by the poles black and white
Cold vs. warm	perpendicular to the bright dark poles blue-green and red-orange
Quality	difference between the degree of "purity" and "saturation" of colors
Simultaneity	based on the attempt of the human eye to generate the complementary color
Complementarity	colors lying opposite in color circle (such as yellow vs. violet)
Quantity	"strength ratio" of colors in an image

For our work we have chosen the classification by ITTEN, because his approach for describing the different contrast classes can be applied directly in computer graphics by interpreting the color models. For the design process the dark vs. bright, warm vs. cold, quality, and complementarity contrasts are essential – they seem to have the strongest influence on the effect. Moreover, these contrasts are comprehensible to the user.

Artists have developed various techniques to change certain qualities of objects in a painting. A painter can "accentuate" or "de-accentuate" details, aspects, or parts of an object in changing their color contrasts.

Definition 7.1
Accentuating characterizes the emphasizing or underlining of a fact, increasing its importance for a certain context. *De-accentuating* characterizes the decreasing of the importance of a fact, and is therefore the opposite of accentuating.

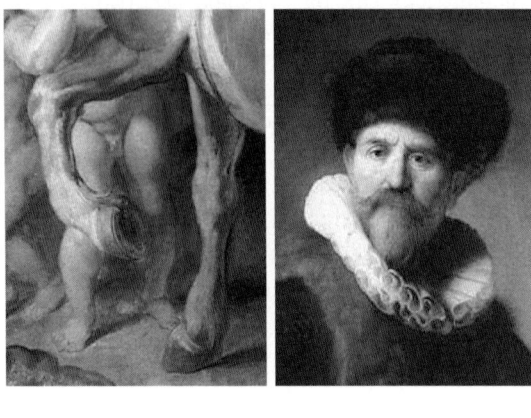

(a) accentuated   (b) de-accentuated

Figure 7.3: Examples of using techniques for emphasis in art

Such special techniques are described in detail in text books about painting techniques or art. Techniques to realize an accentuation of objects in a painting based on changing the quality of color contrasts are:

- *Color phenomena.* Contours of an object or its details are penciled over, producing a colored aura in a color corresponding to a certain impression like warmth (mostly an orange or brown color tone is used), coolness (mostly a blue color tone is used), and harmoniously embedded using a predominant color tone in the environment of the object. Figure 7.3(a) shows a detail of an oil painting. We see an example of emphasis: The artist penciled over the contours of the foot.
- *Increasing contrasts.* The shadowed areas of an object appear darker and the illuminated parts appear brighter than those of neighboring objects.

Techniques used for de-accentuating objects are:

- *Decreasing contrasts.* Shadowed areas of an object appear brighter, illuminated parts appear darker than parts of objects in the neighborhood.
- *Coloring.* The color values of an object are shifted toward a unique color tone. An example is shown in Fig. 7.3(a) – objects in the background appear in a brown tone.
- *Partial brightening.* Used for a region or group of objects in the background. An area around a foreground object is brightened to make this dark object better perceptible. An example is shown in Fig. 7.3(b).
- *Partial darkening.* Used for a region or a group of objects in the background to make a bright foreground object better perceptible.

A software tool should enable the user to control the parameters of this contrast information. Based on this contrast information we apply the techniques described above to "enhance" photorealistic images.

7.3 Theoretical Background

In our work, we examine an approach to analysis and an assessment of the different contrasts in color images produced by rendering systems for an additional utilization in the modeling and post-production process. First, we introduce basic terms and definitions for further explanations.

For a computer-based assessment of color contrasts we have to find a way to make the phenomenon of color understandable to a software tool. Image processing science provides such methods to approach rendered images. According to the description of images used in digital image processing (like in [Hab95, Abm94]), we define an *image* B as a matrix with R rows and L lines:

$$B = (b(x,y)) \tag{7.1}$$

Thereby x represents the line index and y is the row index:

$$0 \leq x \leq R-1$$
$$0 \leq y \leq L-1$$

The *picture element* contains the value $b(x, y)$. The rendered images we will regard in this chapter are color images. A color value c can be interpreted as a combination K of N color channels v according to a given color model V:

$$c = K(v), v \in V \tag{7.2}$$

Therefore, we can conclude for color image C:

$$C = (c(x,y))$$

Certain analysis methods require a description of the values in separate channels of the color model. In addition to equation (7.1) we introduce a counter n for the channels based on a chosen color model V:

$$B = (b(x,y,n)) \quad \text{with} \quad 0 \leq n \leq N-1 \tag{7.3}$$

To describe a sequence of images we can enhance the mathematical model used in equation (7.1). A *sequence* S of images can be described as three-dimensional matrix

$$S = (s(x,y,t)) \tag{7.4}$$

where x and y are the coordinates and t with $T_{start} \leq t \leq T_{end}$ represents the index along the time axis. To estimate a color channel in time we can conclude by analogy with equation (7.3) that

$$S = (s(x,y,n,t)). \tag{7.5}$$

Because of the internal structures of the common file formats, the color images are RGB-encoded. For our approach, the most appropriate mathematical model to describe the different color contrast classes is the HSI color model [Abm94]. The HSI model is more oriented on human perception and can be used directly to describe ITTEN's contrast classification mathematically.

The following development of image and animation analysis is based on information taken from an enriched model (refer to Chap. 3) and based on G-buffers. G-buffers were originally introduced by SAITO and TAKAHASHI [ST90]. A G-buffer is an intermediate rendering result and a special image containing in each pixel a certain property of the visible object.

The model enrichment and the G-buffer technique enables us to use additional knowledge about the model and its objects for extracting contrast relations and for an exact object observation over time.

7.4 Measuring Color Contrasts

In image processing, contrasts are mostly regarded as a local change in brightness, defined as the ratio between the brightness average of an object and its background brightness (see [SHB93]). However, this definition is insufficient for a description of the complex relationships between the colors in an image. The internal relationship of the individual color channels must be depicted, too.

Definition 7.2
We define a contrast Δc between two color values c_1 and c_2 as:

$$\Delta c = c_1 - c_2 \tag{7.6}$$

Its sign represents the relation "less than" or "greater than".

Based on equation (7.2) and the HSI color model with $V = \{h, s, i\}$, where $h \in \{0°, \ldots, 360°\}$ and "red" is at $120°$, $s \in \mathbb{R}, 0 \leq s \leq 1$ and $i \in \mathbb{R}, 0 \leq i \leq 1$, we can now determine selected contrast classes of ITTEN's classification.

The bright vs. dark contrast Δc_b is determined by the intensity channels of the given color values:

$$\Delta c_b = i_1 - i_2 \tag{7.7}$$

The cold vs. warm contrast can be described by its poles red-orange (position $120°$ on the color circle) and green-blue (position $300°$). After the transformation

$$\begin{aligned} w_{1,2} &= (h_{1,2} + 60°) \bmod 360° \\ &= |w_{1,2} - 180°| \end{aligned}$$

we can calculate the normalized contrast value Δc_w:

$$\Delta c_w = \frac{w_1 - w_2}{180°} \tag{7.8}$$

The quality contrast Δc_q is defined by the saturation channels:

$$\Delta c_q = s_1 - s_2 \tag{7.9}$$

After calculating the complementary hue value k_1

$$k_1 = (h_1 - 180°) \bmod 360°$$

the complementary contrast Δc_k can be calculated and normalized:

$$\Delta C_K = \frac{(k_1 - h_2)}{180°} \tag{7.10}$$

For the calculation of the different color contrasts the following information is needed:
- The image B produced by the rendering system.
- The object structure represented by the set $\mathcal{O}$ of object identification keys.
- The object identification matrix I with: $I = (i(x,y))\quad i \in \mathcal{O}$ as an additional product of the rendering process. This G-buffer is used to determine which pixel in B belongs to which object in the scene.

To determine the contrast relations of a selected set of objects in the scene their mean color value is used. The mean color value $\bar{c}$ of an object I_{obj} is calculated $\forall (x,y)$ with $i(x,y) = I_{obj}$:

$$\bar{c} = \frac{\sum_{y=0}^{L-1} \sum_{x=0}^{R-1} b(x,y)}{LR} \tag{7.11}$$

The mean color values of all objects form the basis for the calculation of the color contrasts between them. Thus, for one contrast a relationship network can be built according to a set of selected objects in the scene.

HOPPE, LÜDICKE, and HAUSMANN present in [HLH96] a software tool KONTRAST for an object assessment based on the contrast classification introduced above. The contrast information per object is the basis for an automatic or user-intended post-production. Thereby, adapted techniques from painters are applied to emphasize or de-emphasize objects in the scene without the need for a complete re-rendering.

7.5 Animation Analysis

For the animation analysis, approaches used in image processing science can be adapted. The G-buffer technique avoids classical problems of the motion picture analysis, such as the correspondence or the blending problem [Jäh97]. Furthermore, the G-buffer technique enables an exact observation of a selected object over time.

The animation analysis is based on the following information:

1. The sequence of rendered images – the animation A, encoded in the RGB color model:
$$\mathsf{A} = (\mathsf{a}(x,y,n,t)) \quad \mathsf{a} \in \{r,g,b\}$$

2. The perspective depth information (the z-buffer) Z:
$$\mathsf{Z} = (\mathsf{z}(x,y,t)) \quad \mathsf{z} \in \mathbb{R}.$$

This G-buffer can be produced by many modern rendering systems, such as Alias|*wavefront* or 3D Studio. In addition, the POV ray tracing system was modified to generate all required G-buffers during the rendering process. An example of the z-buffer can be seen in Fig. 7.4(a) – the depth is visualized as brightness in the image.

3. The object identification buffer I:
$$\mathsf{I} = (\mathsf{i}(x,y,t)) \quad \mathsf{i} \in \mathcal{O}$$

Figure 7.4(b) visualizes the different object keys in the identification buffer as randomly chosen colors. The identification buffer can be obtained either directly from the renderer (for instance the modified POV ray tracer) or by color encoding the objects manually.

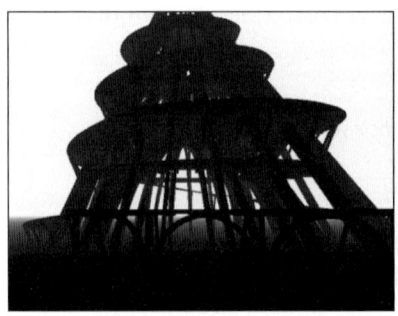
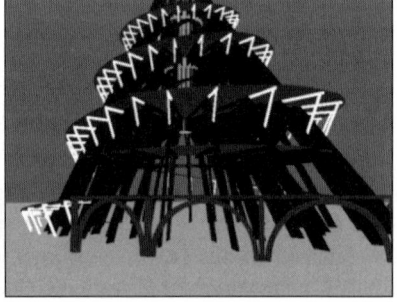

(a) z-buffer (b) Object id buffer

Figure 7.4: Visualization of the G-buffers used as input data

The goal of the animation analysis is to isolate a variety of events in the animation sequence disturbing the continuity of color change or motion. These events can be caused by the user during the modeling process (a cut scene, turning on/off light sources, etc.) or by accident.

Definition 7.3
An *event* $e(t)$ is depicted as a function surveying a particular condition at the point in time t, and returns the truth value *TRUE* or *FALSE*. All events appearing as a discontinuity in color change or motion flow of a selected object or object group *not* being caused by the user are further referred to as *unwanted events*.

7.6 Color Discontinuity

An approach for the quality analysis of an animation is the observation of the color values. In contrast to still images the depiction of the mean color value per object is often sufficient. The color channels are calculated separately. Because of the internal organization of the image data, all color based operations during the postprocessing are carried out on the color channels. An analysis of the separated color channels is therefore reasonable. The mean color channel value $\overline{w}$ can be calculated as follows:

$$\overline{w}(t) = \frac{\sum_{y=0}^{L-1} \sum_{x=0}^{R-1} \mathsf{a}(x,y,n,t)}{LR} \qquad (7.12)$$

The basis for a measurement concerning the discontinuity of the color change is the difference $\Delta \overline{w}(t)$ of the mean color channel values between two adjacent frames.

$$\Delta \overline{w}(t) = |\overline{w}(t-1) - \overline{w}(t)| \qquad (7.13)$$

For the observation of a selected object this operation is carried out only on the picture elements belonging to this object I_{obj}:

$$\forall (x,y) \text{ with } \mathsf{i}(x,y,t) = I_{obj} :$$
$$\Delta \overline{w}_{obj}(t) = |\overline{w}(t-1) - \overline{w}(t)|$$

As a color discontinuity at a point in time t we define the event $e_{col}(t)$, where the difference between (at least) one channel value and the corresponding channel in the previous frame is greater than a given threshold W_{max}:

$$e_{col}(t) = \begin{cases} TRUE & \text{if } \Delta \overline{w}(t) > W_{max} \\ FALSE & \text{otherwise} \end{cases} \qquad (7.14)$$

The threshold is defined by the user. This enables users to input their experiences and knowledge about the animation to the analysis process.

After building the event list according to equation (7.14) for all objects, these events can be compared with an event list provided as context information from the model. This list contains all events that can cause a discontinuity in color changes. A new list can be generated containing all events which are candidates for an unwanted event.

7.7 Discontinuity in Motion

A measurement for object movement is the number of picture elements that have changed since the last frame. We define $\mathcal{P}_t$ as the set of all picture elements belonging to an object I_{obj} at the time t and $\mathcal{P}_{t-1}$ at the time $t-1$

$$\forall (x,y) \text{ with } \mathsf{i}(x,y,t) = I_{obj} \rightarrow \mathcal{P}_t$$
$$\forall (x,y) \text{ with } \mathsf{i}(x,y,t-1) = I_{obj} \rightarrow \mathcal{P}_{t-1}.$$

Then the set $\Delta \mathcal{P}_t$ of points changed relative to the previous frame is

$$\Delta \mathcal{P}_t = \mathcal{P}_{t-1} \setminus \mathcal{P}_t \qquad (7.15)$$

The elements of $\Delta \mathcal{P}_t$ are counted and this number of elements $d(t)$ is the measurement for the movement of the object I_{obj}.

Objects in 3D computer animation not only move along the x or y axis but can also move in perspective. For these movements the z-buffer Z is used. Per object, the mean perspective buffer depth $\bar{z}$ is calculated $\forall (x, y)$ with $i(x, y, t) = I_{obj}$:

$$\bar{z}(t) = \frac{\sum_y \sum_x z(x, y, t)}{\text{number of pixels of } I_{obj}} \qquad (7.16)$$

Now we can conclude that for a discontinuity in motion at a time t, there is the event $e_{mov}(t)$ when the number $d(t)$ of changed pixels or the difference $\Delta \bar{z}(t)$ of the depth values opposite to the previous frame is greater than their appropriate thresholds D_{max} and Z_{max}:

$$e_{mov}(t) = \begin{cases} \text{TRUE} & \text{if } (d(t) > D_{max}) \vee (\Delta \bar{z}(t) > Z_{max}) \\ \text{FALSE} & \text{otherwise} \end{cases} \qquad (7.17)$$

Based on these concepts of motion analysis more information, like relative speed or direction of the object, can be calculated. The method presented above can also be used for comparing different camera models when using various rendering platforms for the same model. The use of different renderers can be necessary to speed up the rendering of a large animation. A sequence of difference images for a selected object I_{obj} can be calculated for two animations coming from different renderers:

$$\begin{aligned} \forall (x, y) \text{ with } i_1(x, y, t) &= I_{obj} \\ \text{or } i_2(x, y, t) &= I_{obj} \\ \Delta I &= |I_1 - I_2| \end{aligned} \qquad (7.18)$$

The picture elements in ΔI can be analyzed to calculate the differences in the camera models. Also, the lists of mean color values $\bar{c}(t_1)$ and $\bar{c}(t_2)$ can be used to estimate the different illumination conditions, etc., in the scenes. These differences can help adjust rendering parameters like surface colors being used in the different modeling or rendering systems.

7.8 Emphasizing Objects

When painters use techniques for emphasis, they have special knowledge about the objects they wish to depict. Besides the information about shape, color, appearance of the surface, illumination, shadows, etc., they have information about an object concerning

- its *importance* for the whole scene,
- its *characteristic aura* (for instance should the object appear "kind of cold", "lively" or "harmoniously embedded"?), and
- its *role* in explaining a context to the viewer (e.g., "should the viewer focus this object?").

This knowledge makes it possible for the painter to decide whether an object should be emphasized, and if so, by which technique.

For applying these techniques to computer graphics and for generating accentuated images in a computer-supported way, it is necessary to pass on such knowledge to a rendering system. Therefore, an enriched model is used to develop emphasizing techniques. For our approach the following information is used:

- *Object name* – used for user interaction,
- *Object identification key* ($id \in I$) – an unambiguous key determined during the rendering process,
- *Assembly hierarchy* – to process the appearance of objects in connection with their environment,
- *Importance* (imp) – representing the importance of an object in the context of the whole scene; we distinguish between five possible categories: "unimportant background object", "unimportant object", "normal object", "important object", and "very important object",
- *Characteristic appearance* (chr) – an index in a list containing methods for changing the effect of an object on the user; appearance of the object when it is accentuated using color phenomena or when it is de-accentuated using coloring can be described as "kind of warm", "kind of cold", or "embedded in color context", and
- *Intensity* (int) – a scaling factor to determine the intensity of applying the chosen method.

We placed this part of the modeling process after the modeling of object geometries, arranging the scene and after the rendering process. This enables the user to control the listed parameters interactively watching their effects on the image. However, also initial context information can be inserted during the process of modeling. The ZOOMSTRUCTOR tool (described in Chap. 3) is used to enrich a modeled 3D scene with context information. AKZENT analyzes this information based on a special database and makes suggestions for accentuating or de-accentuating objects in the scene. AKZENT is intended as a post-production module and is part of independent programs which communicate via file interfaces with a dialog component for interaction with the user and with the rendering data (see Fig. 7.5). Furthermore, a set of values $object(w), w \in \{name, id, int, imp, chr\}$, representing the context information is defined for each object. In this file also the hierarchical information is encoded.

Finally, there is a lookup table including the parameters for the application of the different methods for accentuation/de-accentuation. These meth-

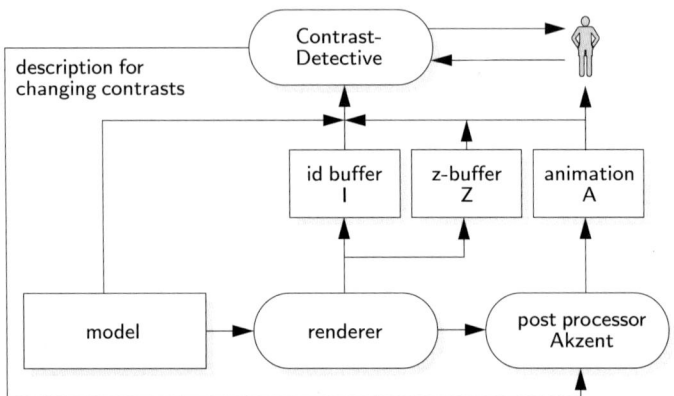

Figure 7.5: Information flow in COLORDETECTIVE

ods are based on a sequence *op_seq* of image processing operations $op(op\_seq)$ on the G-buffers, referenced by the importance *imp* of an object. Furthermore, the color values $c(v), v \in \{r, g, b\}$ for the color tone shifting are defined, referenced by an object's characteristic appearance *chr*.

The files listed above are the initial data for AKZENT. The accentuation process works per accentuated object on the rendered image buffer R: If AKZENT finds objects with the importance "normal object" ($object(imp)$ = NORMAL_OBJECT) the image buffer R is not changed. After finding an object to accentuate or de-accentuate, a temporary buffer is created containing the z-buffer values of this object only. According to the importance and the characteristic appearance AKZENT estimates an index *op_seq* for the accentuation method, and a color value $c(v)$. The sequence *op_seq* defines an order of image processing operations in combination with the value for intensity *int*. These operations are carried out on the temporary buffer creating a mask for the combination of the image buffer R with the accentuation color $c(v)$ to the *accentuated image buffer* R_{acc}. Output from AKZENT is R_{acc} after all combinations and is displayed by the dialog component. Now the user can interactively change the parameters determining the accentuation and can select objects for the accentuation process. The following values per object can be changed by the user:

- importance *imp*,
- the characteristic appearance *chr*, and
- the intensity *int* of the applied method.

After updating the context information the accentuating process starts again and the image is redisplayed.

7.9 Results

For the evaluation of the presented concepts we designed a software tool: the COLORDETECTIVE. This program is implemented in C using the OpenGL library for user interaction. COLORDETECTIVE is organized as a post-production module. The general concept of COLORDETECTIVE is displayed in Fig. 7.5. Input for COLORDETECTIVE are the z-buffer Z, the identification buffer I, and the animation A. The animation can be changed during postprocessing. COLORDETECTIVE needs also additional information from the model. After analyzing the required information, COLORDETECTIVE presents the results. This can be done in different ways:

The color classification and all events which are candidates for unwanted events are listed as values in a table. For a better overview the event list can be presented in diagrams. In addition, the mean color values of selected objects can be animated: The bounding boxes of the objects are displayed depending on their mean depth value $\overline{z}$, filled with the mean color values. This abstraction gives the user an impression of the continuity of the objects' color change. In addition, discontinuities in camera panning can be perceived.

An example of the "BUGA tower" animation may illustrate the detection of unwanted events: In Fig. 7.6 the events based on the color value of the whole scene in the interval $t = \langle 2\,000, 2\,500 \rangle$ are shown. A clear peak of the curve can be seen at position $t = 2\,384$. We found that the postprocessing was not carried out on this frame because of a hardware crash.

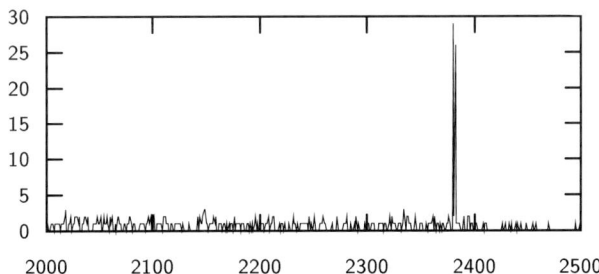

Figure 7.6: RGB values in the "BUGA tower" animation

A second example may illustrate how AKZENT carries out an accentuation process on objects in an image. Figure 7.7(a) shows a model of the monastery in Magdeburg. To let the building appear solid and to give an impression of the material on the object surfaces, side lighting was chosen.

In Fig. 7.7(a) the rendered image buffer R is shown. We notice problems of discernibility of the piers on the left wall. After changing the importance *imp* of these piers to "important objects" and the characteristic appearance to "cold" (corresponding to an impression of air), AKZENT generates the accentuated image in Fig. 7.7(b).

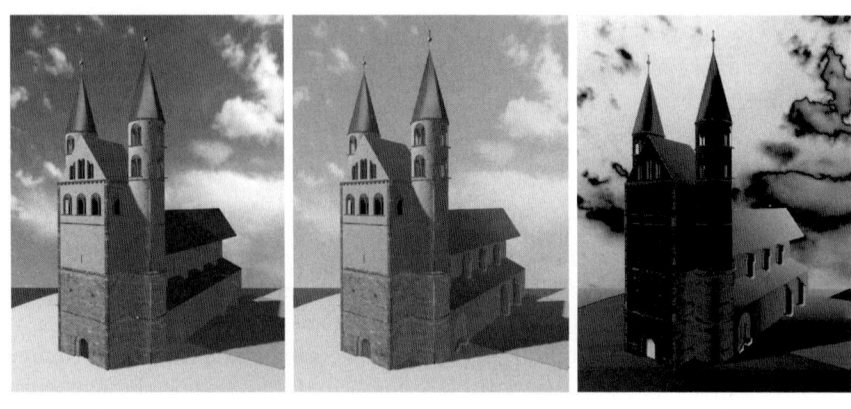

(a) Original (b) accentuated (c) difference

Figure 7.7: An example of an accentuated image – the monastery in Magdeburg

Contributors of Chap. 7: Axel HOPPE and Kathrin LÜDICKE

Part III

Adaptive Zooming and Distorting Graphics

One of the most important attributes of hand-drawn images which makes them look good and makes them more appropriate for specific tasks which users wish to undertake is that they are not drawn entirely to scale. Changes to the scale are often subtle and go unnoticed to the untrained eye, even though they have a marked effect on how useful an image is. To make matters algorithmically difficult, the scale may vary over an image. This part analyzes the phenomenon of distortion in images and introduces methods and tools for incorporating similar effects in computational visualizations.

Maps are perhaps the most widespread kind of visualization to use selective distortions. Indeed, maps for end-users, for example of cities, are rarely drawn to scale, but are adjusted manually by a cartographer so as to encode certain information. Rainer MICHEL and Jörg HAMEL thus begin Chap. 8 by discussing methods of systematically distorting 2D renditions of maps. They introduce a new technique called the *focus line* which is particularly suited to uncluttering maps along line segments which contain too much detail to be visualized adequately.

Chapter 9 moves to a more general method of zooming in graphics. Andreas RAAB and Michael RÜGER devise a method of zooming based on fisheye methods which can be applied to one, two, or three-dimensional data. Their zoom algorithm pays particular attention to empty space in the 2D visualization and adjusts the displacement mechanism to fill the screen space available. Their method is particularly well suited for use in interactive systems, as it is based on bounding boxes of individual objects to be zoomed and is thus highly efficient. The method of zooming introduced in this chapter is drawn on repeatedly in various situations throughout the rest of this book.

In Chap. 10, Michael RÜGER, Bernhard PREIM, and Alf RITTER use the zoom algorithm in a new method of exploring complex information and application spaces. Their method, called zoom navigation, is based on a pluggable implementation of the zoom algorithm. Going beyond the usual degree of interest used in fisheye techniques, they introduce what they call an aspect of interest which guides the selection of attributes of the underlying information space to be visualized. They show how the concept of zoom navigation can be applied to window-based user interfaces and to the exploration of 3D graphics.

Chapter 8

Distortions and Displacements in 2D

Distortions are a common means to present complex information in an expressive and easily comprehensible way. To enhance the viewer's perception, one or more areas of interest to the viewer are emphasized – they are brought to the *focus*. Typically, the areas lying in the focus are enlarged at the expense of their surroundings; they can be shown with more detail. Hence, distortion is a way to cope with the limited space of a presentation area, in general the screen or a sheet of paper.

The "screen real estate" problem becomes even more serious with growing size of the data set to be examined. For the exploration of large information spaces, e.g. , graphs or maps, panning and zooming techniques find their limit when local detail is desired while the global context should be maintained. Displaying graphs in such a way that nodes of current interest are enlarged to reveal their details while the remaining nodes are displaced and shrunk to compensate for the increased space requirements results in a detail and context presentation that aids to solve the "screen real estate" problem.

Early attempts to distort maps systematically date back to the 1950s when the map publishing company Falk (Germany) patented a photo-mechanical method to manufacture city maps with a varying scale. Their maps display the centers of European cities that are usually cluttered with narrow little streets and alleys enlarged while the scale is continuously reduced toward the map edge. Although the scale in the center is up to twice the scale at the edge, the resulting distortion is subtle and usually remains unnoticed.

In general, distortions may be used for maps with a varying symbol density. In order to keep the map size down, cluttered areas can be enlarged at the expense of the sparse areas, resulting in different map scales. Figure 8.1 shows the effect of such distortions for a rural region with several settlements.

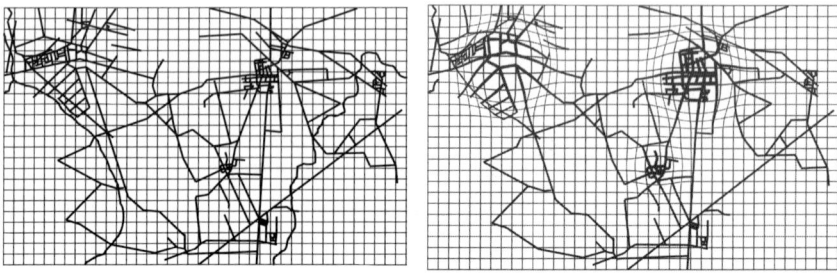

(a) Undistorted, constant scale map   (b) Distorted view using three foci

Figure 8.1: Two maps of a rural area with several settlements: distortion is applied to enlarge the settlements (redrawn after [Lic83])

8.1 Methods for Distortions

In principle, distortions displace points surrounding the focus by adding a *displacement vector* to each point (see Fig. 8.2). For point-shaped foci, the direction of the displacement vector usually points radially away from the focus.

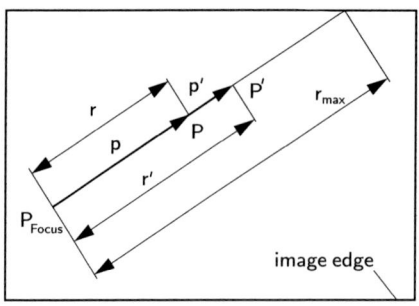

Figure 8.2: General principle of 2D distortions: point P with distance r to the focus P_{Focus} is moved by the displacement vector $\vec{p}$ to P'

In most cases, the strength of displacement is largest in the vicinity of the focus and fades away toward the map edges. In case the method supports multiple foci *(polyfocal distortion)* the displacement vector is usually the weighted sum of the displacements of all foci.

One of the early distortions is the *hyperbolic distortion* [Kad75]. KADMON developed this distortion method to create maps with varying scale. The larger scale m_0 at the center is linearly decreased to a predefined scale m_1 typically at the map edge over a distance d. The x-component of the distortion vector for each point P with distance r to the focus can be calculated as follows (the y-component is determined analogously):

$$x'(m_0, m_1, d, r) = \frac{-m_0 + \sqrt{m_0^2 + 4c_x x}}{2c_x} \quad \text{with} \quad c_x = \frac{m_1 - m_0}{d} \frac{r}{x^2} \quad (8.1)$$

SNYDER manipulates the map layout using the paradigm of a *magnifying glass* [Sny87]. The region underneath the magnifying glass is enlarged and presented with a constant scale. For the surrounding region the scale is either constant but smaller or decreasing gradually to zero at the map edge. The first method results in an abrupt change at the border of the magnifying glass, an effect which is reasonably reduced by the latter method. However, since the scale in the inner region remains constant, discontinuities are still visible.

In the realm of interface design a different paradigm has been established – the *fisheye*. SARKAR and BROWN describe a graphical fisheye distortion that continuously displaces the area around the focus similar to fisheye lens for cameras [SB94]. Unlike the optical solution their method is also applicable for several foci. The distortion is controlled by an empirical parameter that has no direct geometric equivalent.

While the distortions mentioned above were restricted to point shaped foci, SARKAR et al. present an approach using closed convex polygons as foci [SSTR93]. This method is based on *morphing* which is typically used for raster image manipulation and has an unrestricted global impact on the image.

Following the rubber sheet paradigm more directly, CARPENDALE et al. developed an interactive distortion method allowing the user to lift the image surface in 3D [CCF95]. The resulting hills in the surface are bell-shaped with steep slopes, visualized as a shaded landscape. The bell shapes originate from the use of the Gaussian curve and, hence, are characterized by the standard deviation.

8.2 Distortions Along Linear Features

A common property of the approaches to 2D distortions so far is a more or less radial distortion in all directions. In the few cases where linear or polygonal shaped foci were used, these were treated as stretched points, i.e., polygonal foci displaced their surrounding radially to their center and linear foci displaced them perpendicularly along the sides, but behaved like point-shaped foci at the end points.

However, to increase the applicability of distortions a more general focus model is required that goes beyond the current rubber sheet model. In a number of cases, there is a specific need for a limited area only to be subject to distortions and, furthermore, only in a few directions. Thus, in areas with a highly varying feature density, it is preferable to use the space from sparse areas only. Consider, for example, a densely settled coastal region with a bay on one side and a desert on the other. When focusing on a city, it seems best to borrow the necessary space primarily from the water or the desert, rather than from the surrounding cities.

In addition, linear structures are a typical domain where a distortion displacing in all directions is often unintentional or even disturbing. In cartography, a well-known example is a valley formed by a river and with roads and railway tracks running along the river. Reducing the map scale very soon leads to these features overlapping, which can be counteracted by a perpendicular displacement. However, an additional lengthwise displacement is not only ineffective but would result in unmotivated distortions that might confuse the reader.

Another example showing the need for a direction-dependent distortion method is the anatomical depiction of a limb. In this case, bones, muscles, veins, and sinews lie roughly parallel to each other. Focusing on, say, a sinew requires a perpendicular displacement of the surrounding muscles and veins to gain an unobstructed view. Again, a lengthwise displacement is completely unnecessary.

In summary, a simple radial distortion displacing evenly in all directions as has been the practice so far is ineffective or even unintentional in a number of cases and should thus be replaced by a more general approach allowing direction-dependent distortions.

Besides direction dependency, other properties are necessary for a distortion method supporting detail and context displays. In particular, the resulting distortion should be continuous, smoothly integrate the focus area, and run to zero at the image edge to preserve the image size. Furthermore, a focus should distort just as much as needed to show the feature in enough detail without any further distortion beyond what is absolutely necessary. For this purpose, it is essential that the space allocation can be precisely controlled. This calls for a distortion function which is adjustable by parameters that have a geometric interpretation.

8.3 The Focus Line Distortion

In keeping with the requirementss formulated in the previous section we have developed a direction-dependent distortion method – the *Focus Line*. So far our application area is symbol displacement in maps in the context of cartographic generalization; therefore, all the following examples will be maps.

The two significant aspects of the Focus Line are the shape and the amount of displacement of objects in its vicinity. While the shape determines the direction-dependency of the focus, the amount characterizes the efficiency and continuity of the distortion. Both together have an impact on the smoothness of the distortion and determine how well it can meet the requirements formulated above.

8.3 The Focus Line Distortion

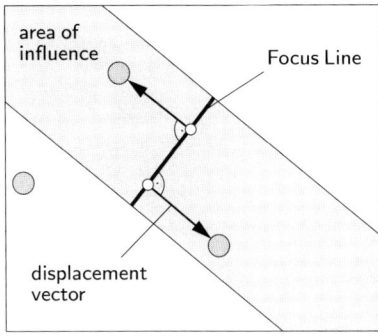

Figure 8.3: A primitive Focus Line placed on an image: points inside the *area of influence* are about to be displaced, the others not

8.3.1 Defining the Shape of the Distortion

As described in the previous section, the shape of the distortion introduced by a linear focus should be such that it displaces the surrounding objects symmetrically and perpendicular to itself. The area of influence has to be adjustable; for a line focus it is defined by the area between two lines drawn perpendicular (to the line) through the end points of the line. The influence in one dimension is hence controllable by the length of the Focus Line.

The Focus Line can, therefore, be imagined as a set of point foci on a line from which each point in the area of influence selects the one nearest to it. Note that the point focus thus selected displaces objects perpendicular to the line.

Decisive for the shape of the displacement is how points are treated at the outer limits of the area of influence. For example, Fig. 8.4(a) shows an undistorted map; clearly, if the influence of the Focus Line is cut off as sharply as in Fig. 8.4(b), unwanted distortions are induced, caused by a discontinuity at the edge of the area of influence. Simply extending the Focus Line across the edges of the image, such that the whole image is in the area of influence, would remove the discontinuity but also cause other unwanted distortions along the Focus Line, as shown in Fig. 8.4(c). We refer to this unwanted distortion as the *corridor effect*.

Obviously, space must be defined where the displacement introduced by the Focus Line is allowed to fade out. We call this space the *damping section* in contrast to the *core section*, where the displacement is applied fully. The damping section is an extension of the original focus line, so the area of influence is prolonged, such that there are no discontinuities on its outer limits. The amount of damping *DMP* is, in its simplest form, a function of the distance t of the point focus from the core section.

Demanding continuity at the outer limits requires the fading function to be C^1 continuous. Therefore, cubic spline interpolation has been used to determine the fading function, enforcing C^1 continuity and a decrease to zero over a distance a from each end point. The resulting function is given in equation 8.2 and depicted in Fig. 8.5.

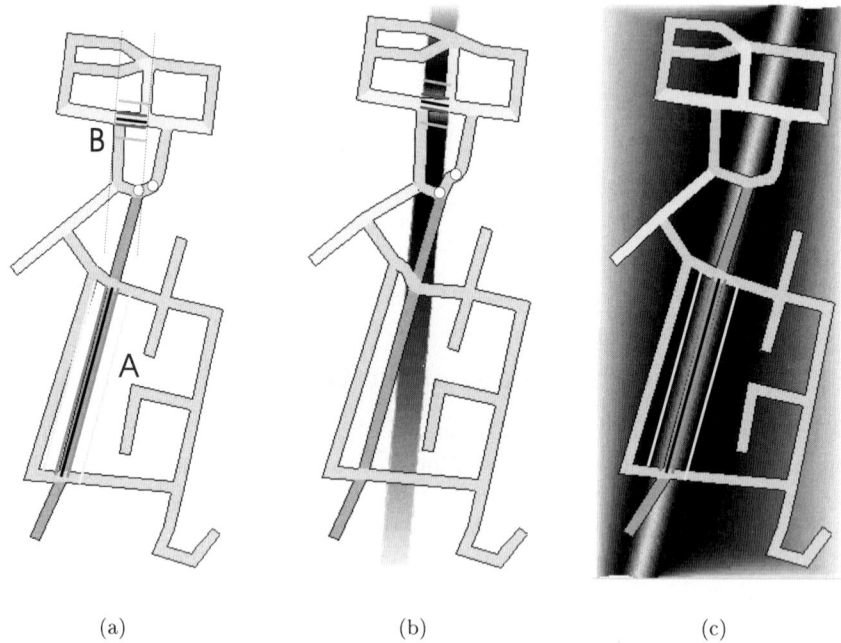

(a)   (b)   (c)

Figure 8.4: Straightforward solutions to the behavior of the Focus Line at the end points. The original image with two Focus Lines marked A and B can be seen in the left image. Cutting the displacement introduced by Focus Line A leads to a highly distorted orientation of the street segment between the marked points (middle). In the right image unintentional distortions are visible due to extending the displacement of Focus Line B to the map edges; note in particular the roundabout in the upper part

$$DMP_d(t) = \frac{2}{a^3}t^3 - \frac{3}{a^2}t^2 + 1 \qquad (8.2)$$

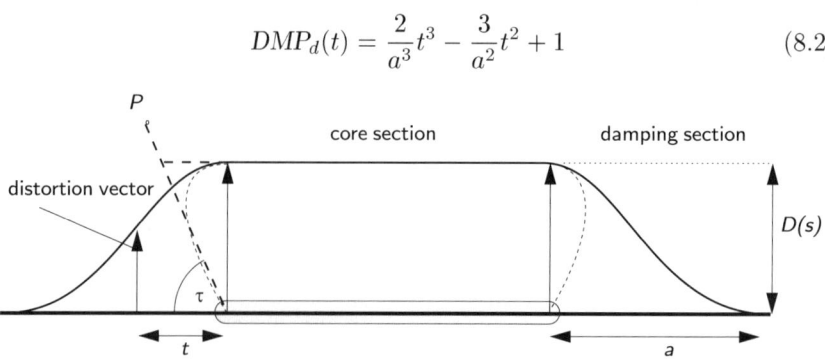

Figure 8.5: The Focus Line with core and damping sections: the displacement vector for a point P in the damping section is calculated depending on its distance to the core section and the angle τ

8.3 The Focus Line Distortion

The impact of the introduction of the damping area is illustrated in Fig. 8.6. Note that the distortion to the whole image is reduced. However, since the distortion is strongest near the Focus Line, objects in the damping area can experience an unintended large displacement, if their offset to the extended Focus Line is small. This leads to orientational distortions as shown in Fig. 8.7(b).

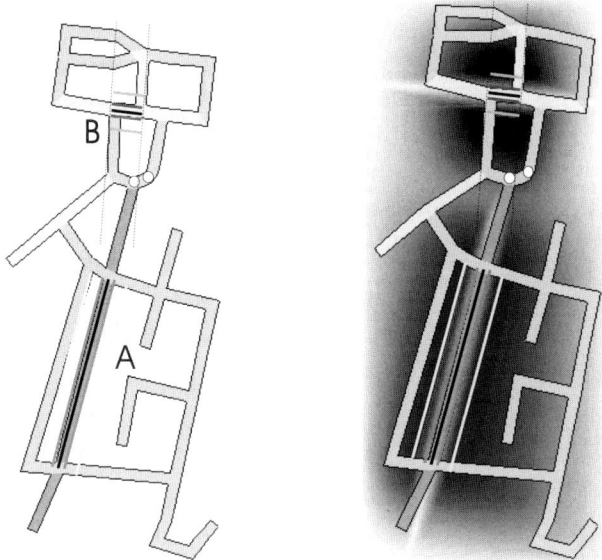

Figure 8.6: Effect of using the Focus Line with the damping area (cf. Fig. 8.4). The original image with two Focus Lines is shown on the left. The right image shows how the displacement is slowly faded out in damping areas on both sides of the Focus Lines

The important characteristic of this situation is that the remaining part of the feature makes a small angle relative to the focus line. In fact, the larger the angle, the less the amount of orientational (or angular) distortion caused by the displacement. Therefore, we consider in addition the angle τ (see Fig. 8.5) as a parameter controlling the damping. Equation 8.3 proved to be appropriate for these means.

$$DMP_a(\tau) = |\sin \tau| \qquad (8.3)$$

Figure 8.7(c) shows the result when both damping functions are combined. It is apparent that the angular damping reduces the amount of unintentioned distortions further. Collecting the results of the previous reflections we can therefore define equation 8.4 to describe the shape of the Focus Line distortion.

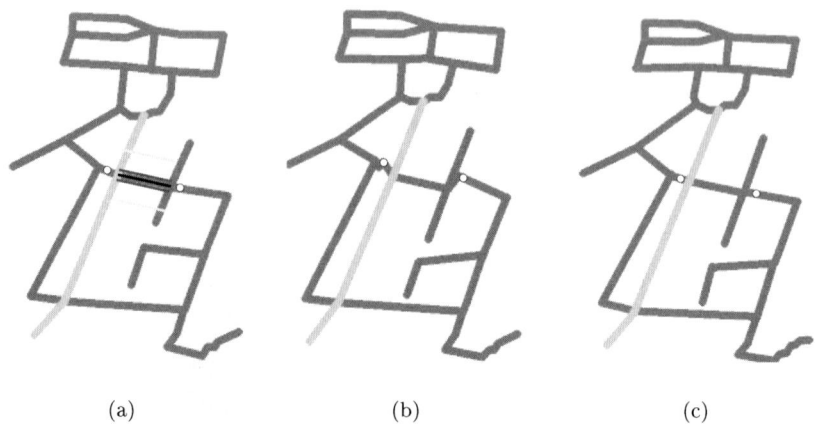

(a)   (b)   (c)

Figure 8.7: The use of angle damping: The Focus Line used in the left image leads to a highly distorted orientation of street segments close to the focus line (see middle image), whereas angle damping, as shown on the right, treats segments in the vicinity more carefully.

$$\vec{p}' = \begin{cases} \vec{p}\left(\frac{D(s)}{s} - 1\right), & \text{if } P \text{ in core section} \\ \vec{p}\left(\frac{D(s)}{s}\, DMP_d(t)\, DMP_a(\tau) - 1\right), & \text{if } P \text{ in damp section} \\ \vec{o}, & \text{otherwise.} \end{cases} \quad (8.4)$$

with $s = r/r_{max}$, the normalized distance r in respect to the image edge. The function $D(s)$ determines the amount of distortion and will be derived in the next section.

8.3.2 Defining the Amount of Distortion

As stated in Sect. 8.2, the space allocation of the displacement must be precisely controllable. Therefore, we now split this quite general request into a few more specific requirements which, mathematically formulated, lead us to the function required. The function shall fulfill the following requirements:

1. It shall map the available space to the required one.
2. It shall not distort more than necessary, i.e., it should magnify only where there is a need for space (if that actually is the problem) and demagnify outside that area.
3. It shall not induce discontinuities and thus unwanted distortions in the image. Therefore, it should be at least C^1 continuous.

The situation is shown graphically in Fig. 8.8. All objects outside distance s_0 from the focus line shall be displaced to lie outside distance s'_0, thus making

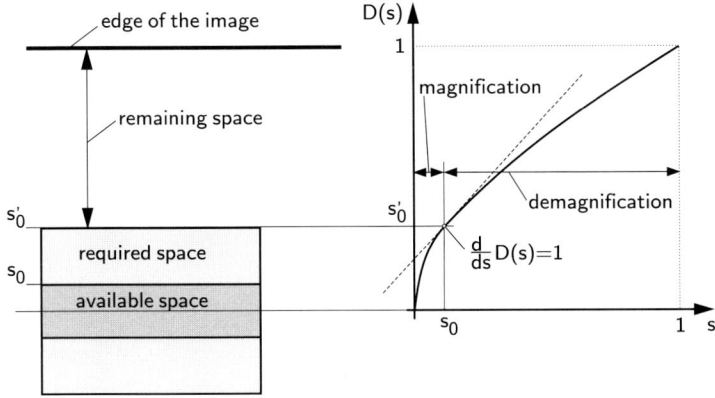

Figure 8.8: Customizing the displacement function

space for the objects within s_0. Magnification and demagnification are determined by the first derivate. From this we derive the following requirements:

$$D(s_0) = s_0' \tag{8.5}$$

$$\frac{d}{ds}D(s) \begin{cases} > 1 & \text{for } s < s_0 \\ < 1 & \text{for } s > s_0 \end{cases} \tag{8.6}$$

$$\lim_{s \to s_0} \frac{d}{ds}D(s) = \frac{d}{ds}D(s_0) = 1 \tag{8.7}$$

Equation 8.8 was derived to meet these conditions:

$$D(s_0, s_0', s) = \begin{cases} es^2 + fs, & \text{for } s \leq s_0 \\ \frac{1}{2g}\left(h - \sqrt{h^2 + 4g(1-s)}\right) + 1, & \text{for } s > s_0 \end{cases} \tag{8.8}$$

where e, f, g and h are auxiliary variables defined as follows:

$$e = \frac{s_0 - s_0'}{s_0^2}, \; f = \frac{2s_0'}{s_0} - 1, \; g = \frac{s_0 - s_0'}{(1 - s_0')^2}, \text{ and } h = \frac{2(1 - s_0)}{1 - s_0'} - 1.$$

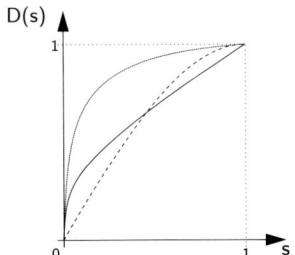

Figure 8.9: The function used for the amount of distortion

Within the interval $[0, s_0]$ the function is quadratic, and in the interval $[s_0, 1]$ it is a quadratic root function. While both are obviously C^1 continuous (in their respective intervals), C^1 continuity at $D(s_0)$ is forced by equation (8.7).

The use of quadratic interpolation guarantees that the function does not oscillate, which is a good payoff for the higher computational cost of the square root compared to a cubic spline, for example. Figure 8.9 shows plots for three different (s_0, s'_0) pairs.

8.4 The Interactive Focus Line

The Focus Line distortion function has been developed to be controllable by two parameters that have a geometric correspondence. This property lays the foundation for the design of direct-manipulative tools for point-shaped and line-shaped foci. Although originally developed to aid in displacements perpendicular to lines, the Focus Line distortion function can also be used for point-shaped foci.

In both cases the foci are easily placed and adjusted by defining their centers and two distances representing s_0 and s'_0. For point foci, a user may click to define the central point of the focus and then move the mouse to define two concentric circles. The inner circle represents s_0, i.e., the border of the area to be enlarged, while the outer circle corresponding to s'_0 marks the destination size of area enclosed by the former. The amount of enlargement is directly visible through the difference between the two radii (see Fig. 8.4).

The displacement from line foci is defined analogously. In this case, a central line determines the length of the core area of the Focus Line. Depending on whether the displacement is expected to work in one direction or in both directions of this line, another line or a pair of lines on either side of the central line is drawn setting s_0. The other parameter s'_0 is set similarly by a line or a pair of lines farther away from the central line. As in the point focus case, the inner line marks the border of the area that will be subjected to the enlargement, while the outer line marks the final size of this area; the difference between these represents the amount of distortion (see Fig. 8.4). The length of the damping area is set to multiples of the amount by a user-defined factor a.

For the integration of the Focus Line distortion in an interactive system it is important to give the user a feeling for the amount of the resulting distortion and its global impact. A first impression can be gained from observing the results of a regular grid exposed to the distortion. Figure 8.10(a) shows the resulting image for a point focus and two line foci.

However, while it is very expressive for the point focus and the horizontal line focus it is confusing for any line focus that is not parallel to the x or the y-axis. An alternative is to fill each grid cell with a gray shade that corresponds to the local amount of distortion this cell was subject to. The color index

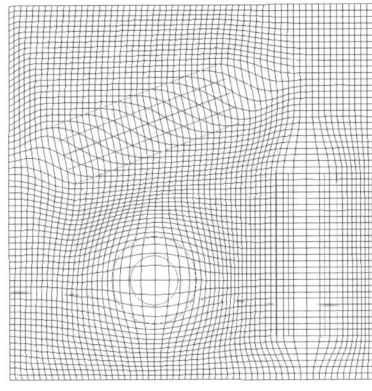 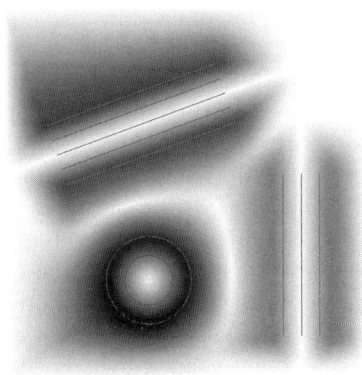

(a) Visualization using a regular grid

(b) Visualization using shades of gray

Figure 8.10: Visualization of the impact of the distortion

c_i for the i-th cell can be calculated as the displacement between the old position of the cell center P_i and the new displaced position P_i' normalized to the number of gray values supported by the output device c_{max}:

$$c_i = \frac{|P_i' - P_i|}{\max_j |P_j' - P_j|} c_{max} \qquad (8.9)$$

The color is assigned such that the gray shade darkens with increasing displacement. This is easily calculated and yields expressive depictions that can be regarded as landscapes with hills having light tops and dark slopes. Figure 8.10(b) shows such a landscape model for the same focus configuration as Fig. 8.10(a). Note that the valleys describe areas where two or more foci interact resulting in an area where almost no distortion is noticeable.

The resulting image is similar in appearance to the landscapes created by CARPENDALE et al. [CCF95]. However, while their image is the result of a rendering process of a 3D plane, our image is simply a by-product of the distortion process and needs no real 3D interpretation.

8.5 Concluding Remarks

This chapter has presented Focus Line displacement as a tool to create detail and context displays. It goes beyond previous approaches by offering a more sophisticated model for the control of space allocation. Two parameters allow the definition of the beginning and the amount of space of allocation. These have a direct geometric counterpart and allow thus precise control of the enlargement. Unlike a simple radial displacement, Focus Line displacement is designed to be applicable when space is needed along linear features. For this purpose a special shape was developed for the distortion ensuring a smooth integration of the enlarged region in the wider context. To facilitate use in an interactive environment, Focus Line displacement offers visual cues about the distortion applied.

Focus Line displacement extends the earlier cartographic approaches (see [Kad75] and [Sny87]) by offering more precise control of the enlargements using direct-manipulative parameters and direction-dependent displacements. Unlike SNYDER's magnifying glass approach [Sny87], it ensures a smooth integration of the focus in the context.

While SARKAR's and BROWN's fisheye technique [SB94] remained restricted to point-shaped foci, Focus Line displacement allows, in addition, the use of line-shaped foci. It also allows a more flexible space allocation in contrast to their approach where the distortion function is controlled by a distortion factor that influences the function's curvature.

The polygonal stretching method of SARKAR et al. [SSTR93] based on morphing allows the use of polygonal foci, but results in a global impact on the whole image. By contrast, the Focus Line allows an adjustable distortion where the size of the area subject to the distortion can be limited preventing regions far off the focus from being drawn into the displacement process. Thus, the Focus Line avoids the corridor effect and ensures a fading to zero of the displacement at the map edges.

Unlike previous work, the 3D pliable surfaces approach of CARPENDALE et al. [CCF95] allows the use of arbitrarily shaped foci. However, their bell-shaped distortion model always causes a more or less radial displacement. The Focus Line extends this approach by offering a direction-dependent displacement. The use of the Gaussian bell curve causes a narrow compression zone around the focus, resulting in a strong distortion in the immediate vicinity. The Focus Line, by contrast, ensures a gentle fading of the enlargement. In addition, while the bell curve is parametrized by the standard deviation and the height, the Focus Line offers more intuitive parameters for the control of the displacement.

The Focus Line allows distortions to images with response times that allow its integration in interactive systems. It has been integrated in a system for the creation of tactile maps for blind people where it is successfully used to allocate presentation space in a flexible way. This application will be discussed in Chap. 20.

Contributors of Chap. 8: Rainer MICHEL and Jörg HAMEL

Chapter 9

Zooming
in 1, 2, and 3 Dimensions

The advantages of 3D computer graphics are being exploited in an increasing number of interactive applications. This not only includes classical fields of 3D graphics (such as CAD or geometric modeling) but also fields in which static 2D images have been used so far (e.g., interactive illustration systems and online catalogs).

While typical end-users have learned how to cope with graphical (2D) user interfaces, surprisingly little work has been done on the interaction with 3D graphics. Virtual reality applications use the metaphor of a virtual world in conjunction with 3D input devices. However, the typical user's equipment is still dominated by the computer monitor. This, in turn, raises the question how users can interact with 3D presentations if limited to a 2D screen. Classical techniques use the metaphor of a virtual camera which can be moved and turned in the 3D scene. Interestingly enough, this resembles the commonly known pan-and-zoom navigation technique from 2D interfaces. This technique, however, has a number of disadvantages from a cognitive point of view. It has been shown (see [SZB+93]) that pan-and-zoom often requires a tremendous amount of memorization since only part of the overall information can be seen at any given time[1] although it was actually intended to examine only part of the information in its surrounding context. If this is true for 2D applications, how much more is it true for 3D applications? Here, we have in addition to the tunnel vision syndrome the problem that data may be arranged in depth, so finding a particular piece of information can result in a difficult "fly-through" of the scene.

---

[1] One could even say that the computer monitor imposes a tunnel vision effect on the user!

Obviously, there is a need to support the user in navigating through information spaces arranged in three dimensions. However, this should not be done without referring to navigation techniques already known to the user such as pan-and-zoom in 2D versus camera movement in 3D. This is because, first, a considerable amount of work has been done on 2D user interfaces, showing which techniques and metaphors are appropriate for certain actions. The results of user studies should be carefully examined to adapt these techniques to 3D interaction. Second, users already knowing a certain technique will learn and accept much more easily a 3D interaction technique if this is based on familiar principles.

In this chapter, we present a technique for navigating in information spaces of arbitrary dimension. While the practical applications are typically restricted to 2D or 3D interfaces, it is possible (and often useful) to apply the technique to information spaces of different dimensions. The next section will describe the basic technique and the goals behind its development. Next, we will discuss some extensions which are imposed by spatial constraints in certain applications. Finally, we will show the application of this technique to different interface problems illustrating the usefulness of our approach.

9.1 Fisheye Zoom Technique

Based on the work of FURNAS [Fur86] (see Chap. 2), several new developments were reached. The *variable zoom* presented by SCHAFFER et al. [SZB+93] is designed for viewing large hierarchical networks in a real-time application of network supervisory control. NOIK [Noi93] combined fisheye views and hierarchically nested graphs for visualizing hypertext documents. *Tree Maps* presented by JOHNSON and SHNEIDERMAN [JS91] use a space filling algorithm to fit a complete strict hierarchy into a window. The first approaches to 3D fisheye views were presented by MACKINLAY et al. [MRC91] using a linear transformation of a 1D space onto a *perspective wall* and by ROBERTSON et al. [RMC91] using *cone-trees* to visualize hierarchies in 3D space.

9.1.1 The Continuous Zoom Approach

Since the work presented in this chapter has been heavily influenced by the continuous zoom [SZB+93, BOD+94, SZG+96] we will briefly review the ideas behind it. The continuous zoom manages a rectangular 2D display space by recursively breaking it up into smaller rectangular areas, creating a hierarchy of nested rectangles. Since it was designed for network supervisory control the display hierarchy generally resulted from the hierarchical organization of the network nodes. The leaf nodes of the hierarchy correspond to the network nodes and are grouped by the interior nodes of the hierarchy (also called *clusters*).

9.1 Fisheye Zoom Technique

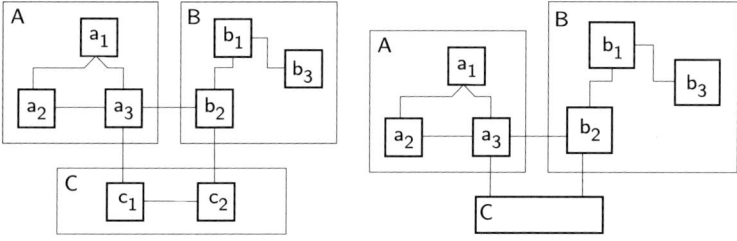

Figure 9.1: Graph layout from the continuous zoom (left) and after closing node C (right)

When a user "opens" or "closes" a cluster its contents are displayed or hidden, respectively. Thus, if a cluster is open the user can see deeper (more detailed) levels of the hierarchy. Through opening and closing clusters, as well as resizing nodes, the user has control over the amount of detail presented in each part of the display.

The algorithm uses a "budgeting" process to distribute space among the nodes of a network. It first breaks up the network into intervals by projecting all node boundaries (or edges) onto the x and y axes. *Intervals* are the spaces between the grid lines created by the projection.

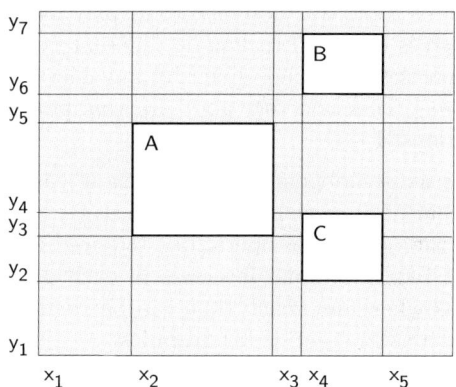

Figure 9.2: Interval structure used in the continuous zoom

When a node is about to change its size a scale factor is defined for this node. Due to the independent projection this factor may be different in x and y which allows simple control by the user.

The algorithm works by calculating a scale factor for each interval which is defined as the maximum scale of all nodes included in the interval i

$$s_i = \max s_i^n$$

where s_i is the scale factor of an interval and s_i^n the scale factor of node n

in the interval i. For empty intervals a scale has to be defined and is set to the maximum scale of its neighboring intervals. The total amount L of space requested in each direction is now

$$L = \sum_{i=0}^{n} l_i s_i$$

where l_i is the length of interval i. To ensure that the space requested does not exceed the initially given screen space the length l_i^* finally assigned to each interval is calculated by

$$l_i^* = l_i \frac{s_i}{S_{root}}$$

where S_{root} defines the scale factor of a root node.

There are a number of extensions to this basic idea (see [BOD+94] and [SZG+96]) allowing the algorithm to work both globally and locally, as well as algorithms to decide when a node is to be opened or closed and what representations to activate.

9.1.2 Dimension Independent Zoom

While the continuous zoom was designed to display hierarchical graph structures, our approach is designed to handle different types of representations uniformly based on the clustering given by any hierarchical structure. Indeed, the *continuous zoom* is a very good starting point for this, due to the following observations:

- It handles the axes independently, making it easy to extend it to an arbitrary number of dimensions.
- It is linear in the number of operations required so far (each node generates at most two additional intervals in each direction), allowing use for applications where not much time can be spent for the actual layout calculation, such as interactive 3D graphics.
- It allows further integration of spatial constraints, which is often necessary in practical applications.

The extension of the continuous zoom to arbitrary dimensions is obvious. Given a k-dimensional object (node), its boundary $B(o)$ can be represented as linear combination of a number of base vectors x_i

$$B(o) = \sum_{i=1}^{k} b_i x_i \qquad (9.1)$$

where b_i is the extent of the object in dimension x_i.

However, for many applications it may be desirable to dynamically restrict the display space, such as in 3D where perspective distortions may reduce the space needed to display an object on the screen. In addition, often better space filling properties are required since empty space typically should be used to allow the enlargement of a node rather than shrinking others. Our evaluation scheme therefore differs from what was originally described in the continuous zoom.

The Basic Algorithm

As in the continuous zoom, we assume a clustering of the objects in an interval structure of a k-dimensional representation (cf. equation (9.1)). The intervals are described by $i = (s_0^i, s^i, N^i)$ with s_0^i the initial size of the interval, s^i the size of the interval, and N^i the nodes contained in this interval. The overall size of the display space of an interval is given by S_{root}^i and may or may not be limited (i.e., $S_{root}^i = \infty$).

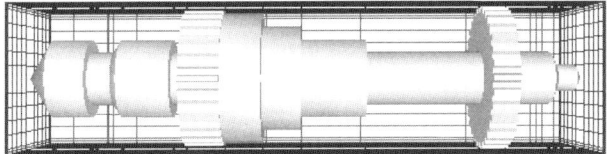

Figure 9.3: A sample interval structure shown in 3D

For an efficient use of empty space, we define the current amount of free space as the sum of the sizes of all intervals containing no nodes.

$$E^i = \sum_{i=1}^{n} s^i : N^i = \lambda \qquad (9.2)$$

A size request $\bar{s}_n$ for a node n is now mapped to the intervals containing this node, resulting in size requests for the appropriate intervals:

$$\bar{s}^i = \bar{s}_n : n \in N^i$$

To achieve better space filling properties, the size request is handled in a two-phase process. In the first phase, the algorithm looks if there is sufficient empty space to allow the request to succeed. This can be easily computed by

$$e^i = \sum_{i=1}^{n} \bar{s}^i s^i - E^i \qquad (9.3)$$

If e^i is less than or equal to zero we do have sufficient space for this request. Note that in the case $S_{root}^i = \infty$, we will always have sufficient space because the nodes are surrounded by an infinite empty interval. If there is sufficient empty space available, it can be allocated by different schemes. We do this by allocating the nearest intervals first, because this will avoid movements of nodes far away from current focus point:

$$e^i = e^i - s^j : |i - j| = \min \qquad \forall j : s^j \neq 0 \qquad (9.4)$$

If, however, there is not enough empty space to fulfill the requested change in size, e^i will be positive and include the amount of space still required after all empty intervals have been occupied. In this case, the size of each interval is normalized to the given maximum amount of display space:

$$s^i = \bar{s}^i s^i \frac{\sum_{i=1}^n \bar{s}^i s^i}{S_{root}} \qquad (9.5)$$

leading to the same behavior as in the continuous zoom. By the evaluation scheme illustrated above we extend the continuous zoom in three ways:

- We allow any number of dimensions.
- Empty space is efficiently handled.
- The algorithm is usable in the case of limited space as well as in the case of unlimited space.

While these extensions may look marginal at a first glance, they allow us to use the very same algorithm in completely different application domains, as shown in Chaps. 13 and 16.

Reversibility of the Algorithm

Typically, it is highly desirable to have a zoom algorithm which is reversable, i.e., a number of operations can be undone by simply doing the inverse operations in reverse order. It is easy to show that given a finite interval structure containing no "holes" (empty intervals) this can be achieved by applying the inverse size requests in arbitrary order [RR96].

Essentially, reversal can be done by shrinking the nodes according to the sum of growth requests they had before. In the case of optimal space filling properties, however, this would not lead to the desired result because empty intervals are shrunk more than non-empty intervals in the structure. Recalling equation (9.3) we can see that to achieve uniform and predictable behavior we have to take into account the case where e^i is larger than E^i. In this case equation (9.3) would not work correctly due to possible zero length intervals. However, we can easily replace equation (9.3) by a somewhat more general formulation:

$$e^i = \begin{cases} e^i - s^j : |i - j| = \min & \forall j : s^j \neq 0 \\ e^i + (s^0 - s^j) : |i - j| = \min & \forall j : s^j < s^0 \end{cases} \qquad (9.6)$$

Applying this formula not only allows reversal of the zoom operations carried out so far, but also serves as a basis for how to deal with empty intervals if many objects become particular small.

9.2 Visual Constraints

While the technique presented so far is useful in its own right, there are a number of constraints which are often useful in the practical application of our method. These constraints are typically imposed by aspects of recognizability (the information has to be presented such that it can be clearly perceived) and by dynamic aspects of interaction (big changes between two subsequent presentations should be avoided). However, many of these constraints can be easily included in the existing approach by a somewhat more sophisticated handling of underlying interval structure.

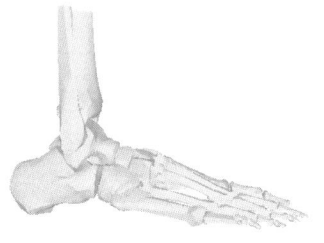

(a) Initial Model

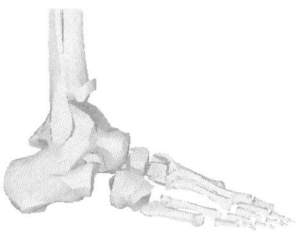

(b) Zoomed State

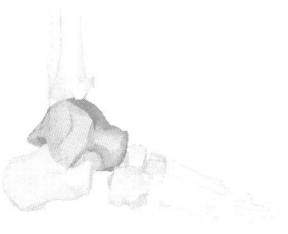

(c) Zoomed with transparency

Figure 9.4: Application of transparency for visualizing a 3D model (a). In (b) the enlarged object is partially hidden, whereas in (c) it is fully visible

9.2.1 Recognition Constraints

Many applications require that even if an object may become small in size it must not shrink below a certain threshold (such as in windowing systems). Indeed, given the original algorithm, the only chance to enlarge an object which becomes very small due to the enlargement of other objects is to shrink these objects again. However, this has turned out to be non-intuitive and difficult for users to understand.

Therefore, the objects are given a *minimum size* which is used to update the new interval sizes accordingly. Given a set of intervals and its associated scale factors we can redefine the actual scale factors according to equation (9.5) as

$$s^i = \bar{s}^i s^i \frac{\sum_{i=1}^n \min(\bar{s}^i s^i, s^i_{min})}{S_{root}}. \qquad (9.7)$$

Equation (9.7) actually redistributes the available space around the minimum required sizes of objects. But note that this may lead to a "deadlock" situation in the algorithm if there are many objects with its minimal size.

9.2.2 Shape Constraints

A particular problem arising when working with general models is that of keeping neighboring relations. Given a general model (such as in Fig. 9.5) the algorithm should not separate its parts because they are perceived as a unit. However, due to the structure of the model this may happen if the aspect ratio of the object is held constant. We therefore use an automated scheme to decide initially which parts may keep their original aspect ratio and which parts have to be distorted due to the internal constraints of the model.

Figure 9.5(b) gives an example in which the object is highly separated due to the constant aspect ratio of its parts. By contrast, in Fig. 9.5(c) the

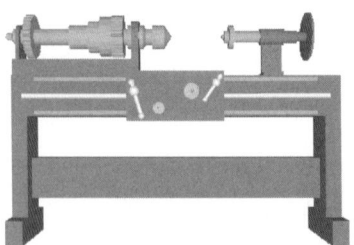

(a) Original Model

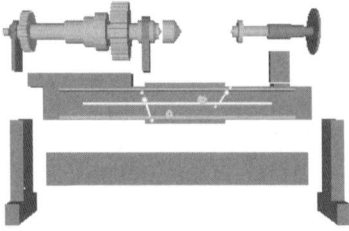

(b) Zoomed with constant aspect ratio

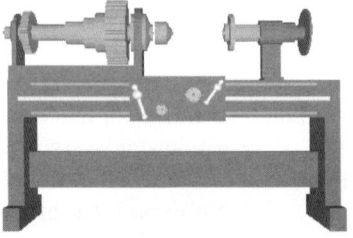

(c) Detection of neighboring constraints

Figure 9.5: Geometric model (a) zoomed with constant aspect ratio (b) and with automatic detection of neighboring constraints (c)

auto-detection algorithm has been used to find neighboring objects which could be perceived as one compound object.

9.2.3 Transition Constraints

While our technique allows a smooth transition (animation) between different sizes of nodes, it is often desirable to have some other ways of visualizing the change of the internal state of an object. So, for instance, it would be desirable to have a continuous transition between an open and a closed node (see Fig. 9.1) in a hierarchical structure.

Transparency can also be used to de-emphasize objects with a small size compared to its original size. This allows us to present the objects currently in focus with a higher emphasis than others while guaranteeing that the objects in the current focus can be clearly (and completely) perceived. This classical technique is particularly useful for 3D applications, as can be seen in Fig. 9.4.

9.2.4 Connectivity Constraints

So far, we have treated objects through their boundaries only. However, in many cases it is far more desirable to treat objects as being non-rigid, such as, for instance, edges in a graph. The connection points of such objects can be treated as separate nodes (in the case of graph edges or lines possibly with zero extent). It is possible that these edges cross other nodes in an unpredictable manner, in particular when the algorithm is used with geometric models.

There are basically two approaches to this problem. The first (and less time-consuming) is to use intermediate points for edges in a graph representation (see Fig. 9.6).

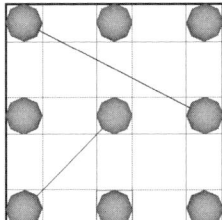
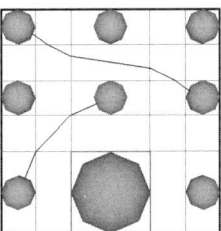

Figure 9.6: An example of edge deformation for topologically correct behavior in 2D: the interval boundaries show where intermediate points are added. Graph representation of an object (left); Zoomed model with edge deformation (right)

It is difficult to define such a graph in a general geometric model, however. Another approach here is the definition of complete parts of the model as non-rigid. Those parts can be re-defined by their relative position in the interval structure. Shape and position are recomputed each time a size request is initiated. While the process is relatively time-consuming, it leads to visually pleasing results, as can be seen in Fig. 9.7.

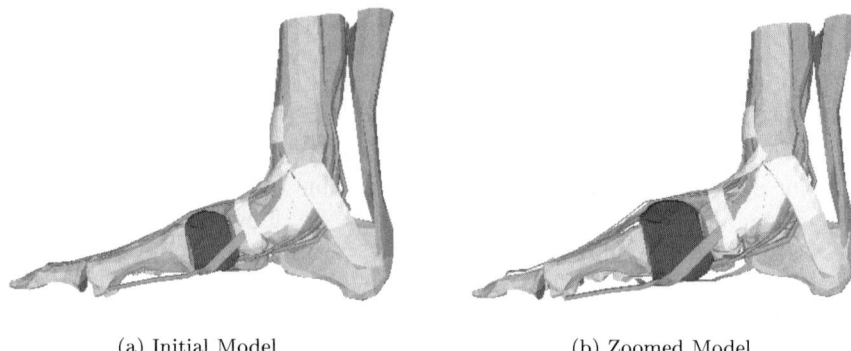

(a) Initial Model (b) Zoomed Model

Figure 9.7: Non-rigid object treatment in a model of the human foot: note the slight change in the course of the muscles around the enlarged bone

9.3 Conclusions

This chapter has focused on the actual zooming technique rather than on possible applications. The most obvious application domain of our zoom techniques are 2D applications, because many objects on the computer screen are represented as rectangular areas.

Although not that obvious, the use of 3D fisheye zooming can help a lot in 3D applications, such as interactive computer graphics. Examples of this can be seen in Chap. 3 (the ZOOMSTRUCTOR) or in Chap. 13 (the ZOOMILLUSTRATOR) where the potential of 3D fisheye zoom can be seen. In particular, the applications mentioned above exploit the power of using the same techniques in different dimensions (i.e., in 2D for textual information and in 3D for graphical information) and therefore allow uniform behavior throughout the interface, in 3D as well as in 2D.

While our technique is general, independent of dimension and fast there is still a way to go to make it to a uniform interaction method. Simply spoken, there is more to do than just enlarge or emphasize objects in its context. Application-specific aspects have to be taken into account as well as the general structure for transmitting and receiving data for the zoom algorithm.

The next chapter will address these problems. It will introduce "Zoom Navigation" as a uniform method for exploring and navigating large information spaces based upon the algorithm described in this chapter.

Contributors of Chap. 9: Andreas RAAB and Michael RÜGER

Chapter 10

Zoom Navigation

Research on reducing the interaction effort when navigating in large information spaces has utilized FURNAS' generalized fisheye view [Fur86] in a variety of techniques (cf. Chap. 2). Existing approaches apply filtering and distorting techniques or both (recall NOIK [Noi94]) according to the degree of interest (*DOI*) at a certain point in the information space (node). "Classical" fisheye views, as described by SARKAR and BROWN [SB94], distort an existing layout to enlarge the view at the point of interest (focus). Distorting fisheye views stick more to the photographic nature of fisheye lenses by applying a non-linear distortion to the display transformation. Filtering fisheye techniques display or suppress the rendering of nodes according to their *DOI*. Hybrid techniques, like the *Intelligent Zoom* as described by BARTRAM [BOD+94], make use of both, applying fisheye distortion to the display transformation as well as choosing an appropriate representation for each node not only depending on its *DOI* value, but also using reasoning techniques to exploit additional contextual information. Semantic zooming as described in [PF93] changes the appearance of objects, too, although only depending on the level of detail (*LOD*).

While the strategies described above deal with navigation in large *information spaces*, we are also interested in navigation among a set of applications. For the latter interaction task we coin the term *navigating in application space*. Navigation in large information and application spaces imposes the same problems of managing detail and context. Therefore, we attempt to develop an approach to unify navigation in an information space within an application as well as navigation between several applications.

Existing approaches to ease shifting between applications which have not been integrated strive to reduce the number of windows by performing in-place editing. The concept of visual editing realized in Microsoft's OLE2 (MEYER and OBERMAYR, [MO94]) enables applications to invoke other applications so as to let the user edit some foreign document part in place without additional navigational effort. This concept is much more flexible than IDEs because all applications which "understand" the OLE protocol can communicate in this way. Within OpenDoc [IBM95] this becomes the basic interaction paradigm, so the user is not forced to switch between different application windows at all.

The interaction effort is already reduced with these techniques, but the limitations imposed by the available screen real estate are not handled with in-place editing.

We introduce a solution which integrates navigation and visualization based on user interaction, as realized by the focus point in fisheye techniques for the application space as well.

10.1 Zoom Navigation

Previous work on navigation in large information spaces concentrated on optimizing distorting functions and filtering techniques for *one* domain. We search for common principles of interaction to establish a framework toward the unification of fisheye-based navigation over several applications. This implies the need to look for generic factors in the definition of *DOI* functions which is the heart of fisheye navigation. Furthermore, we aim at a uniform approach to select appropriate representations (to generalize the filtering aspect). These considerations lead us to define an integrated concept which we refer to as *Zoom Navigation*.

The problem of selecting an appropriate representation is crucial in information spaces which are not only large, but very heterogenous. This is true, for example, in the network supervisory control system, developed by BARTRAM et al. (recall [BOD+94]). Their "Intelligent Zoom" incorporates a context-based selection of an appropriate representation, e.g., whether to show a video of a part of the network, or to present a bar chart with the numeric representation of the traffic within the network. Inspired by this work, we look for a more generic scheme of how to organize representations and how to select the most appropriate one.

Our work aims at the definition of a generic framework and its realization in different domains. The realization helps to better differentiate between generic and application specific parts.

The first step towards a uniform selection of a representation is to formally organize the available representations. Representations differ in their level of detail, but also in their *aspect*. The representations available are not necessarily the same for all nodes (elements of the information space). Therefore, we need a subdivision of the information space into categories. These are by their nature application-specific, but the concept itself can be transferred. In an anatomical context, nodes are classified as to their membership of an organic system (e.g., bones, muscles, and nerves). The representations available depend on the categories. In anatomy, we have muscles for which the location, the supply of nerves, and the shape are interesting. For a node of the bone category the representations are different. We still have a location, but the shape is usually not complex and not described textually. The supply of nerves does not exist at all.

A given point in the information space belonging to an application-specific category or node class is defined by the aspects for which information is available. The user is confronted with additional interaction when choosing between one of the aspects. As a consequence, the selection of an appropriate representation is more than merely adjusting the level of detail. The user's information and navigation needs have to be determined, too. In addition to the *DOI*, whose computation is based on the geometric and conceptual distance to the current focus point, an aspect of interest (*AOI*) is introduced. The computation of the *AOI* is based on the history of the user's interest in aspects of the information space.

An implementation of this concept is described in Sect. 10.4 for a complex simulation environment and in Sect. 10.5 for an interactive anatomical illustration system.

10.1.1 Degree of Interest

The user's current interest is quantified via the *DOI* function. Factors influencing the *DOI* value can be classified into static versus dynamic, and generic versus application-specific ones. Static factors are those which remain unchanged in the process of interaction and are computed via the a priori interest (*API*) function. The dynamic factors of the *DOI* calculation represent distance (spatial and conceptual) functions to one or more focus points. The *API* and *DOI* functions consist of a generic and an application-specific part, balanced by weighting factors.

The generic *API* function part is made up of the size of the objects and their position in the hierarchical structure of the underlying information space. In some cases, the *API* has an identical value for all nodes, if none of these is distinguished in a particular way. The application-specific factors used in the two case studies are described later (see Table 10.1). This leads to the formula for the calculation of the *API*:

$$API = f(size, hierarchy, \langle application\text{-}specifics\rangle) \qquad (10.1)$$

The calculation of a node's *DOI* is influenced by its *API*, the previous *DOI*, and its conceptual and spatial distance to a focus point. Taking the previous *DOI* into account leads to incremental changes of the *DOI*. These changes are easier to comprehend, as the resulting layout is not exposed to radical changes.

The conceptual distance to a focus point is application-specific. Nodes which belong to the same category are less conceptually distant from each other. One indicator for conceptual distance is, for example, the occurrence of hypertext links within the text just displayed. When a node is zoomed up, the *DOI*s of other nodes with hypertext links to this one increase, too.

The spatial distance is of less importance here. Navigation in information and application spaces is ruled rather by logical connections, as with the hyperlinks mentioned above, or by the underlying semantics, as expressed in the categorization and its aspects. However, it may still have an influence on the relative importance of nodes, so it is included in the calculation.

Summarizing the considerations described so far, we come to a definition of a *DOI* as a function of the *API*, the previous *DOI*, and some distance function to focal points:

$$DOI' = f(API, DOI, conceptual\ distance) \qquad (10.2)$$

There is no unit to the *DOI* and the *API*. The numbers representing the *DOI* and the *API* are of secondary interest, and are just used to compare the importance of nodes in a dialog situation. Such a comparison can be used, for example, to filter nodes. The *DOI* and the *API* represent weighted sums of heterogenous parameters, which contribute to the importance of a piece of information. The weights determine the importance of the factors influencing *DOI* and *AOI* and must therefore be chosen as carefully as the set of factors itself.

10.1.2 Representation

The category to which each node in the information space belongs determines the possible aspects to be studied. Each aspect has representations, differing in the level of detail (see Fig. 10.1). This leads us to define a two-dimensional matrix with the rows representing different *LODs* and the columns representing aspects.

To illustrate what we mean by categories, let us follow two examples which we will describe in more detail later. In the description of logistic systems objects belong to either a (physical) material flow or a (logical) control flow. In anatomy, objects belong to different systems, e.g., blood vessels, nerves, and muscles. Note that not all fields in such a representation matrix are occupied. There are levels of detail with no representation for the given aspect. For low levels of detail, especially, there is often only one aspect. An example for this is a label which exists for many categories.

10.2 Aspect of Interest

The definition of the *DOI* is based only on the current focus point(s), the set of nodes currently opened, and on whether the node itself has been zoomed

10.2 Aspect of Interest

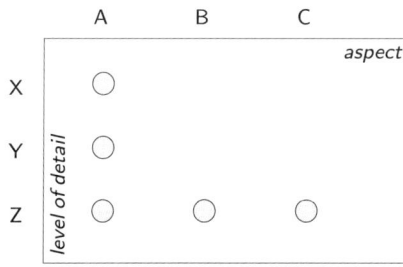

Figure 10.1: Representation matrix

up before. If there are several representations for one LOD (see Fig. 10.1), then the selection of an appropriate representation just using the DOI is not sufficient. Among all representations with the appropriate level of detail, the AOI is used to decide which one to activate.

To define the AOI, operations changing a node's presentation are logged. For each aspect k we record:

1. How often it was presented, N_k
2. How long ago it was presented, T_{1k}
3. How long it was visited, T_{2k}

These values are combined to produce a numerical value for each aspect in a category. The formula of each category's AOI can thus be written as:

$$AOI(\text{aspect}_k) = AOI_k = f(N_k, T_{1k}, T_{2k}). \tag{10.3}$$

The AOI calculation is carried out for each category (node class), whereas the DOI calculation is carried out for each single node (node instance). Based on the AOI calculation we select the aspect with the maximum AOI value as the most appropriate one:

$$\text{Index}(\text{selected aspect}) = k, \quad \text{with} \quad AOI_k > AOI_i, \ \forall i \neq k. \tag{10.4}$$

The representation is selected according to the level of detail using the DOI and the aspect returned by the AOI function. To emphasize this, we call the process of mapping a representation to a presentation "activation".

This AOI calculation and its influence on the presentation is roughly similar (at least in the goal) to the "contextual assistance", which guides the presentation in the "Intelligent Zoom". Yet, there are two main differences to their technique.

First, we use statistics about previous user interaction as a basis for our decision. By contrast, the intelligent zoom (recall BARTRAM et al. [BOD+94]) is controlled by external messages of a security system, which is far more domain-specific.

Second, we rely on straightforward numerical calculations and comparisons and renounce complex AI techniques, such as intelligent agents, which provide the reasoning process in the intelligent zoom. Although we are aware of the advantages of such AI techniques, we restrict ourselves to numerical *AOI* calculations which embody a more general approach and facilitate fast interaction.

Table 10.1: Generic and application-specific factors

generic	application-specific	
	ZOOMILLUSTRATOR	ZOOMNAVIGATOR
size, hierarchy	visibility	—
API, DOI	spatial and conceptual distance	
history	—	—

Our approach for the *AOI* calculation is related to HILL et al. [HHWM92] who analyze how often parts of a textual document have been read and edited. HILL et al. concentrate on visualizing this information which they achieve by superimposing bar charts on scrollbars which correspond to the read or edited document. By contrast to their effort we use statistics on how often aspects were visited not just to visualize it but to improve navigation.

10.3 The Pluggable Zoom

Using the variable zoom algorithm as just described (see Chap. 9), our goal was to implement a reusable software component. The term *pluggable* describes a reusable object-oriented component which can be easily adapted to different application interfaces by connecting the *plugs* with the appropriate *callbacks*. There were several issues to be dealt with while developing this structure:

1. to support different degree-of-interest strategies without changes to the zoom algorithm itself, and
2. to cope with changes to the application data like insertion, deletion, and movement of nodes.

With the Pluggable Zoom we aim at a flexible implementation of the principles of zoom navigation to be applied in different application domains.

The Pluggable Zoom contains a data structure holding a topological representation of the application model. The zoom algorithm itself uses this graph structure for its computations. In order to achieve a wide range of possible application models to be used with zoom navigation, the necessary callbacks are limited to a minimum set: fetching the application model's nodes and the children for each node and thereby recursively traversing the complete graph of parent–children relationships, the application-specific *DOI* and *AOI* values and the initial size and position for each node (see Fig. 10.2).

10.3 The Pluggable Zoom

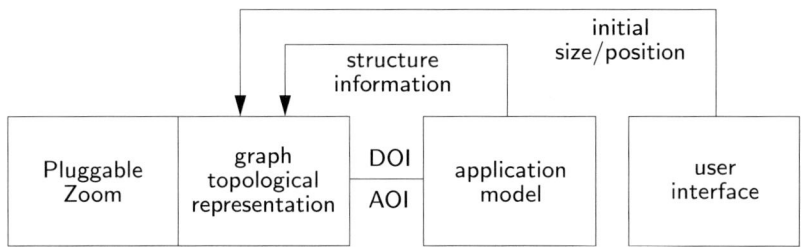

Figure 10.2: Setup of the zoom structure: the Pluggable Zoom fetches the information about the structure (nodes, parent–child relations) and geometric properties (size, initial positions) and constructs its internal graph topological representation of the application model

Modifications as a result of user interaction (zoom step) are propagated back by plugs supplying the modified size and position of nodes and the resulting *DOI* and *AOI* values (see Fig. 10.3).

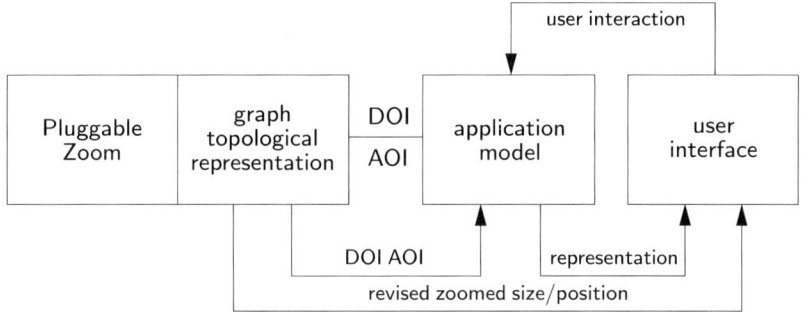

Figure 10.3: Interaction with the Zoom: the user initiates a zoom step (e.g., by mouse click), the zoom algorithm computes the changes of *DOI* and *AOI*, resulting in changes in the nodes' sizes and positions, which are propageted back to the application model

Introducing the extra layer of an internal topological representation within the Pluggable Zoom allows us to deal with application domains which are not aware of their graph properties. Windows and their subviews are an example for such a structure: each window may be seen as a node, with the subviews as its children. Graph-related algorithms, like recursive traversal and propagation of values, are implemented inside the Pluggable Zoom and do not need to be implemented within the application model.

While keeping the variable zoom as the initial zoom step, we decided to introduce a postprocessing step. Postprocessing enables us to fix up undesired effects caused by the algorithm, like unused space between nodes or violation of minimum or maximum sizes without changing the zoom algorithm itself. The *AOI* is also calculated in this step. At the end of the postprocessing, the new *DOI* and *AOI* values (*DOI* and *AOI* in Fig. 10.3), as calculated in the zoom algorithm, are propagated back to the application, which in turn chooses an appropriate representation for the user interface.

10.4 The ZoomNavigator

We used the pluggable zoom to realize the concept of zoom navigation in the ZOOMNAVIGATOR on top of the CREATE! environment. This simulation development environment provides a number of tools for building and running discrete event simulation models as well as tools for modifying the environment itself (RÜGER and BEHLAU [RB95]). It formed an ideal platform to experiment with, as we had full access to the application code.

Within CREATE!the information space consists of a management system containing projects, subprojects, experiments, and the simulation models. The simulation models are built using a graphical model editor for placing and connecting the simulation elements. The application space is divided into the data needed for a simulation run (parameter), the code executed in the elements, and the structural data like interface definitions and variables. Zoom navigation was integrated into the two-dimensional graphical model editor with the model elements mapped onto nodes in the pluggable zoom structure. We currently do not provide a way to zoom list or text widgets as in the flexible window system (see KANDOGAN and SHNEIDERMAN [KS96]).

Figure 10.4 illustrates the different aspects associated with model elements at different levels of detail. The level of detail corresponds directly to the node size in the graphical model editor.

Figure 10.5 shows the default graphical representation of an element in a CREATE! simulation model. After zooming it up to an appropriate size (approx. 200 pixels) additional representations become available. The computation of the *AOI* estimated the editing or viewing of parameters as the user's most probable estimated interest. Within the environment, a potential user interest might have been viewing the component's code or icon definition.

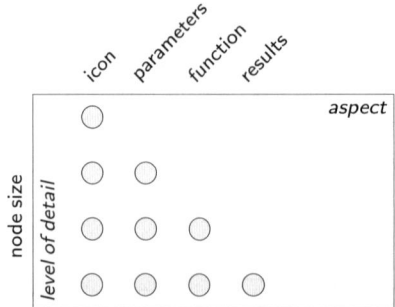

Figure 10.4: ZOOMNAVIGATOR representation matrix

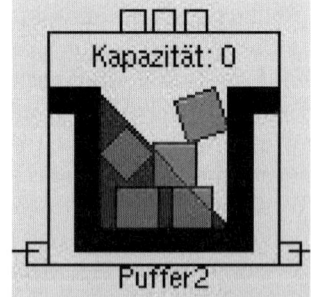

Figure 10.5: Screenshot of a graphical model element

Figure 10.6 shows on the left a zoomed node with its parameter dialog as the current representation activated. An alternate representation visualizing the parameter definition as used in coding the element functionality is shown on the right.

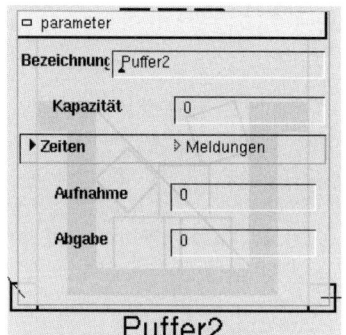
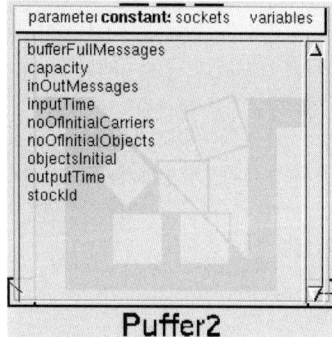

Figure 10.6: Nodes with activated presentations: in the left image the parameter dialog was selected, in the right image the list of constant definitions was determined as the most appropriate representation

10.5 The ZoomIllustrator

In order to verify the principles and to test its general applicability, we also applied the pluggable zoom tool to a quite different application, the ZOOM-ILLUSTRATOR (see PREIM et al. [PRS+95] and [PRS97]). The ZOOMILLUS-TRATOR is a flexible tool which reads scene descriptions of geometric models and related textual descriptions to integrate them in interactive illustrations (see Fig. 10.8 for sample output and Chap. 13 for a detailed description).

It is quite natural to employ the Pluggable Zoom in this application. In the illustration process the problem consists of arranging labels and explanations around an image. This is problematic because the overall number of labels and explanations to illustrate complex phenomena is by far too large to be displayed all at once. Usually, interactive systems like this allow the user to request explanations which are subsequently presented in a new window and hard to mentally integrate with the image they refer to. The Pluggable Zoom, by contrast, allows the immediate integration of explanations in the illustration. Zoom techniques can be used to place and scale information entities based on the *DOI* and to activate appropriate representations based on the *DOI* and the *AOI*.

Although this application is very different from the ZOOMNAVIGATOR described above, the general application scheme of the variable zoom and the procedure of adjusting the presentation in a postprocess remain the same.

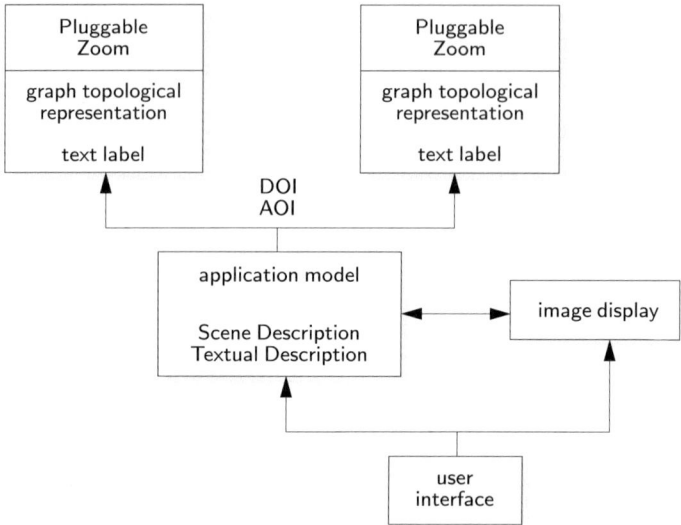

Figure 10.7: The basic principle for the application of the pluggable zoom in the ZOOMILLUSTRATOR

Again, static and dynamic factors influence the calculation of the DOI. The precise functions need to be redefined, however.

Both the geometric model and its textual description are structured into objects. These objects are hierarchically organized, where this hierarchy corresponds to whole-part relations. If we transform this into the terminology of Fig. 10.1, we come to the following analogies.

The application model consists of the scene description and related textual description. The object hierarchy delivers the "structure information" from which the graph topological representation is derived. The textual description for each object is mapped onto each node in the topological representation. The architectural scheme shown in Fig. 10.7 illustrates the integration of the zoom component.

What is the most important artifact in this application? For the illustration of complex phenomena as found, for example, in anatomy, textual information must not occlude parts of the image. Therefore, textual information is arranged in separate areas. This implies that several networks for the zoom are necessary on different sides of the image. We restrict ourselves to arranging textual information on the left and on the right side of the rendered image in two different networks.

To translate this into the terms of Fig. 10.1, we have two topological representations and two pluggable zoom structures (see Figs. 10.8 and 10.9 for the layout).

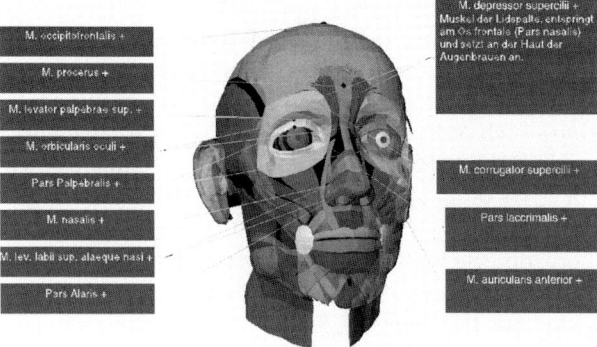

Figure 10.8: Initial layout

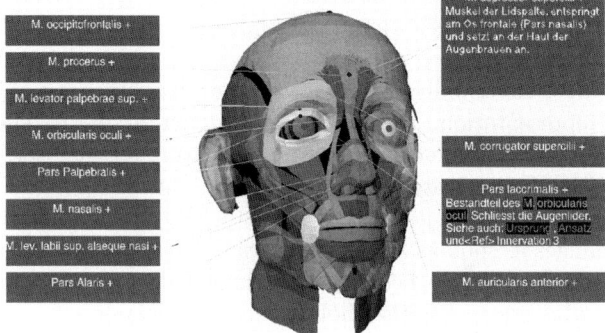

Figure 10.9: After zooming

The assignment of a node to one of the networks is a compromise between the desire for a balanced layout of labels and the wish for recognizable relations between labels and parts in the geometry. To be more exact, those labels which refer to objects on the left side are labeled on the left, others on the right. However, this strategy is adapted to make sure that the number of labels on each side is approximately the same.

10.5.1 Definition of API, DOI, and AOI in the ZoomIllustrator

The initial layout of an illustration is based on the calculation of the *API* which guides the filtering of the available objects. The *API* is a function of the *size* of the objects in the geometric model and the position of the object in the object *hierarchy* (which corresponds to Table 10.1). Besides this generic *API* we have several – application-specific – geometric criteria which influence the *API* and thereby the initial layout.

The most important of these geometric criteria is *visibility*. Objects which cannot be seen do not necessarily need to be referred to in a label. This is obvious, because such objects cannot be pointed to by reference lines.

For the application at hand we define relative visibility, which determines the relation of parts of an object which are visible to the extent of the parts which are occluded.

Furthermore, objects with their center point located far away are regarded as less important than those close to the observer. This leads to the consideration of *depth*. For this purpose, the distance in the z-dimension from all objects to the camera (which is placed in the xy-plane) is registered. These considerations lead to the formula for the initialization of the *DOI*:

$$API = f(size, hierarchy, visibility, depth) \tag{10.5}$$

In contrast to size and position in the hierarchy, visibility and depth factors are exposed to changes due to user-initiated rotations. In this case, a reconfiguration is necessary because new nodes should be labeled according to these changes in visibility. This leads to a reconstruction of the graph-topological representation. However, a reconstruction and its effects on the presentation are both time-consuming and irritating for the user. Therefore, this function is only activated after major rotations.

In the initial layout, objects are simply labeled (not explained). The *DOI* of a node changes as soon as zooming occurs. When a node is zoomed up, its *DOI* is increased. If it reaches a certain threshold value, an explanation is placed inside this node. The threshold value has a default setting, but can be changed by the user in order to control the amount of information presented.

The spatial distance to the opened node is one factor considered in the *DOI*. This makes sense because the vicinity of a label corresponds to the vicinity of the objects referred to in the 3D model. With this factor it is possible to explore a certain region in detail.

For our system with several networks belonging to one domain, another factor should be taken into consideration: if interaction in one network takes place this has consequences for the *DOI* of the nodes within the other network, too (these nodes differ in their conceptual distance to the node zoomed up). However, it is irritating if nodes are closed or opened on one side of the image due to interaction on the other side. Therefore, this network distance is incorporated in the calculation of the spatial distance, resulting in a large spatial distance between nodes of different networks – reducing changes in one network due to interaction in the other.

In addition to the spatial distance we define a conceptual distance. This conceptual distance from one node to another is small if the explanations related to one node contain hypertext links to the other. Correspondingly, the *DOI* of all nodes mentioned in this explanation is increased. The second factor included in the conceptual distance is the agreement of group attributes.

Each node has – besides its category which defines the aspects available – group attributes, which summarize nodes belonging to the same region or having a similar function.

$$DOI = f(size, zoomed\ size, spatial\ distance, conceptual\ distance) \qquad (10.6)$$

10.5.2 Selection Using the AOI

The choice of a representation is based on the DOI and again the AOI. The DOI determines, for example, whether or not an explanation is displayed, that is, the level of detail. If there are several representations with the same DOI, e.g., several detailed explanations, we consider the AOI of all these representations to decide which one to activate. We will give an example of how the DOI and AOI calculations relate to each other and influence the selection of an appropriate representation.

The user zooms into a detailed explanation of a certain muscle. This increases the DOI of other muscles with low conceptual and spatial distance. If their DOI is high enough, these muscles are also zoomed up to accommodate an explanation. Which of the available explanations (which aspect) actually is displayed depends on the AOI. Depending on the interaction history, the probability is high that the same aspect is chosen as for the muscle explained before.

Let us compare the ZoomIllustrator with the previously described ZoomNavigator. The zoom in the ZoomIllustrator relates to the placement and scaling of textual information within *one* window. For this reason the application of the zoom is more restricted than in zoom navigation, which standardizes navigation within one single window with the navigation within several windows and even applications. Topological correctness is important for a very practical reason; changing the sequence of labels leads to crossing lines. Furthermore, the vicinity of labels would not correspond to vicinity within the rendered image. The separation between two zoom networks prevents irritating changes in one network due to interaction with the other.

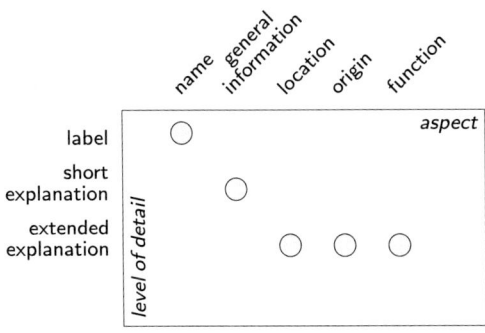

Figure 10.10: ZoomIllustrator representation space

10.6 Conclusion and Future Work

We have presented zoom navigation, a framework for the application of fisheye views in large and heterogenous information spaces. Zoom navigation exploits the advantages of fisheye views while abstracting from the application domain. This framework consists of generic functions for the *API* and *DOI* functions. Furthermore, the concept of representation matrices enables a uniform organization of the available representations.

Our concepts have been realized in pluggable zoom, an object-oriented component which is reusable through a variety of domains. The adaption process necessary is mainly a redefinition of the functions for the *API* and the *DOI*. This redefinition involves a careful selection of parameters and their influence on the importance of pieces of information.

Our approach is based on a classification of nodes as to their membership in categories. On the basis of the categorization we developed the notion of representation matrices which formally organize the representations available for one category. Thus we introduce the term *AOI* which we calculate for each representation based on previous user behavior. The *AOI* allows us to choose one of several possible representations for display.

Note that we try to estimate whether or not a user will be interested in a certain part of information, but this estimate is a comparison of simple numerical values computed in a generic, application-independent way. While we are aware of the advantages of a sophisticated planning scheme, including backtracking mechanisms, we prefer this simple strategy because it is effective in terms of speed, which is crucial for interactive systems.

To prove that our concepts are widely applicable, we incorporated pluggable zoom into two quite different applications, the ZOOMILLUSTRATOR (see Chap. 13) and the ZOOMNAVIGATOR (see Chap. 16).

Contributors of Chap. 10: Michael RÜGER, Bernhard PREIM, Alf RITTER

Part IV

Textual Methods of Abstraction

Using pictures to convey information inevitably also means working with language somewhere along the line. Indeed, there are a variety of situations in which pictures and language meet one another. Some of these are:

- *Image generation*
  Practically all images generated by computer stem from an expression in one kind of formal language or another. For 3D graphics, such expressions are produced by the modeling software (some users even type in models using text editors, claiming this to be more efficient a way of modeling).
- *User transcription*
  When a user has viewed an image or an animation, he or she sometimes "takes notes," i.e., writes down in language key conclusions drawn.
- *Collaborative work among users*
  In scientific and engineering applications, more than one user will often examine a graphical presentation of data. Such users will then typically talk to one another about what they have seen.
- *User response*
  After viewing an image or an animation, users will typically respond to the system with the goal of obtaining more images. In most commercial systems and research prototypes, user input is in the form of an expression in a formal language. Often the language is disguised by the use of pull-down or pop-up menus, but this does not change the linguistic nature of the input.

Thus users make heavy use of language and linguistic expressions while working with pictures. Indeed, different images will tend to lead to different linguistic formulations. In particular, by virtue of its very definition, the process of abstraction affects what users have to say about the images. We therefore conjecture that effective methods of abstraction will also take into account linguistic formulations of images. This means that ways must be sought in which images and text can be linked closely to one another in interactive systems.

To push the concept of verbalization of images to the limit, Ian PITT describes in Chap. 11 how a particular kind of image, those arising when working with graphical user interfaces (GUIs), can be converted into a textual representation for users to explore as an alternative to visual inspection of the image. While such textual presentations are clearly inappropriate for most people, blind computer users are forced to rely on this form of presentation and interaction. Besides its practical value for disabled users, the topic provides an excellent testbed for studying linguistic expressions whose aim it is to convey the same meaning as images.

Short of trying to replace an image by text, images may be in need of some amount of explanation before they can be understood or their significance be fully comprehended by users. Bernhard PREIM and Rainer MICHEL take up this topic in Chap. 12 in the design of concepts and a prototypical system for producing figure captions to go along with rendered images. They show what information should be encoded in such captions, and how a rendering system can gather and organize this information. It turns out that such captions are of vital importance in connection with the process of abstraction, as users need information pertaining to what has been changed in an image over and above the "normal" view. A particularly interesting turn of events is the authors' suggestion that users can edit the (automatically generated) figure captions; consistency between the image and its caption is maintained by the system, resulting in a new image to fit the modified caption.

Another step toward linking images and their verbalization more closely together is to include labels and short textual descriptions within the images themselves. Bernhard PREIM studies methods and tools for managing such labels in Chap. 13. In particular, he uses the zoom methodology introduced earlier both for the individual objects within the image as well as the labels, and pays particular attention to the correspondence between the two kinds of information. Finally, he shows how the user can interact with the image, the labels, and figure captions. The concepts are demonstrated in the ZOOM-ILLUSTRATOR, an interactive illustration system for anatomical models.

Chapter 11

From Graphics to Pure Text

This chapter will concentrate on the relationship between images and text, and in particular on the use of text to present nominally graphical information to blind people. The following chapter will then consider the role of text within images. First, we look at the role of text, both as a component within graphical images, as a complement to graphical images, and as an alternative means of conveying information.

11.1 Giving Blind People Access to Graphics

Computer manufacturers and software developers have seized upon the possibilities offered by high-resolution graphics and have developed interfaces which use visual interaction and organization to make computers easier to use, or to present complex data in more easily accessible forms. Unfortunately, while such systems may help sighted people, they place blind and visually impaired people at a greater disadvantage. If the use of graphics enables sighted people to work more efficiently, blind people who cannot benefit from the improvements in efficiency will be left even further behind and will be correspondingly less attractive as employees.

The problem is not confined to the use of computers. As visual displays become cheaper and more sophisticated they are being employed in an ever wider range of products. Many devices which once posed no problems for blind people are now routinely equipped with visual displays, offering new facilities and ease of operation to sighted people but leaving blind people at a greater disadvantage than before. An example is the telephone, which for many years has been a valuable aid to blind people. Now telephones, too, are being equipped with visual displays, and soon many services currently accessible through speech may require visual communication, too.

Thus it is essential that blind people are able to gain access to information in graphical form. If this can be done, the steady computerization of tasks in education, industry and leisure will open up new opportunities for blind people. If, on the other hand, computers continue to be made such that blind people cannot use them, or can only use them with limited efficiency, blind people will not only miss out on new opportunities but may also find themselves excluded from activities which were open to them in the past.

11.1.1 Blind People's Understanding of Graphical Concepts

Before considering how best to present graphical information to blind people, we should consider what sort of information is likely to be of use to a blind person. Is it reasonable to expect that someone who has no vision – particularly someone who was born without vision – will understand visual concepts in the same way as someone with normal sight?

The question "how do blind people visualize the world around them?" has exercized philosophers for several centuries. It has formed part of a much wider debate on the role of knowledge and experience in human development and on the role played by the various senses in bringing individuals to an understanding of their environment.

In considering this question, two radically different theories of human development have been proposed. The Rationalists argue that the form of knowledge, including spatial understanding, is innate and unaffected by the sensory channel through which it is obtained. Empiricists, by contrast, argue that all understanding originates with sensory experience and that spatial ideas must differ depending on whether they were obtained by touch or by sight. Blindness has provided an important testing ground for this debate since blind people so obviously differ from sighted people in the sensory means through which they experience the world. LOCKE [Loc90] wondered how someone blind from birth who was suddenly restored to sight would view the world – would they be able to recognize by sight objects which they had previously explored only through touch, or does tactile exploration by someone with no visual experience produce a mental image which is wholly different from that obtained by sight?

A great deal of research has been carried out since LOCKE first pondered this question, and the evidence suggests that in most respects blind people (including congenitally blind people, those who are born blind) organize visual information in much the same way as sighted people. It has been found that blind people are aware of factors such as perspective and visual occlusion, can perform mental operations on visual material with roughly the same levels of ease and success as sighted people, and even have a good understanding of wholly visual concepts such as color.

Evidence that blind people can understand perspective and visual occlusion has been produced by, among others, the Canadian researcher KEN-

NEDY [Ken80]. He suggests that blind people do not differ significantly from sighted people in their understanding of such concepts, but differ in their reporting of such images because they have not learnt the accepted ways of representing 2D objects in a 3D space.

To test this theory, he conducted a number of experiments in which blind subjects of various ages were asked to identify tactile images or to produce images themselves on German film.[1] Several of his subjects were asked to draw a table, commenting on the drawing as they produced it (see Fig. 11.1). All recognized that the table would appear differently depending on where the observer was positioned in relation to it, and most realized that some parts of the table might be obscured by others when viewed from certain positions. A number of the subjects began by drawing the table in plan view with legs radiating out from the four corners, but all realized that this was just a way of representing the table and not necessarily what it would look like. One drew the table from the side with the two nearest legs attached correctly to the bottom of the table and the two farthest legs rising upwards from the table, again commenting that this was just a way of representing the relationship between the parts. When asked to draw the table as it might be seen from the side, all were able to produce a reasonable representation. Some illustrated the table with four legs visible, usually grouped into pairs, while others drew only two legs and indicated that the remaining two would be hidden behind the visible legs. One subject clearly indicated that two of the legs would appear to be longer than the others and when asked about this commented "I think the back legs should be shorter", although she could not explain why [Ken80, pp. 281–289].

Other researchers have compared the use of mental imagery by blind and sighted people. Much of this research has centered upon the role of mental imagery in recall. NEISSER and KERR [NK73] argued that if mental imagery is an aid to recall, items which cannot easily be visualized will be recalled less readily than others. KEENAN and MOORE [KM79] tested this theory by presenting a group of subjects with a series of broadly specified scenes. In some cases all of the elements in the description were visible (i.e., they would appear on a drawing of the scene) while in other cases a number of elements were present which did not form part of the image and could not easily be incorporated within it. Subjects were questioned about

---

1 German film is a translucent plastic sheet material used for the production of tactile illustrations. In use, it is placed on a soft surface (usually a rubber mat) and then embossed using a stylus which is pressed hard into the film and the backing material. This produces a distortion of the film's surface which is readily discernible by touch. A particular advantage of German film over other embossing materials is that the image can be felt on the same surface of the film as that on which it was embossed. On most other films the stylus produces an indentation which can only be felt from the underside of the film, thus requiring that the illustrator draw the intended view in mirror-image and then turn the film over before presenting it to a blind person. German film removes the need to draw a mirror-image and also makes it easier for a blind person to inspect the illustration as it is being created.

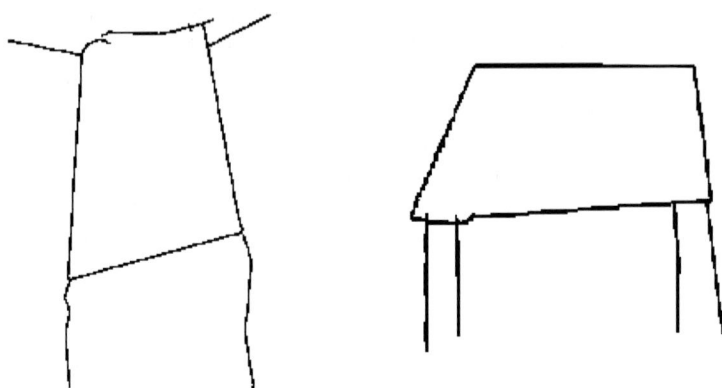

Figure 11.1: Examples of tables drawn by blind people [Ken80]

the mental image they had created (to make sure that the extraneous items had not been incorporated in any way) and were then asked to recall the contents of the image. KEENAN and MOORE found that the non-visible items were remembered significantly less well than the visible items. ZIMLER and KEENAN [ZK83] conducted a similar experiment using both blind and sighted subjects and produced similar results. Both groups found it more difficult to remember items when they were absent from the mental image. Thus it appears that not only does mental imagery aid recall, but blind and sighted people do not differ significantly in their use of imagery in this respect.

In another experiment in the same series, ZIMLER and KEENAN attempted to find out how blind people perform when dealing with visually referenced concepts which could only have been learned by verbal means. They used a free-recall task involving groups of words linked by a common, modality-specific attribute. One group was based on the visual/tactile attribute *round* (for example, wheel, clock), another group was based on the auditory attribute *loud* (for example, scream, thunder) and the third group was based on the non-tactile, visual attribute *red* (for example, cherry, blood). The subjects were not told what the linking attributes were. Zimler and Keenan found that blind people performed at least as well on the *red* words as they did on the *round* words and in each case there was no significant difference between the performance of the blind subjects and the sighted subjects. In line with earlier findings, however, the blind subjects performed significantly better than the sighted subjects on the *loud* words.

If congenitally blind people learn about color by verbal means, then it might be expected that they would acquire this knowledge more slowly than sighted people. Accordingly it had been predicted that congenitally blind children would lag behind their sighted counterparts in color awareness. This was only partially borne out by the results: the blind children among the sample achieved similar scores to their sighted counterparts on the *red* words, but it was noted that while the congenitally blind adults were consciously using *red* to link these words, the blind children were often unsure what the link was even though they recognized that a link existed.

As had been found in many earlier experiments, the most significant differences between the blind and sighted subjects were in their handling of non-visual material. The sighted adults performed significantly less well on the *loud* words than did the blind adults, and the difference was even more marked among the children. The blind children also performed better than the sighted children on the *round* words (which have both visual and tactual referents) although this difference was not apparent among the adults. In short, sighted children show at least as great a "developmental lag," if not a greater one, in acquiring tactual and auditory knowledge as blind children do in acquiring knowledge of the visual world.

MARMOR [Mar78] examined blind people's understanding of color concepts in more detail. She asked 48 college students (sixteen congenitally totally blind, sixteen who were born with sight but later became totally blind, and sixteen with normal sight) to consider pairs of color names and comment on how similar or dissimilar they felt them to be. Nine different color names were used, giving a total of 36 pairs, and subjects were asked to rate similarity on a nine-point scale. The results were analysed using a multi-dimensional scaling program which converted judgements of similarity into distances across a 2D space. The results from each group of subjects yielded a color wheel with the individual colors arranged in approximately spectral sequence around its rim. Contrary to expectations, the results from the congenitally blind subjects were not greatly dissimilar to those of the sighted subjects, with the late blind group falling somewhere in between. Marmor concluded that good knowledge of color relations can be developed in the absence of visual experience.

In summary, it appears that both congenitally blind people and those who become blind later in life are comfortable with visual concepts and use mental imagery in much the same way as sighted people. The evidence reviewed here suggests that blind people understand the concept of viewing a scene from a single point and appreciate that this will give rise to occlusions and perspective distortion. Blind people can perform mental operations (such as recall) on words which are largely or wholly visual in content with much the same efficiency as sighted people, and show similar patterns of forgetting when prevented from using mental imagery. Blind children show a developmental lag compared with sighted children in acquiring knowledge of color, perspective, etc., but eventually acquire virtually the same level of skill as their sighted counterparts. Blind adults make better use of sound and tactile information than sighted adults, and this combined with their skills in visual manipulation enables them to perform recall and processing tasks at least as well as sighted people and sometimes better.

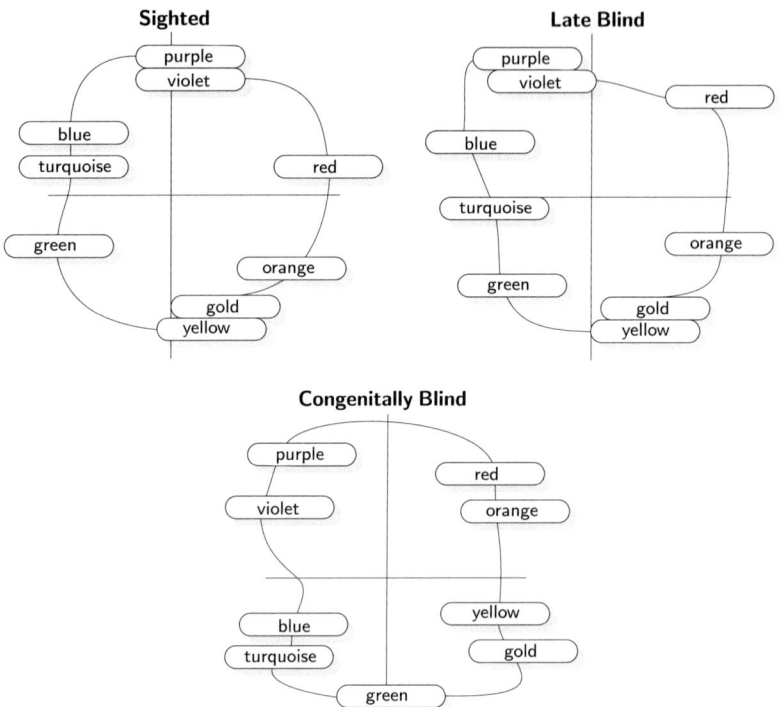

Figure 11.2: Color wheels obtained by MARMOR [Mar78] from congenitally blind, late blind, and normally sighted subjects

11.1.2 Text Versus Tactile Graphics

Given that blind people need access to graphical material and have a good understanding of visual concepts, what is the best way of presenting graphical information?

An obvious solution is to reproduce a screen image directly on a tactile display so that blind users can feel the image with their fingers. This is possible and has been done, but the approach has a number of drawbacks.

Tactile displays can take several forms, but all are based on the same basic principle. A flat panel is drilled with a pattern of closely spaced holes, into each of which is placed a small pin. A mechanism under the panel allows individual pins to be raised or lowered so that they either protrude above the surface of the panel or lie flush with it. In this way tactile patterns can be formed. Unfortunately, tactile displays tend to be both expensive and mechanically unreliable. Various methods are employed to move the pins, among the most common being miniature solenoids, piezo-electric crystals (which distort when a current is applied to them) and bi-metal strips (which flex when heated by a current). All have particular benefits in terms of response time, current consumption, etc., but all are expensive to produce and involve moving parts which are subject to wear. Tactile displays are also hard to protect against dust and dirt, which can cause pins to stick or prevent them moving over their full range. All these factors combine to make tactile displays an unattractive choice for many applications.[2]

Another drawback of tactile displays is that the user must have a reasonably high level of tactile sensitivity in order to be able to perceive the image. However, many blind people have relatively poor tactile sensitivity. This is partly because the blind population includes a high percentage of elderly people, and the sense of touch, like vision, tends to decline with age. In addition, many younger blind people suffer reduced tactile sensitivity because premature blindness is often the result of a condition (such as diabetes) which can affect other senses as well as vision. This may be one of the reasons why such a small percentage of blind people read Braille (the figure for most Western countries is between 2 and 5 percent).

A further problem is that there is no guarantee that a screen image which includes perspective, shading, etc., will make sense when translated into tactile form. MERRY and MERRY [MM33] considered the question of 2D versus 3D representations while investigating the problem of teaching blind children about objects using embossed diagrams. They compared "two dimensional" diagrams (simple raised diagrams giving a 2D symbolic view) with "tri-dimensional" diagrams (simplified 3D diagrams in which attempts were made to indicate perspective, base line, visual occlusion, etc.) and concluded that neither type of diagram was of much value. 2D diagrams could be interpreted if the child was given sufficient instruction, but there was some doubt that their meaning generalized beyond the specific taught instance. Tri-dimensional diagrams were even less effective since they could not be understood at all without considerable training.

Similarly, LOWENFELD [Low80] describes the difficulty a blind child faces in recognizing a tactual representation of a dog. The child, who is presumably familiar with dogs, views the legs as being placed at the "four corners" of the animal and cannot relate this to their representation in one plane on the diagram. This may be because, as Kennedy argued, blind people understand the concepts associated with a 2D view but have not learned the accepted

---

[2] This situation may change in the not-too-distant future. A great deal of research effort has been directed towards the improvement of tactile displays, and a number of promising non-mechanical systems are currently under development. One such system is that developed by Texas Instruments and described in US patent 5,580,251. It makes use of an organic gel which expands when an electrical current is passed through it. The patent describes a display which consists of a network of tiny holes, sealed on the underside and covered with a flexible membrane on the upperside. Each hole contains electrodes and is filled with the gel. Activating the electrodes causes the gel to expand, creating a "bulge" in the membrane above it. The authors of the patent claim that this system will be both cheaper and more reliable than existing tactile displays, but emphasize that considerable further development is needed before such a display can be offered commercially.

ways of representing 3D objects in a 2D space. LOWENFELD concludes that tactual diagrams can be effective in representing essentially 2D data such as geometric shapes, maps, graphs, etc., but less effective in representing 3D objects.

Taken together, these findings suggest that tactile diagrams have a role to play in the presentation of graphical images to blind people, but that they suffer from a number of drawbacks which limit their usefulness. These include the relatively high cost, the requirement that users have a high level of tactile sensitivity, and the problems involved in choosing suitable tactile representations for some types of image.

11.2 Graphics Versus Text

Given that tactile presentation of graphics has certain drawbacks, is text a valid alternative?

Assuming an image can be converted into text, presentation to blind people poses few problems. Systems which can convert text into synthetic speech are readily available and cost relatively little. For those blind people who can read Braille, text can also be made available by means of "soft" Braille displays. These are a form of tactile display designed specifically for presentation of Braille text, and while they share many of the disadvantages mentioned earlier they require fewer pins than a display designed to present images and are therefore cheaper. In the hands of an experienced Braille user they allow faster access to text than is possible through speech. Soft Braille displays also have the advantage that they can be used by people who are deaf as well as blind.

There is little difficulty, then, in presenting text to blind people. The real issues concern the relationship between graphics and text and the technical problems involved in converting from one to the other.

11.2.1 Fundamental Differences Between Graphics and Text

LARKIN and SIMON [LS87] consider the differences between diagrammatic representations and what they call sentential representations – sequences of elements analogous to strings of text or speech. They identify the following differences between the two types of representation:

- Sentential (elements arranged in a single sequence, with each item adjacent only to the next item in the list)
  - Generally best at preserving information about temporal and logical sequence relations.
  - Usually has to be searched linearly, unless an index exists. Thus search time is strongly influenced by the size of the data structure.

- Diagrammatic (elements indexed by two-dimensional location)
    - Generally best at preserving information about topographical and geometric relations.
    - Often cannot be searched linearly but may, depending upon its nature, allow faster searches (e.g., because related data is placed at adjacent nodes with direct links). Thus search time is strongly influenced by the organization of the data structure.

LARKIN and SIMON compare the value of sentential and diagrammatic representations as sources of data for someone trying to solve problems typically found in physics, geometry, and economics. They note that two representations may be *informationally equivalent* (i.e., all the information in one is also inferrable from the other, and vice versa) but that this does not mean that the two representations will be equally easy to use in a problem-solving task. Rather, the suitability of a representation for a particular task will be determined by the number of *transformations* that have to be performed upon the data before it yields the required information. A transformation occurs when a user finds it necessary, for example, to create a diagram (either physically or mentally) in order to make sense of verbally presented data. To take a very simple example, if one of the steps in solving a problem requires that the user determine whether a particular parameter is rising or falling in value relative to some other parameter (e.g., time) the answer will be obtained most quickly from a diagram which represents the parameter as a rising or falling line against time. Obtaining the same information from a list of parameter pairs expressed numerically will require more effort. However, if the information required is the absolute value of one parameter at a certain point, this may be easier to obtain from a list of numerical values.

Thus the principal factor in determining whether a particular type of representation is suitable for a particular application is the amount of transformation which has to be performed on the data before it can be used. The best representation will be the one which requires least transformation. LARKIN and SIMON note that for most of the problems they considered, diagrammatic representations are most appropriate, and that the most significant problem which arises when using sentential data to solve problems of this type is that it places an enormous demand on the user's memory.

Work on the relationship between graphics and text was also undertaken as part of the GUIB project (Graphical User Interfaces for Blind People, a multinational collaborative project funded by the European Union). It was suggested [The95] that images can usefully be divided into two types:

- Topographical images, which rely on the spatial relationship of points to convey meaning, and in which spatial distortion changes meaning. An example of a topographical image is a map, on which changing the position of a point changes the information presented regarding the location of the place represented by that point.

- Topological images, which do not rely on the spatial relationship of points to convey meaning, and which may therefore be spatially distorted without changes of meaning. An example of a topological image is a calendar, in which changes of absolute position and distance between points do not change the meaning provided relative positions are maintained.

11.2.2 What to Translate, What to Ignore

The distinctions identified above enable us to make some important decisions regarding what kinds of graphical data we should try to translate and what kinds to ignore.

Clearly, it is not appropriate in most cases simply to present sets of coordinates or lists of graph values. While these might be informationally equivalent to the original graphic (in the sense defined by Larkin and Simon), they are unlikely to be of direct use to a blind person who wishes to interpret the image. Rather, the type of data provided must reflect the task being performed, whether that demands a number, the name of a parameter, a description of a shape, a statement of a trend (e.g., "rising" or "falling"), or some other form of output.

It is also clear that topographical data is extremely difficult to present to blind people other than by means of a tactile diagram or display. Textual or verbal descriptions which retain all the topographical data (i.e., are more or less informationally equivalent to the map) will almost certainly be long and detailed and will require extensive transformation before useful data can be extracted. Trying to build up anything other than a very superficial mental image of, for example, a map, from a verbal description is likely to prove both frustrating and time-consuming. However, it should not be too difficult to extract and present non-topographical data from a topographical representation (for example, "Town A is 25 miles South-East of Town B").

It seems then, that in most cases it will be necessary to convert all the data in the original graphic into some other form, and then to provide a means of exploring this data interactively, allowing the user to inspect the information in different ways according to the requirements of the task. An example of how this might work can be seen in the SOUNDGRAPH system [PE93]. The SOUNDGRAPH software is designed to allow blind people to examine and create line graphs. It accepts graph descriptions in various forms (scanned, downloaded from a spreadsheet, created internally, etc.) and stores the results as a table of coordinates. The user can then explore this data in a number of ways. The overall shape of the curve can be represented as a musical tone which varies in pitch over time, and the user can vary the speed so as to allow anything from a rapid musical "glance" at the overall shape to a more detailed examination of the way the line varies over time. The user can hear the whole graph played from end to end or, if preferred, interrupt it at any point in order to explore interactively, moving backwards and forwards along the curve as desired. It is also possible to select portions of the graph and enlarge them, thus increasing the relative pitch range and making small variations in gradient more apparent. In all these modes, the user can also obtain further information via synthetic speech. The x and y coordinates at any point can be obtained, as can the slope of the graph, the maximum and minimum x and y values, and much else. Two graphs can be loaded simultaneously and compared through a combination of musical tones (using a different timbre for each graph) and speech. If desired, the user can attach a personal comment or description to each graph, making it possible to store the most pertinent data for later analysis or for comparison with other graphs.

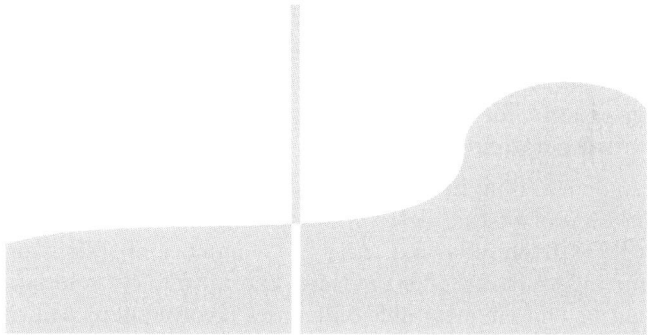

Figure 11.3: A simple line graph, as displayed by the SOUNDGRAPH system. The auditory display comprises a musical pitch which rises and falls to represent the height of the graph. The visual display presents the graph as two areas of highly contrasting color, allowing users to make maximum use of any residual vision they may possess. The vertical bar moves across the visual display in synchronization with the changing musical pitch. All other information, such as x and y values, location of the origin, etc., is available through synthetic speech at the request of the user. (Slightly modified for printing.)

A similar approach to the presentation of graphical material through sound has been taken by other researchers, for example [KSP+95].

The features described above provide a high degree of flexibility in exploring graphs, allowing the user to select different types of information according to current needs. The challenge is to find similarly flexible methods for making other types of graphical data available to blind people.

11.3 Translating Graphics to Text – Technical Issues

Deciding what information to present to blind users is, of course, only part of the challenge. The practical issues surrounding the conversion of graphical material into non visual forms are even more challenging.

In recent years there has been considerable progress in the field of computer recognition of graphics. This process, often known as image understanding, allows objects within a composite image to be identified and labeled. The process typically involves scanning the image in order to identify discrete elements within it, translating these elements into a semantic model (after filtering to remove distortion cause by perspective and angle of view) and finally attempting to match the semantic description against a series of "standard" descriptions held in a library. Thus an image understanding system faced with an image of a table and chairs might use edge detection to separate the individual objects, then reduce the resulting shapes to simple semantic descriptions which can be compared with descriptions of typical tables and chairs held in the library. The result could be expressed as a simple textual description (e.g., "table" or "chair"). Once the elements have been identified it might be possible to identify simple spatial relationships between the objects, for example, noting whether the chairs are close to the table or quite separate from it.

Image understanding methods offer considerable potential for the automatic generation of textual descriptions from graphics. However, the technique is still relatively new and there are a number of serious problems to be overcome before it can offer anything like a complete solution. Particular problems include the inevitable difficulties involved in recognizing objects which are partially obscured in the image, and the vast range of images which are encountered in everyday life and the consequent difficulty of creating a comprehensive library. Another problem is that some images have more than one semantic representation, making it difficult to select a meaningful text label by automatic means.

One solution to these problems is to use a human moderator to perform at least part of the graphics-to-text conversion process. Work carried out as part of the GUIB project [KRS94, KSP+95] focused on the task of gaining access to certain types of pictorial representation, namely numerical diagrams (e.g., graphs), computer-generated images, photographs, and line drawings. It was concluded that these could not be handled automatically but were best dealt with in a two-stage process. In the first stage a human moderator examines the image and uses an interactive tool to build up a model of it. This model is then given to the blind user who examines it using an interactive presentation tool. The presentation tool can have various outputs. For example, it can present tabular representations drawn from graphs as musical tones, either discrete or continuous.

A better, longer-term solution is to encourage interface designers to produce applications which can easily be extended to provide both visual and non visual interfaces. One way of doing this is to create applications with separable interfaces, perhaps by using one of the many User Interface Management Systems (UIMS) now available. UIMS allow a designer to create an application and interface which are entirely separate but communicate using standardized protocols. This makes it a relatively easy task to replace the existing interface with a new one which is fully compatible with the underlying application but handles input and output in different ways, perhaps replacing visual interaction with tactile and auditory interaction. A UIMS designed specifically for the task of creating parallel interfaces for blind and sighted people is described in [SS95].

In addition to the problems posed by graphics themselves, there is also the issue of how to handle textual labels and captions attached to graphics. Many graphics, particularly technical diagrams and graphs, have text labels which indicate the functions or values of individual parts. In some cases these are quite short, while in others they can be as long as a paragraph. On some anatomical diagrams, for example, the label attached to each bodypart includes both the name of the part, a description of its function, and information on its relationship to other parts illustrated in the diagram.

Such diagrams can be quite daunting for sighted users, and some recent attempts have been made to use interactive presentation techniques to improve their usability. The ZOOMILLUSTRATOR [PRS$^+$95] allows graphics to be rotated and viewed at different levels of abstraction (e.g., in the case of an anatomical diagram one might be able to view the skeleton, the circulatory system, musculature, etc.). Only visible elements are labeled, so if a picture is rotated such that a particular element of the picture moves out of view, any labels associated with that element will also disappear. The quantity of text shown in a label may also change as the orientation of the illustration changes, for example, if a formerly peripheral element is moved to the center of the view or vice versa. When a text area is progressively expanded, labels which provide higher-level descriptions (such as summaries) appear first, with lower-level, more detailed labels appearing later. A further refinement is the use of an aspect of interest (AOI) value to determine whether a particular text element should be made visible or not. This makes use of predetermined values for the relative "importance" of each element but also takes account of the history of the current interaction, noting which views the user spends most time examining and using this information in an attempt to match the information provided to the user's area of interest.

Some aspects of this approach might be useful when presenting labeled graphical material to blind people. The notion of presenting only high-level information (part names, summaries, etc.) in the first instance and then progressively offering more detailed information in response to user requests lends itself well to the relatively narrow focus of text or speech presentation. This can be compared to the concept of information scoping in speech-based interfaces [Yan94].

The use of AOI values and selection of labels based on the history of the interaction are also interesting. We have noted that the information required by the user may vary enormously depending upon the task in hand, and that an interface for blind people should offer as much flexibility as possible in the choice of presentation method. A system which notes the types of information being requested by the user and attempts to match further interaction to the user's probable requirements may, if carefully designed, offer benefits in terms of speed and usability.

11.4 Presenting the Text

As has already been pointed out, the two principal methods of presenting text to blind people are through soft Braille displays and synthetic speech.

Most Braille terminals comprise 20, 40, or 80 cells, allowing them to represent up to one line of an 80-column display. However, the larger displays are very expensive and most blind people are forced to make do with one of the smaller sizes. The Braille display is normally placed just above the keyboard so that the user can alternate between typing input and reading output with the minimum of movement. Means are provided to scroll from one line of the screen to the next, but interaction is inevitably faster if this can be avoided and all messages accommodated within one line of cells. Unfortunately, this can be difficult to achieve, particularly with the smaller displays, because there may not be a one-to-one correspondence between text characters and Braille cells. Standard Braille uses six dots and can therefore represent up to 64 different characters, but this is not enough to handle the full range of letters, numbers and punctuation characters in general use. For this reason some text characters have to be represented by two Braille characters. Some modern Braille displays attempt to overcome this problem by providing eight dots per cell, allowing them to represent the full range of characters in the ASCII character set. However, the patterns used to represent characters in eight-dot Braille (often called Computer Braille) vary widely and no standard has yet emerged [Web95].

The conversion of text to speech is a relatively straight forward process, and a wide range of systems of varying levels of sophistication are available to perform this task.

The speech synthesizer itself may consist either of a piece of software which drives the internal sound circuits of a computer or, more commonly, a hardware device located on a plugin card or connected externally via one of the output ports. The quality of electronic speech has improved enormously in recent years, and this, coupled with the parallel development of speech recognition technology, has opened up new applications for sighted people as well as for blind people. The result is that speech synthesis is fast entering mainstream computing. Speech synthesis chips are now available on popular brands of plugin sound cards, and it seems likely that within a few years speech synthesis will become a standard feature on most general-purpose computers. This has brought the price of speech synthesis down sharply and has also removed an important psychological barrier – a blind person who wishes to use a computer no longer needs special equipment, merely a standard sound card with speech synthesis and the appropriate software to drive it. A typical text-to-speech system will offer the following features:

- Rules which ensure correct pronunciation of most commonly used words in the target language and also permit the system to handle novel words (for example, proper nouns) with reasonably acceptable results.
- A mechanism for overriding the pronunciation rules where necessary, for example, in the case of words which are frequently encountered in a particular application but which the existing pronunciation rules do not handle correctly. Such mechanisms usually take the form of a "dictionary" file which contains the words whose pronunciation is to be modified along with the preferred pronunciations expressed in a standard phonetic code.
- For languages other than tone languages, rules to determine the correct intonation pattern for most commonly used words. In English, for example, most words have a particular intonation pattern associated with them, and sound quite wrong if spoken with a different intonation pattern.
- Rules to determine the correct stress pattern for most commonly used words in the target language. In English, for example, the word "April" takes its stress on the first syllable ("*A*-pril") and the word "July" takes its stress on the second syllable ("Ju-*ly*"). As with most other English words, they would sound quite odd if spoken with the stress on the wrong syllable.
- User-presettable options governing the speed of the speech, average pitch, length of pauses, etc.
- Rules for the expansion of common abbreviations, such as "Mr." and "St.", into acceptable spoken form.
- User-presettable options governing the handling of numbers (for example, to determine whether "12" is reproduced as "one, two" or "twelve"), strings of capitals (for example, to determine whether "USA" is reproduced as "oosa" or "you, es, ay"), and certain other types of input text string.

It can be seen that many of the basic difficulties involved in converting text to speech are already taken care of by the speech-synthesis system, and therefore need not trouble the system designer. However, effective speech communication relies on much more than good pronunciation and appropriate pausing and speed of delivery. If spoken messages are to be of real value, thought must also be given to the content of the message.

There is not space here to discuss this issue in depth, but a brief outline will be given in an attempt to indicate the significance of these factors for effective presentation of data through synthetic speech.

When choosing the text of a spoken message, the major determining factor is the limitation imposed by human short-term memory. Speech, unlike visually presented material, is transient and must be held in memory while its message is absorbed. Thus it is important to keep the messages as short as possible without sacrificing clarity. Long passages of speech can also be very distracting because speech is difficult to ignore – whether we wish it to or not, speech tends to enter our consciousness and demands attention, leaving fewer resources available to handle other cognitive processes. Speech is also a relatively slow medium of communication, and keeping messages short will help to increase the speed of interaction.

It is difficult to formulate rigid guidelines on this, but a good rule of thumb is to ensure that each speech string contains just one item of information which is new to the listener. Analysis of spoken language suggests that human beings normally parse speech into a string of clauses, separated from one another by pauses and further delineated by a characteristic rise and fall in pitch. Within each clause there is typically one item of information which the speaker judges to be new to the listener, sometimes accompanied by supporting information which the speaker assumes that the listener will already know or could readily infer from the context. To take an example, in response to the question "How many did we sell in July?", one might give the answer "July sales were 2 830." In this case, "2 830" is new information while the remainder of the response is not - it would have been perfectly acceptable had the answer been given as "2 830" and the remainder of the clause omitted entirely.

In other cases the given information might be more important. If one were presenting a table of monthly sales figures, it would be helpful to state the month each figure relates to as well as giving its value, so that the listener knows which point in the list has been reached. If one merely reeled off a list of numbers the listener could easily become confused. However, it is usually neither necessary nor desirable to present the same supporting information repeatedly. For example, it is unlikely that someone asked to read out a list of sales figures would respond by saying "January sales were 1 982, February sales were 2 008, March sales were 2 074, April sales were 2 193..." It is much more likely that the speaker would respond by saying something like "January sales were 1 982; February's were 2 008; March, 2 074; April, 2 193..." In this case, the supporting information is included only until the structure of the response and the purpose of each element has been established, after which it is omitted. This reduces the time taken to read the list and also removes extraneous speech which might make it harder for the listener to focus on the required information.

When deciding how much data to provide in response to each request, it is important not only to distinguish between new and supporting information but also to determine how much detail the listener requires. There is no point in overburdening the listener's memory by giving numerical values correct to four or five significant digits when one or two significant digits would suffice. For example, if someone is listening to a set of sales figures with the aim of gaining a broad, overall impression rather than precise details, they may prefer to have the figures expressed to the nearest hundred rather than in units.

11.4 Presenting the Text

It is also important to note that one would not present a long list of dates and figures in this way if the listener needed to store them in memory or to perform some operation on the data. The amount of material presented would far exceed that which most people can hold in their memory. If recall is necessary, the list would have to be presented in smaller chunks and a means provided whereby the listener can explore the list interactively at his or her own pace.

An example of how this might be done can be found in [Pit96], which includes a description of an interactive tool which allows users to examine lists of items – such as the filenames in a computer directory – through speech. In order to ease the task of examining such a list (which may be quite long), the tool uses an algorithm which sorts the names into groups of related items.

The operation of the tool is illustrated in Fig. 11.4. When it is started up, the user is told how many files the directory contains. Moving down to the second level (by pressing the DOWN cursor key), the user is told how many groups the directory has been sorted into and what those groups are called. If the directory is very large and has been sorted into a correspondingly large number of groups, the list is not read out in full but divided into shorter lists. In this case, the prosody of the synthetic speech (i.e, the rhythm and intonation) indicates that there are more group-names to be heard, and the user can hear them by pressing the LEFT or RIGHT cursor keys. Repeated movements in one direction will take the user back to the start of the list, whereupon the prosody of the speech makes it clear that the full list has been heard and that the user is now hearing parts of the list again. Pressing the

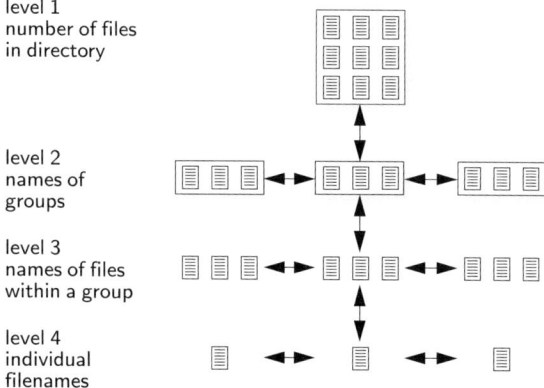

Figure 11.4: Organization of data (in this example, the names of files in a directory) to allow exploration using speech feedback. At the top level, the user is merely told how many files are in the directory. At level 2, the files are placed in groups and the user hears a list of the group names. Selecting a group and moving down to level 3, the user hears the names of the individual files within that group. Moving down to level 4 allows a single file to be selected for use in subsequent operations.

DOWN cursor key at any time takes the user to the third level and to the group whose name was last spoken, whereupon the names of the individual filenames in that group are spoken out. Again, if the list is long, it is divided into smaller sections which can be reached using the LEFT and RIGHT cursor keys, and prosody is used to indicate the limits of the list. Moving down to the bottom level, the user is presented with a single filename, that of the file whose name was last spoken at the previous level. Moving left or right selects other files in the same group. Using single-key commands, the file can be examined further (e.g., to determine its size or date of last modification) or selected for use in a copying or moving operation.

As well as being of use in indicating the start and end of spoken lists, prosody may be of value in helping listeners to grasp the relationships between files within a group. Consider, for example, the names of a group of files associated with a programming project:

diary.im
diary.cha
zoomDiary.im
zoomDiary.cha

When reading such a list aloud, a human speaker would almost certainly use rhythm and intonation to mark those elements of the filenames which appear more than once. The first two filenames – diary.im and diary.cha – would probably be spoken with the words "diary dot" at the same pitch each time, but with the syllable "im" at a higher pitch and the syllable "cha" at a lower pitch. This highlights the fact that the words "diary dot" are the same in both filenames but that the final syllables differ. When the next two filenames are spoken, the syllable "zoom" will probably be placed at the highest pitch. This may alert the listener to the fact that this is where these filenames differ from the previous two. The role of prosody in speech communication is not well understood, but patterns such as these are widely observed in natural speech and it is generally accepted that they are of value to the listener. Studies have shown that where intonation and rhythmic cues are missing or inappropriate, listeners will have more difficulty extracting meaning from the speech. These difficulties may be reflected in increased response times, reductions in recall rates, increases in error rates, and reduced ability to identify and resolve ambiguities (see, for example, [Rei80]).

In view of this, the interactive list reading tool identifies repeated syllables and similar features within lists and uses prosodic variation to highlight them. The nature and extent of the variations sounds somewhat coarse and exaggerated compared with natural prosody, but tests have shown that listeners still found the prosodic cues helpful.

Through the use of prosody and by allowing interactive exploration of a hierarchical structure, the interactive list reading tool greatly eases the task of recovering information from long lists using speech. When evaluated in comparison with a conventional list-reading utility (which allows only sequential, linear exploration), it was found that subjects performed a practical task more than twice as quickly using this tool and also reported lower levels of effort and fatigue.

11.5 Conclusions

We have seen that graphics are a useful tool in many human information processing activities because they present the required information in the most immediately accessible form. We have also seen that blind people are capable of understanding most if not all of the concepts embodied in graphical representations, but that providing access to graphics (for example, by tactile means) poses considerable problems. Textual representations are far easier to present to blind people, but while it may be possible to create a textual description which is informationally equivalent to a graphic it does not necessarily follow that the text will be as easy to use. Therefore, considerable thought needs to be given to the way in which graphics are represented as text. Some elements (for example, those which are purely decorative) may be better ignored, while of the reminder, some may be far more important than others. Ultimately, the decision as to which information is important and which not may be determined by the way in which the end-user employs the information. This is usually beyond the control of the designer, so it is necessary to build interfaces which are as flexible as possible, allowing the user to view the data in whichever way is most appropriate to the task at hand. Further research may also help to identify better ways of analyzing and categorizing graphics and so aid this process.

When presenting text as speech, it is also necessary to bear in mind that speech is harder to ignore than vision and makes much heavier demands on cognitive resources such as memory. More research is needed into the design of good spoken-dialog systems, particularly into the relationship between semantic content, syntactic structure, prosody, etc., and the cognitive effort required to assimilate speech.

Contributor of Chap. 11: Ian PITT

Chapter 12

Figure Captions in Visual Interfaces

Visualizations are produced to enable a viewer to extract information. For this purpose, visualizations are not merely a straightforward rendering of the data. Limited presentation space imposes restrictions on the visualization, resulting in omissions, exaggerations, or displacements. Moreover, viewers may wish to explore the data under a thematic focus. Thus, portions of the data may be presented in more detail or more comprehensively, while others may be simplified, shrunken, or even left out.

As a result of sophisticated manipulations, complex images may arise which are difficult to interpret. In traditional print media, an image is therefore often accompanied by a figure caption which describes verbally how the image has arisen, what message it should convey, and which details may be important, particularly when these are difficult to recognize.

Textual information to enhance the interpretation of images is sometimes neglected because images are thought to be descriptive on their own. This is not entirely true, as the art historian GOMBRICH pointed out: "No picture tells its own story" [Gom84]. WEIDENMANN, an educational psychologist examining how to learn with images, builds on GOMBRICH's work and argues that figure captions are in fact crucial in a learning context [Wei89]. They enhance the interpretation of images [Wei89] and make it easier to remember the contents of an image over a longer term [Nug83].

In this chapter we show how the potential of figure captions can be employed for the enhancement of *visual interfaces* – interactive systems which produce images based on an underlying model. We discuss the generation of figure captions with reference to medical illustrations (see Chap. 13) and geographic information systems (see Chap. 20). Furthermore, we discuss how to maintain consistency between visualizations and their captions.

Besides the content selection (what to describe), the generation of figure captions requires phrases to verbalize this content appropriately. This incorporates a linguistic analysis of the domain and some text generation. Because figure captions are rather concise and follow a fixed structure, acceptable results can be expected with simple text-generated approaches.

This chapter is organized as follows. First, we analyze figure captions in print media to derive the basic structure of descriptive figure captions (Sect. 12.1). A look at related work is presented in Sect. 12.2. After this, we discuss issues of figure captions specific in interactive systems in Sect. 12.3. In Sect. 12.4, we show how figure captions can be used to manipulate an image: we present *interactive figure captions*, captions with sensitive parts the user can modify. With interactive figure captions a bidirectional connection between images and their captions exists. Based on these observations, in Sect. 12.5 we develop a concept for the integration of figure captions in interactive systems. This includes a generic architecture and a sequence of steps to prepare the integration of figure captions. The concluding Sect. 12.6 contains an extensive look at future work.

12.1 Figure Captions in Print Media

In traditional print media, diverse kinds of figure captions can be found. By no means all of them can be generated automatically or can be regarded as role for interactive systems. To clarify the figure captions to which we restrict ourselves, we propose the following classification. Following BERNARD [Ber90], we refer to *descriptive figure captions* if the content of an image is described verbally.

We shall use this definition in a broader sense. Descriptive figure captions describe a view on a model or a section of the real world. This definition also comprises phrases describing not only what is visible in the figure but also what is hidden, what has been removed, or what important objects are close to the depicted portion. Consequently, descriptive figure captions describe an image and its (spatial) context. Descriptive figure captions are employed, for example, to explain the construction of complex objects.

By contrast, *instructive figure captions* describe either how to interpret an image (typical phrases include "Look carefully at ...") or what to do in the real world with the depicted objects. Instructive figure captions, for example, explain how to operate, repair, or maintain technical devices. These captions are often employed to describe different stages of a complex operation. The images and their description explain how to use objects and assume that the construction of these objects is known.

This classification covers a large portion of captions in reference materials, text book and repair manuals. Other figure captions, such as those naming people in a photograph in a journal, are beyond the scope of this classification.

In this chapter we deal with descriptive figure captions only. We show how the content of these captions can be derived automatically based on *structured models* and user interaction with it. Structured models refer to models that consist of distinct objects together with some semantic information, at least the names of objects and the affiliation to categories.

By contrast, the generation of instructive figure captions requires not only semantic information about object names and categories, but also a considerable amount of information on the application domain, for example, on possible complications in the maintenance of objects, and on alternative ways to perform an operation under difficult circumstances.

In the following we analyse the use of descriptive figure captions in two application fields – anatomical atlases and maps. While figure captions in anatomy have developed over a long period of time, similar comprehensive descriptive texts are less widespread in cartography. Only in rare cases have legends been extended to describe artifacts of the image generation process (see also SCHLICHTMANN [Sch97]). We review this work briefly and compare the results later.

12.1.1 Figure Captions in Anatomical Atlases

Anatomical atlases consist of large, often complex images which are not surrounded by textual information as in textbooks (hence the name "atlas"). Figure captions are the only form of textual information available and do not interfere with other references to an image. We conducted a series of interviews with medical students; these revealed that figure captions are studied carefully to get an orientation when studying complex images. Our analysis is based mainly on the widely known atlas of SOBOTTA [Sob88] and the book by WALDEYER [WM92].

Figure captions in anatomy follow a rather fixed structure. The first items mentioned in figure captions are generally the name of the depicted contents, the viewing direction and the important aspects (e.g., "muscles and sinews of a foot, lateral view"). This information is essential if an unfamiliar picture of organs inside the human body is depicted.

After the information about the image as a whole, important parameters of single objects are usually described. Among these parameters, manipulations that affect the visibility of objects are most important. Typical phrases include "[$object_1$] has been removed to show [$object_2$]" or "[$object_1$] has been removed in the area of [$object_2$]". Obviously it is important to mention certain objects that are omitted. In addition to the removal of objects, it is common to pull an object aside to expose another one. This technique is applied, e.g., to muscles which can be moved in reality due to their elasticity. Such manipulations affect the visibility, too, and are often mentioned.

If small objects are important in a specific context, they must be enlarged to emphasize them. In this case the context is preserved for better orientation, so that the surrounding objects cannot be enlarged. Such changes in the relative sizes are reflected by phrases like "[object] slightly enlarged" in the caption.

Besides geometric manipulations, *presentation variables* like colors and textures are often adapted to a specific context, e.g., to show spatial relations more clearly and to communicate structural relations. In anatomy, objects of certain organ systems are colored uniformly according to accepted conventions.[1] The assignment of colors is described once in the preface of a book. In figure captions, the use of colors therefore needs to be described only if it differs significantly from the conventions or even conflicts with them.

An interesting facet is the generation of one figure caption for several images, for instance when images show the same model from different directions. Furthermore, visualizations may exploit the symmetry of anatomic objects and show different aspects in both halves. In both cases, the similarities between the images are mentioned first, while the differences are described later. If horizontally arranged images are described by one caption, it is important that the left image be described before the right one, because there is a natural sequence of "reading images" from left to right.

Figure captions also depend on other textual components. In order to refer to objects via their name, they must either be labeled or circumscribed by characteristic features which are easy to recognize in the image.

12.1.2 Figure Captions and Legends for Maps

Maps are an abstract visualization of a part of the real world, usually of objects on the surface of the earth. Instead of presenting geographic objects as they appear on aerial photographs, symbols are used to present categories of objects. Depending on the map scale, legible symbols may become larger than the objects they represent. Resulting conflicts are resolved by removing, simplifying, or repositioning symbols. This abstraction process is referred to as *cartographic generalization* [Mon96]).

Color is used independently of the appearance of the objects in the real world. Instead, it is employed so as tu ensure the discriminability of the symbols. In thematic maps, more than one thematic variable (e.g., population density and net income) usually needs to be presented, but size can only represent one. Therefore, color is often used as an additional degree of freedom to encode another thematic variable.

Maps are, thus, constructed of symbols which do not resemble the objects they represent, either in shape or in size or color. Hence, maps are not interpretable as they are but need an explanation. For this purpose, legends are usually provided along with maps that explain the use of the symbols. Besides this interpretational purpose, legends may serve more functions. SCHLICHTMANN identified major functions of map legends [Sch97]. From his enumeration we derive the following:

---

[1] Muscles are depicted red, nerves are yellow, and bones are white

- *Provision of additional information about mapped objects*
  A legend may contain information that is not shown in the map itself. For example, in a map that shows the value of a thematic variable for each region, the legend may give an explanation of the symbols and in addition present them with their value for the whole area.
- *Presentation of the underlying structure*
  Sometimes a structure is inherent in the data that is not easily conveyed in the map. For example, in maps for bedrock geology the temporal sequence of the sediments is not encoded in the map and, thus, needs to be presented in the legend. This can be accomplished by describing their age as well as explaining the textures or colors used for each sediment.
- *Information about the underlying classification scheme*
  If a variable may represent a large number of values, or even continuous values, it is not feasible to code all of them as different colors. Instead, categories are formed using domain knowledge (e.g., an income below $200 is under the poverty line). Each category is assigned a color value, and the legend can be used to reveal the underlying classification scheme.
- *Provision of information about the visualization*
  This is probably the most interesting aspect of a map legend's functionality, as it reveals what has happened in the abstraction process that transformed the real world data to the map. It covers in particular all aspects of presentation fidelity. For example, in a map about farm sizes in Canada you may find statements like "Values are rounded to the nearest five farms" indicating the error for the rendering of the number of farms. Another example for this kind of information can be found in a nautical chart from Australia with a longer textual legend [oRAN94]. Here omissions in the map are mentioned in the legend, stating that certain aids could not be presented but may be found in a larger-scale map. The same legend informs the reader of the presentation accuracy by saying that the sand banks are not necessarily where they are depicted in the map as they are shifting.

In consequence, map legends are an important part of maps. Besides providing information about the coding scheme for the symbolization they may also contain information about the data structure and aspects of fidelity. Restrictions to the map fidelity are usually a consequence of the visualization process and may be extremely important to the map reader; recall, e.g., the relevance of the existence of shifting sand banks for cruising ships.

Map fidelity usually lessens with decreasing map scale. Small-scale maps need a more comprehensive generalization to display all symbols with sufficient size to be legible and to resolve graphical conflicts between them (see MÜLLER et al. [MLW95]). Through these processes, objects of minor importance are removed and symbols are repositioned to prevent overlapping; this is an instance of the process of abstraction as defined in Chap. 1 of this book. Hence, the maps thus obtained no longer reflect the reality in full detail –

they mislead with respect to completeness or distances between objects (see "How to lie with maps" by MONMONIER [Mon96]).

When maps are no longer created manually, the data about fidelity can be gathered as a direct by-product of the visualization process. Hence it may be used to generate legends that reveal the inaccuracy that was introduced in the map and help the reader to determine which operations are still performable on the map and which no longer yield trustworthy results.

Considering the various functions of map legends it becomes apparent that they should be structured in different ways according to their purpose. For the most widespread use of map legends – symbol explanation – a schematic legend is suitable and commonly used. This is a table-like legend where in the first column the symbol is displayed, and in the second column its meaning is explained.

However, for the extended functionality this simple approach is not feasible. The information to be presented is more complex and not as easily structurable. For these cases, textual descriptions ought to be used. We refer to these natural language descriptions as figure captions, which is in accordance with the widespread use of the term outside the area of cartography.

We will focus on the generation of figure captions for maps describing the visualization process, i.e., the operations that have been performed on the data to obtain the map and their impact on its reliability.

12.1.3 Generalized Structure of Figure Captions

In order to derive a common approach to the generation of descriptive figure captions, a generalized structure is presented in the following.

Figure captions describe the depicted content and the view of an underlying model. This model may be three-dimensional, as in anatomy, or two-dimensional, as in cartography. The view of the model is characterized by a viewing direction (in 3D) or by the visible portion (in 2D). Besides this, a view is determined by thematic aspects on which the visualization focuses (e.g., water ways in maps or the human skeleton in anatomy).

Since visualization is a sophisticated process, manipulations that restrict the image fidelity ought to be described in the caption. This covers the mentioning of single objects whose visibility or position was modified during the visualization process.

Often, there is no uniform scale in the whole visualization. Instead, the scale is adapted to the density of symbols and objects or their size. Since these modifications usually remain unnoticed to the untrained eye, their existence needs to be described in a figure caption.

Conventions, e.g., for the use of colors, reduce the need for comments in figure captions. The variety of the formulations in figure captions is high, but the basic structure is fixed and some typical phrases dominate in each domain.

12.2 Related Work

The incorporation of figure captions in interactive systems is a new approach to enhance the usability of visual interfaces. Figure captions in a narrow sense, that is, captions that describe images previously generated, were first developed by MITTAL et al. [MRM+95]. This work has been carried out in the context of the SAGE project, where complex diagrams are generated. MITTAL et al. argue that users can deal with more complex diagrams if they are complemented by explanatory captions. To put it in other words: complex relations that must be depicted in several images (without captions) can be integrated in one diagram when explained appropriately.

Some systems produce what we have introduced as instructive figure captions (recall Sect. 12.1). In particular, in the WIP project (Knowledge Based Information Presentation, see WAHLSTER et al. [WAF+93]) and in the COMET project (Coordinated Multimedia Explanation Testbed, see FEINER and MCKEOWN [FM93]) technical illustrations and textual descriptions are generated to explain the repair and maintenance of technical devices. The textual components are generated based on large knowledge bases.

The selected content is presented within different media (graphics, animation and text) which are used either in a complementary or redundant way. For example, a verbal description can complement a graphic by conveying information which is hard to visualize. Presenting redundant information aims at reinforcing the message, e.g., by appropriate cross-references. In this *media selection* process, the suitability of a medium to convey information is considered. Moreover, sophisticated *media coordination* facilities are employed.

This situation is considerably different from the problem we describe in this chapter. In WIP and COMET, graphics and text generation mutually influence each other – the textual expressions generated affect the graphics generation and do not only comment on them. The content of the figure captions often goes over and above the content of the figure.

12.3 Dynamic Figure Captions

For enhancing interactive systems by using figure captions, ideas can be borrowed from print media. This orientation, however, is limited to static aspects. The incorporation of figure captions in interactive systems raises some fundamentally new questions. Figure captions describe images exposed to changes and therefore must be updated. Furthermore, incremental changes of figure captions are useful for easy identification of changing parts. It must be decided whether a figure caption should be legible in its entirety or, for example, be embedded in a dialog with scrollbars. This section discusses possible answers to these and other related questions.

12.3.1 Layout Considerations

Different opportunities exist for arranging a caption relative to other components, especially to the image(s) they describe. Usually, figure captions are arranged immediately under an image (see TURTSCHI in [Tur95]). This, however, is not necessary in an interactive system. If the overall distribution of screen space becomes unsuitable they can be placed beside the image to which they refer.

Furthermore, it is important to present the content in a pleasing and legible way. Colors, fonts, and their sizes are important parameters to achieve these goals. Figure captions have a higher priority than other textual components, e.g., labels, which refer only to parts of an image, and the layout should convey this importance.

These observations are also valid for static figure captions, but some additional issues arise in interactive systems. Figure captions may contain sensitive parts for selection and even invalid parts – these features must be communicated with an appropriate layout. The sketch in Fig. 12.1 presents a suggestion for this visualization.

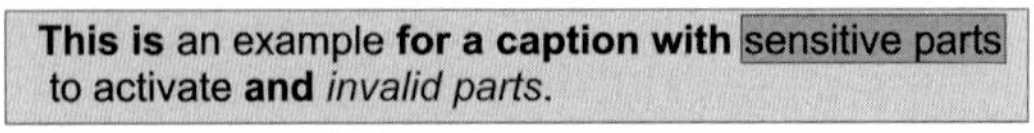

> **This is** an example **for a caption with** sensitive parts
> to activate **and** *invalid parts*.

Figure 12.1: A caption has sensitive parts (with an underlying rectangle) and invalid parts (light gray and italic). Bold parts represent fixed phrases which are based on the templates (see Sect. 12.5.1).

Moreover, figure captions in interactive systems may change in length over time. On one hand, it is desirable that the caption is changed incrementally, so that those parts of a caption which do not change remain at their positions. On the other hand, this strategy may conflict with a well-balanced layout with captions centered under an image.

Figure captions in interactive systems are thus exposed to various changes. Their position, their presentation, and even their content may change. We therefore refer to them as *dynamic figure captions*.

12.3.2 Adaptable Figure Captions

While figure captions in print media are necessarily static, dynamic figure captions can be tailored to the needs of the current user. Such an adaptation is useful because the overall amount of information to mention in a figure caption can become quite large. Adaptation facilities should enable users to control the content selection. Several parameters are particularly important for adaptation:

Content Selection. The caption generation process can be adapted to what kind of information is to be presented and to which level of detail. The information selection option (see the top left part of Fig. 12.2) allows a user to request a notification when a certain property of the image has changed, i.e., when a presentation variable (like visibility or color) has been altered or when geometrical aspects of the image (like the size or the shape of a single object or its relative position) have been manipulated (see the bottom left part of Fig. 12.2).

In addition, a user may control the amount of information by specifying the level of detail (see the upper left part of Fig. 12.2). Selecting short figure captions means that only the most important changes in each selected category are presented, whereas long figure captions inform the user about every modification to the selected property.

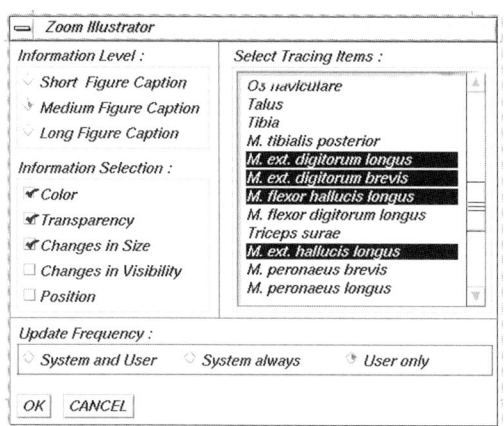

Figure 12.2: Adaptation of figure captions. In the left part, the content selection is customized. In the right part, the user selects objects for monitoring

Object Monitoring. Users should be able to express their interest in specific objects or regions (parts of the underlying model). Based on such a specification, the user will be informed of all changes that affect the objects or regions traced and of their current state (see the list in the right part of Fig. 12.2). For instance, if an object becomes hidden, the system comments on the visibility of such objects (e.g., "the traced [$object_1$] is currently hidden by [$object_2$] and [$object_3$]"). This is similar to debugging tools which allow the user to monitor certain variables.

12.3.3 Updating Figure Captions

Nearly all interactions on images lead to incomplete or even invalid figure captions. This raises the question of when the caption is to be updated and who initiates the update process. In any case, the system should detect whether changes in the image affect the figure caption. In this case, the system or the user can initiate an update. Between these two variants, hybrid approaches are possible where the system initiates an update only after major changes and the user can always initiate an update.

- *Update on explicit request only*
  The caption is updated only upon the user's request. The system indicates invalid parts (recall Fig. 12.1).
- *Automatic update*
  Compared to the other variants, automatic updates by the system require fast generation of captions. This may confuse users because of the high frequency of changes in the corresponding area of the screen. However, the advantage of this approach is that captions remain consistent with the image at all times.
- *Hybrid variant*
  The caption is updated automatically only if radical changes in the image occur. Examples are considerable changes in the viewing specification (e.g., via a rotation) leading to a change in the visibility of a large number of objects or the removal of a class of objects due to filtering operations. Another example is the incorporation of an additional view which requires the figure caption to describe both views.

As there is no optimal variant that is suitable for all application domains, leaving the decision on the initiation of an update up to the user seems to be the preferable option (see the bottom line in Fig. 12.2).

12.4 Interactive Figure Captions

Figure captions, as we know from a variety of printed material, comment on an image. They provide background information about the creation of an image and its context.

So far, we have described the incorporation of *dynamic* figure captions in visual interfaces. Although specific issues like the update and adaptation emerged, the basic function of figure captions remains the same – to guide the interpretation of images.

As we show here, figure captions can be used for a very different purpose; they can be manipulated and cause an update of the image. With this approach, figure captions serve as input for the graphics generation process. Therefore, we refer to these captions as *interactive* figure captions.

Usually, an image can be manipulated with different handles. There are dialogs or handles to invoke transformations, material editors to change presentation variables and other dialogs to initiate filtering operations, to modify rendering styles and lighting conditions. The interactive manipulation of the corresponding parts of a figure caption, unifies these interaction facilities.

Interactive figure captions are also attractive in another respect – a figure caption does not only describe an image but also makes it possible to modify it. The image is no longer superior to the caption in that the caption is dependent on the image, but both stand on the same level and offer interaction facilities.

12.4 Interactive Figure Captions   207

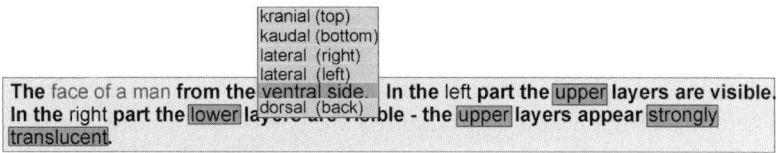

Figure 12.3: Interactive figure captions. The selection of "lateral" causes a pop-up menu to appear containing the six main viewing directions

In this section, we demonstrate first results of this attempt. Note that this approach differs from the graphics and text generation in WIP and COMET (recall Sect. 12.2). In our concept, either the caption describes an image *or* the image is guided by the caption. The generation processes are still autonomous.

It is necessary to guide the user through this interaction. An unrestricted editing of the caption may lead to the specification of unfeasible or ambiguous commands. Moreover, the user may not be aware of what interaction options are available. Guiding the user also avoids the enormous problems coming along with natural language understanding.

Therefore, sensitive regions are provided (recall Fig. 12.1) which display simple dialogs with alternative choices for this item when selected. These can be pop-up menus, sliders, or text edit fields for the specification of numbers (see Figs. 12.3 and 12.4). Pop-up menus, which are used for the selection out of a small number of items, can be derived from the specification of the lexical mappings of the corresponding template variable. Using this approach, a modification of the external mapping specification is always kept consistent with the pop-up menu.

However, using these interaction facilities is not always convenient: 3D widgets allow more direct control of 3D transformations, while WYSIWYG color editors may be more intuitive for selecting colors than a list of color names. On the other hand, it is important that the selection of a sensitive part in a caption leads to a uniform reaction. As a trade-off between

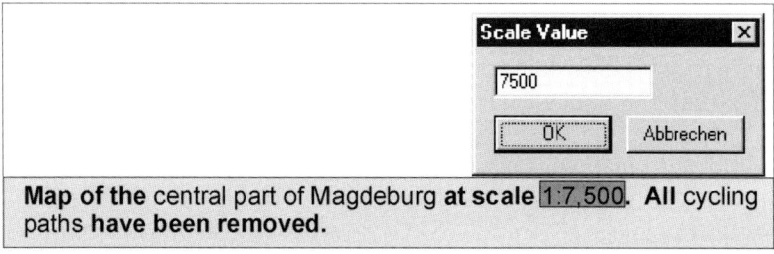

Figure 12.4: Interactive figure captions. Using a text edit window to modify the scale value

dedicated interaction facilities and consistent feedback, the pop-up menus displayed after the selection can contain an item that invokes a dedicated editor, tailored to the interaction task.

The application of interactive figure captions reveals that it is not desirable to modify all variables of a figure caption. In particular, it is questionable whether modifications should be possible which would invalidate large portions of the caption. If the user, for instance, can alter the subject of the visualization the rest of the caption becomes useless. As a rule of thumb, parts of the caption that describe *how* something is depicted should be interactive while parts that describe *what* is depicted should not.

The interactive usage of captions is also limited by the fact that the figure captions must correspond to generable images. The system can only offer attributes for manipulation if it can actually handle an alternative specification for this attribute. If the system states that "[object$_1$]" is hidden by "[object$_2$]", the user cannot be allowed to delete "[object$_2$]" or to replace it by another object, because it may be impossible to generate such a visualization.

12.5 Integration of Figure Captions in Interactive Systems

In this section we develop a concept for the integration of figure captions in interactive systems with respect to the issues discussed above. In particular, the generation of figure captions and the update process are considered.

12.5.1 Template-Based Generation

In the field of text generation there are basically two approaches which differ considerably in the implementation effort, on the one hand, and in the quality of the textual descriptions generated, on the other: *template-based generation* and *natural language generation.*

The template-based approach is a low-cost and low-quality approach, based on prepared phrases, called *templates*. A popular example of template-based text generation is the APPLE MACINTOSH BALLOON help system [Rei95]. Templates contain variables as place-holders which are substituted by the current values (e.g., colors, viewing directions). This replacement requires that the numerical values representing the state of an interactive system are converted into verbal expressions. In its simplest form, there are straightforward mappings of numerical values from an interval to a word or phrase.

Natural language generation (NLG) does not rely on prepared phrases but generates the whole expression from a semantic representation. Obviously, NLG is much more flexible, as it can consider many parameters. Thus, documents can be generated in different languages and different styles (concise or verbose, informal or polite) based on the same semantic representation.[2] The generation of sentences takes into account what has already been generated. Furthermore, similar expressions are merged. This flexibility is gained at the expense of a higher effort, but that pays off especially in larger texts.

Templates, on the other hand, can be generated with less computational effort. They are appropriate for shorter texts that follow a rather fixed structure. Figure captions are an application for which acceptable results can be expected with templates.

12.5.2 An Architecture for Figure Captions in Visual Interfaces

The generation of figure captions that remain consistent with the image requires that all changes to a visualization (e.g., an illustration, a map, or a diagram) are represented explicitly in data structures. As we pointed out in Sect. 12.1, figure captions also depend on textual components, e.g., on the availability of labels. Therefore, the *visualization component* consists of a text and graphics display (compare the architecture in Fig. 12.5).

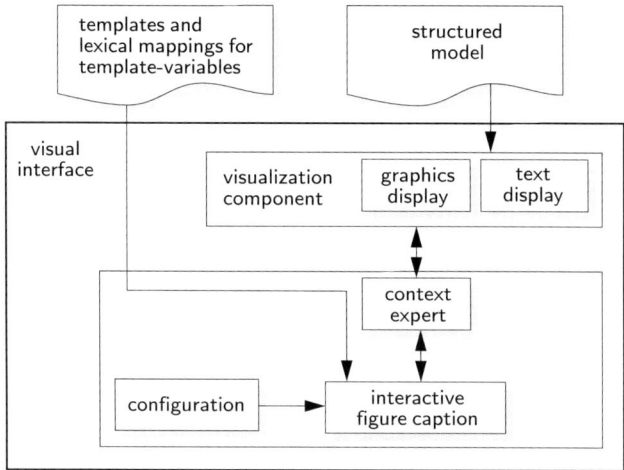

Figure 12.5: Architecture of a visual interface with dynamic figure captions

In order to describe the modifications that have been applied to the visualization, it is necessary to represent not only the cumulative state of an image and the corresponding textual elements, but also the interaction history. For this purpose, an agent is required which is informed whenever the visualization changes. This agent manages the context of the interface and is therefore called the *context expert*.

---

[2] For a comprehensive comparison of both approaches refer to [Rei95] and [RM93a].

The context expert[3] communicates with the *graphics display* and the *text display* and with the *interactive figure caption*. It analyzes the changes and initiates the text generation based on the user's specification (recall Sect. 12.3.2). The generation is also supplied with a separate description of sentences (templates) and the lexical mappings for template variables (often numerical values).

If figure captions are manipulated to control the visualization, a message is sent to the context cxpert (representing the requested changes) and the visualization.

12.5.3 Basic Scheme

The incorporation of figure captions in interactive systems requires, in general, a number of steps to be carried out. Based on our experience, we consider this to be:

1. a task analysis,
2. an analysis of the visualization algorithms,
3. an event analysis,
4. the content selection, and
5. the linguistic realization.

(1) Task Analysis. This step entails the identification of typical visualizations in a specific domain including groups of visualizations that are often viewed at in unison with one another. The analysis is performed with respect to the operations that viewers usually perform on these images in order to extract the requested information. As a result, the operations are identified that should be supported by a class of visualizations. This yields directly the properties of the image that must be preserved, in order to achieve a presentation that fulfills a viewer's demands.

(2) Analysis of the Visualization Algorithms. Based on the properties to be preserved, visualization algorithms are examined as to whether they may conflict with the above mentioned information extraction. Such conflicts may emerge from several constraints that affect the visualization process, e.g., legibility, visual discriminability, screen resolution, or limited presentation areas. As a result of the application of these algorithms, important properties may be violated which should be signaled to the viewer. Hence, the application of such algorithms yields candidates for the content selection for a verbal description of the visualization.

---
3 This terminology is related to the reference model for Intelligent Multimedia Presentation Systems; see [BFM$^+$97]. This reference model has been established as a joint effort of researchers. The core of the reference model is an architectural scheme of the key components of multimedia presentation systems.

(3) Event Analysis. In the third step, an *event protocol* is established comprising the events that may effect the verbal description. In general, these events reflect the operations identified in Step 2 that may restrict the extractable information. The events are sent to the *context expert* (recall Fig. 12.5) and analyzed with respect to the actual results of the operations, i.e., whether any preservable properties of the visualizations have been violated globally or locally. Note that user-initiated operations, which usually need no further comment from the system, may have side effects that do require a notification.

(4) Content Selection. In this step, the events that have actually lead to modifications in the image are prioritized, sorted, and filtered according to their impact and the user's specification (recall Sect. 12.3.2). Related events may be combined, events of minor importance may be removed, and user-initiated events may be ignored if they have no severe side effects. As a result, a subset of the original events together with information about causal and temporal order is used for the content selection.

In order to ensure consistency between the figure caption and the image, the statements already generated must be checked as to their validity. This applies also to the validity of lexical mappings for template variables. This process involves an analysis of the effects of events generated, e.g., about the visibility of objects after a rotation of a 3D model. As a result, it may be sufficient to indicate what is no longer valid (recall Sect. 12.3.2).

(5) Linguistic Realization. Based on a linguistic analysis to identify typical phrases in the domain, the text generation is prepared. This analysis includes figure captions and other kinds of textual information related to the description of images. This covers three steps:

(5a) Text Structure Analysis. The sequence of text blocks is analyzed resulting in a description of the contents of each block, e.g., the existence of a title at the beginning, giving a concise description of the depicted contents and a description of the single modifications in the following text blocks.

(5b) Sentence Structure Analysis. If the template-based approach is taken, the result of this analysis is a set of templates (natural language expressions) together with conditions as to how templates should be selected. The templates should consist of typical phrases and be as concise as possible. They are grouped into categories from which no more than one is selected in the generation process. It is surprising that even similar parameters, like viewing directions or positions, may be expressed differently in different domains.

(5c) Lexical Realization of Template Variables. The final step is the mapping of numerical values to template variables. In the case of the template-based approach, for each attribute a numerical value interval is directly mapped to a sequence of words. With this approach, a value is always described in the same way. Colors are an example where this is useful. For this attribute, a widely accepted color naming system has been developed by BERK et al. [BBK82] which can be used to describe colors objectively.

In some cases, absolute mappings using fixed intervals are not suitable. Values are considered differently depending on the range of the values for this quantity in a given visualization; what is large in one context may be very small in another. These issues are discussed in more detail in [SH97].

12.5.4 Representation of Events

All operations that affect the textual or graphical display emit an event notifying the context expert. Operations can affect the whole model, single objects, objects of a region, or a certain category. So, the range of an operation is an important parameter.

As described earlier, modifications may be caused by the system, e.g., to adapt the visualization to the context. For the viewer's comprehension it is crucial whether something changes at his or her request or by an automatic process. Therefore, all events include a parameter indicating who initiated the change: the *user* or the *system*. If the system initiated a manipulation, its reason is also recorded. An event, therefore, has a name and several parameters:

- the range of the event,
- the initiator of the event, and
- the reason for the event and additional parameters enabling the evaluation of the degree of change.

12.6 Concluding Remarks

Descriptive figure captions contribute to a correct interpretation of complex images as they arise in interactive visualization systems. This has been discussed for applications as different as medical illustrations and maps. Descriptive figure captions describe the view of a model. They are crucial to make users aware of important manipulations such as objects which have been removed and thus to make complex image generation processes transparent. Figure captions explain system-initiated manipulations and their reasons as well as complex user manipulations. Dynamic figure captions have some peculiarities compared to their counterparts in traditional media:

- They should be consistent with the image they describe. So the system must analyze whether captions become invalid or incomplete. As a reaction, figure captions are updated or their invalid parts are tagged.
- They can be tailored to the user's needs with appropriate configuration facilities.
- They can be used for the parameterization of the images they describe (interactive figure captions).

The generation of figure captions must be carefully adapted to the availability of other kinds of textual components. They enrich an illustration with information which cannot be conveyed by schematic legends and labels alone.

The incorporation of figure captions is not that cumbersome to accomplish. Using the template-based approach and restricting it to the application domain at hand, only a small number of typical phrases and lexical mappings must be prepared. Furthermore, an internal representation of the state of the interface is required. This representation is not an extra effort exclusively for the generation of figure captions but can be used in a number of ways, e.g., to undo operations, to allow a reset to an earlier stage in an interactive session, or to adapt the system's behavior to the discourse of human–computer interaction.

As a result of the development of interactive figure captions, not only have new interaction facilities emerged but interactive access has also been extended to attributes inaccessible so far. Interaction facilities with captions have been restricted to the replacement of single values until now – additional interaction facilities, like the insertion and removal of items in figure captions are worthy of study.

Although figure captions are just emerging, they serve to accomplish some widely recognized usability goals (see for example NIELSEN [Nie94]): *Make the system's state visible* and *Speak the user's language*. Figure captions present important information about the state of a system. While this effect could partly be achieved with a formal output in the form of spreadsheets (e.g., viewing direction: [Direction], displacements: [List of Displacements]) figure captions are more strongly related to the terminology users are familiar with. The terminology employed is carefully adapted to users who are not programmers, e.g., to students of medicine or cartographers.

The concept of generating, updating, and interacting with figure captions has been derived based on two application areas which are elaborated further in this book. In Chap. 13 examples of figure captions are discussed for anatomic illustrations. Figure captions for cartography are presented in Chap. 20. These discussions follow the approach discussed in Sect. 12.5.

Figure captions in visual interfaces are new and therefore require careful validation. The linguistic approaches employed so far are straightforward. An important area for future work is to refine these approaches, including natural language generation methods. It remains an open question under what circumstances the additional possibilities of natural language generation justify the extra effort compared to the template-based approach.

A possible application of figure captions left for future study is their use as bookmarks. They are used to set landmarks in large information spaces. It would be very useful to generate meaningful names automatically for the organization of bookmarks in visualization systems. Short figure captions can serve for this task. They are consistent with the state of the visual interface and provide the necessary information to recall the generated images.

Finally, if an interactive system makes it possible to produce screenshots, a corresponding figure caption can be saved as well to enhance retrieval tasks. For this purpose, detailed figure captions are required because screenshots are often looked at later in the absence of the interactive situation in which they were generated.

Contributors of Chap. 12: Bernhard PREIM and Rainer MICHEL

Chapter 13

Interactive 3D Illustrations with Images and Text

Interactive 3D graphics have a high potential for the explanation of complex spatial phenomena as can be found, for example, in engineering and anatomy. The interactive exploration of complex 3D models is crucial for spatial understanding. While this is well recognized, not enough effort has been spent on flexibly combining interactive 3D graphics with textual descriptions.

At present the emphasis of the research literature is placed, on the one hand, on the construction and visualization of complex models, and, on the other, on structuring text in hypertext systems in connection with scanned images. The combination of both, however, is necessary to exploit the potential of computer graphics for educational purposes.

The relationship between images and text determines to a large degree whether the depicted content can be extracted. Borrowing from textbooks gives hints on how to combine images and text. Images often are surrounded by labels referring to their parts via reference lines. Explanations refer to the spatial structure and are enhanced by cross references as to spatial relations. In textbooks, however, explanations are generally not integrated in an illustration but are placed under an image or even on a separate page, which complicates comprehension. This is especially true for anatomical illustrations. To study a part of the human body, numerous illustrations with plenty of labels and explanations have to be compared with one another (see, e.g., [Sob88]). This is due to the static character of a book, which makes several viewing directions necessary in order to give an idea of the 3D situation, and due to different aspects (blood vessels, nerves, muscles) which cannot be covered in one image.

Interactive systems can handle this problem and tailor the presentation to the information requested. In current hypermedia systems, however, this often results in the display of multiple windows, the management of which imposes a high burden on the user.

Based on these observations we developed a system to handle interactive illustrations consisting of rendered images and related text. These illustrations are presented within *one* window. Users can ask for explanations which are incorporated immediately in the illustration. To avoid overlapping information and the need to rearrange the desktop, fisheye views, as introduced by FURNAS [Fur86], are used. They simplify navigation because different levels of detail can be presented simultaneously in different parts of an image. To emphasize the importance of zoom techniques, we call our system ZOOMILLUSTRATOR.

With this system the user is able to interact with both the image and the text, while the system is responsible for the *consistency* between these media (see also [PRS$^+$95]). To achieve this consistency, several rules are established which refer to how textual information should relate to an image. Based on these rules material properties and transformations are adapted to emphasize relevant parts and thus ensure their *visibility* and *recognizability*. For ease of viewing, our system aims at continuous transitions between complex views. It turns out that there is a trade-off between this consistency, on the one hand, and the continuous transitions on the other.

Objects of moderate or large size can be emphasized if an appropriate viewing direction is selected and if they are colored in a striking manner. However, to explain a small detail it is not enough to emphasize it or to remove objects which occlude it – it is necessary to scale it to make it recognizable. If the whole model is scaled uniformly it becomes so large that a significant portion must be clipped. From a cognitive point of view it is more useful to scale up the interesting detail only and automatically scale down others. This can be accomplished with a distorting fisheye zoom in three dimensions. The ability of a 3D fisheye view to illustrate local graphical detail in its context is essential for the exploration of complex 3D models. The application of fisheye techniques for label navigation and for the exploration of a 3D model unifies the interaction. We refer to this as *coherent zooming* (see also [PRS97]).

The principles are tested for anatomical illustrations, an interesting area of application, because complex issues are involved which cannot be explained at all without images.

This chapter is organized as follows. Section 13.1 describes previous work on illustration design and on interactive illustrations, in particular from anatomy. In Sect. 13.2 we formulate rules for consistency between rendered images and their textual labels. In Sect. 13.3 the architecture of the system is described. Section 13.4 presents concepts for using zoom techniques in interactive illustrations. In Sect. 13.5 we describe the interactive handling with respect to the rules for consistency. It turns out that conflicts arise. Different strategies are presented to solve these conflicts which differ in the range of users involved. Because our system aims at interactivity but also involves complex transformations, compromises between the quality of illustrations and the rendering times are necessary. The application of figure captions to further assist a user in exploring geometric models is presented in Sect. 13.6. In the concluding section the approach is summarized and future work is discussed.

13.1 Related Work

Our work has been inspired by research on illustration design. As we apply our system mainly to anatomy we briefly survey interactive illustrations in this field. As fisheye zoom techniques are the basic interaction paradigm, previous work on applications of fisheye views is also related to this work. But this work was summarized in Chap. 9.

13.1.1 Generating Illustrated Documents

Work on illustration design concentrated on techniques for illustrating 3D models and on combining images with other media, like text. The IBIS system (Intent-Based Illustration System) of SELIGMANN and FEINER [SF91a] is the pioneering work in the field of 3D illustration design. It is based on an extensive study of what technical illustrators do in order to achieve their intent. Besides techniques to bridge the gap between intent and realization in static illustrations, an interactive component is included. IBIS illustrates complex 3D models using transparency, cut-aways, and insets (small details scaled up in a large image). We learned from their work that *visibility* and *recognizability* of important objects are crucial for illustrating 3D models. With IBIS, excellent images can be produced, but textual descriptions are not included.

In contrast to the IBIS system, the work carried out in the WIP project (Knowledge-Based Information Presentation) by WAHLSTER et al. [WAF+93] targets the coordination of images and text. This includes sophisticated strategies to annotate an image with textual labels. Furthermore, an integrated planning scheme ensures a close relation between the images generated and the verbal comments. WIP has been applied mainly to explain the handling and maintenance of technical devices. To emphasize the use of knowledge-based techniques for the coordination of different media, the term *IntelliMedia* systems has been derived. The knowledge-based approach has been extended to a semi-interactive method to illustration design (see ANDRÉ and RIST [AR94]). The process of generating an illustration has become interactive, but the goal remains to design a final illustration and not to provide an interactive illustrator.

13.1.2 Interactive Anatomical Illustrations

While IBIS and WIP have been applied to technical domains with regular, often convex shapes, anatomical illustrations are characterized by highly irregular shapes. A look at interactive anatomical illustrations reveals systems based on scanned images and those using 3D models. The latter are more advanced because they allow more flexible transformations of the subject being studied. The leading example in this field is the VOXELMAN developed at the University of Hamburg by HÖHNE et al. (see [PPR+94]) and [SNTH96]. The VOXELMAN employs volume models, constructed using imaging approaches (e.g., CT images and MR images) from patient-specific data. The use of volume models offers free positioning as well as the possibility to interactively cut off or take away parts, i.e., literally to operate virtually. For educational purposes it is extremely helpful that parts of the geometric model (voxels in this case) are related to symbolic knowledge (labels, structural information). For the integration of geometric information and symbolic knowledge a special data structure, *Intelligent Voxels*, has been designed. Although the images are labeled and optionally explained, the coherence of pictorial and textual information, the correspondence between these basic components is not managed by the system. For example, users are responsible for the placement of annotations. Explanations are presented in separate windows and are therefore hard to integrate mentally with an image.

Summarizing related work on illustration design and interactive illustrations, we can conclude:

To convey information with pictures (for educational purposes or maintenance) more than mere geometry is necessary. Symbolic information, like labels and textual description, is required. Consequently, interaction facilities should support the exploration of both pictorial and related symbolic information. In the IBIS and WIP projects AI approaches have been exploited for illustration design. Although we target interaction facilities we realize that an interactive system can benefit from high-level support over and above the direct-manipulative handling of an illustration.

The synthesis of an overall layout with areas for images and text, the placement of annotations around an image and the coordination between images and text are candidates for high-level support.

13.1.3 Fisheye Techniques to Explore 3D Models and Related Text

Integrated image-text illustration systems must deal with orientation and navigation in large information spaces. Fisheye views, with their ability to integrate detail and context, are well-suited for this purpose (recall Chap. 2). We are especially interested in a comfortable exploration of textual information and of the underlying 3D model.

FURNAS [Fur86] pioneered the idea of fisheye views. The placement of information is guided by a degree of interest (*DOI*) derived from user interaction. From a cognitive point of view, it is desirable that changes between successive views are animated smoothly. This is accomplished with the *Continuously Variable Zoom* introduced by DILL et al. in [DBHH94]. The Variable Zoom manipulates rectangular areas in which all information to be presented is embedded. If more detail is requested for one piece of information, called a *node*, the corresponding rectangle is enlarged at the expense of others, the sizes of which are reduced accordingly. As a consequence of the scaling, the representation changes depending on application-specific thresholds.

13.1.4 3D Fisheye Zoom

Recently RAAB [RR96] extended the 2D fisheye zoom to the third dimension. The 3D zoom turns out to be very effective for the exploration of 3D models. Graphical objects can be scaled up, while others are automatically scaled down and moved away. With the 3D zoom a similar effect as in exploded views can be realized. The 3D zoom enables the illustration of graphical details because their visibility and their recognizability is improved.

We incorporate the 3D zoom in the ZOOMILLUSTRATOR and apply fisheye views to both the exploration of a 3D model and navigation through text. Thus a uniform interaction is offered.

13.2 Consistency of Rendered Images and Their Textual Labels

Our design is guided by rules for consistency between images and textual information. We derived these rules by an analysis of traditional teaching materials (e.g., [Sob88]) and by following explicit hints in books which describe how to make good medical illustrations (e.g., [Bri90]). These rules guide the creation of an initial illustration as well as the placement of information after user interaction.

1. Labels are connected by reference lines to the objects in an image to which they refer.
2. Graphical objects which are textually explained should be easily recognizable.
3. The labeling of objects should be adapted to the visibility of the objects.
4. The placement of labels should be coherent with the position of reference points in an image in order to avoid long lines crossing each other.
5. The size of labels should vary according to the depth of the object referred to in the image.

While these rules sound simple enough, their strict application results in radical (and therefore irritating) changes of the presentation. We will explain the problems that might arise later in this chapter and show how to solve the problems that do arise.

13.3 Architecture

The generation of an illustration is based on four input sources (see the top four vertical boxes in Fig. 13.1): The first is a *scene description*, containing a polygonal 3D model which is structured into objects. To ensure high-quality images, we rely on commercially available models. The object structure has been tailored using the ZOOMSTRUCTOR as described in Chap. 3.

Secondly, we employ related *textual descriptions* referring to the objects in the scene description. Textual descriptions include labels, short explanations, and extended explanations as to more specific aspects. Short explanations contain pointers to more detailed information. Textual information of different nodes are connected with each other via cross-references. Furthermore, each object has a reference to the category it belongs to. This allows the creation of illustrations with the focus on certain categories. Textual information is the result of the enrichment process as explained in Chap. 3. Textual information tends to be very long, as detailed descriptions for each

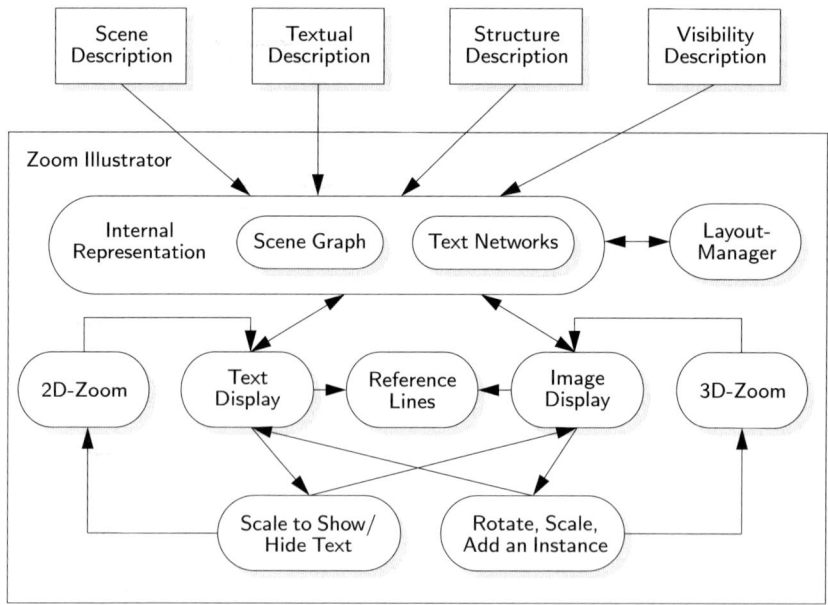

Figure 13.1: Architecture of an integrated image text illustration system

object are involved. For many purposes it is useful to have an extract of this information to find out which categories exist, which nodes belong to a certain category, how many nodes are linked to nodes of a category, and which kind of explanations exist for a category. This extract is summarized in *structure information*. Structure information is like a header-file for textual information.

Finally, we use precalculated *visibility information*. This file contains information on which objects are visible for discrete viewing directions. Azimuth and declination have been increased with a step size of 45 degrees each – resulting in an amount of 26 viewing directions, which turned out to be a reasonable amount of information. For each object an "optimal" viewing direction is registered (optimal in terms of visibility and size). Figure 13.2 illustrates how this information is derived. The information is recorded off-line because it is time-consuming to derive. As we will see, this information is very useful for the interaction.

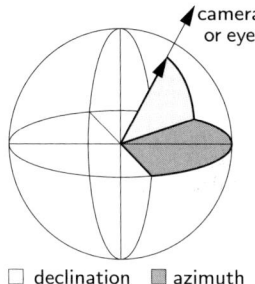

Figure 13.2: Visibility information is derived from several viewing directions

After the sources are loaded, an internal representation is generated using a common identifier for objects in the external sources. This step is followed by the choice of which categories are important. The user can select the available categories from a menu, the content of which is derived from structure information. Such a selection is essential because the whole amount of information for one part of the human body is overwhelming and cannot be presented in its entirety in one view.

Layout synthesis. Based on the selected categories, an initial illustration is created which includes labels, reference lines, and the rendered image. This task is accomplished by the *layout manager*. The decision which objects to label is a two-step process. The first step is to find out whether all relevant objects (relevant in terms of categories selected) can be labeled. Depending on the number of relevant objects, the font size for the labels is determined. A conflict arises when there are too many relevant objects for their labels to be displayed with legible size in their entirety. In this case a second step selects the most important objects according to their *DOI* (recall Chap. 9). The layout manager is also responsible for a well-balanced arrangement of labels around an image.

The application of zoom techniques in textual information requires a concept for the distribution of textual information in different domains. To ensure that the image is not occluded by the text and vice versa, the ZOOM-ILLUSTRATOR's window is subdivided into a central part for the image (covering half of the screen), and a left and a right part for label networks with textual descriptions, each occupying 25 percent of the screen (see Fig. 13.3).

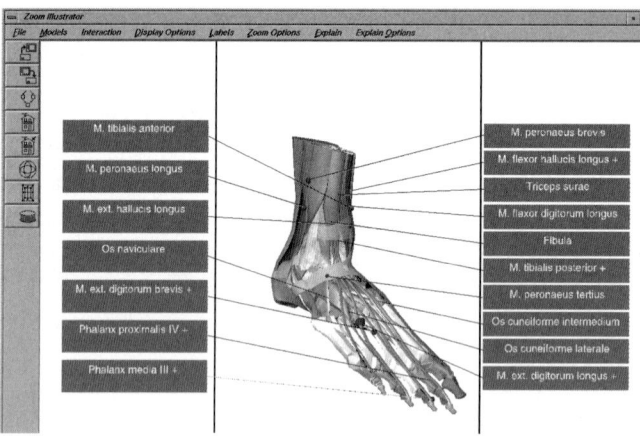

Figure 13.3: Basic layout with text networks on the left side and right side of the rendered 3D model with white lines superimposed to show the separate areas

Annotation. The process of linking labels to parts of an image is referred to as *annotation* (compare [Ris95]). Annotation in our system is realized via reference lines which connect labels to parts of an image. Placing labels directly in an illustration is very unusual in anatomical illustrations. It is ensured that a point of the object's surface near the bounding box center is selected as reference point. This point is marked with a small disk. If an object consists of several distinct parts one reference point is calculated for each part. This annotation is not optimal for the illustration of complex, irregular shaped objects, as they occur in anatomy. To clarify the shape of these objects, a topological analysis is necessary to identify branching structures and calculate reference points which reveal the characteristic shape of these objects.

13.4 Zoom Techniques for Illustration Purposes

Integrated image-text illustration systems deal with very different information domains. On the one hand, we have the graphical domain consisting of a set of scanned or rendered images (the latter being generated from surface or volumetric models). On the other hand, there is a lot of textual information to convey, describing function, relations, and assembly (see Fig. 13.4, which depicts an information space). While there are often limited representations available on the graphical side, the textual information representation can be chosen by several aspects.

The presentation of information is further characterized by *presentation variables*, as there are fonts and colors for the text display as well as color, transparency, and textures for the display of graphical objects. Therefore, a coherent illustration system needs to select uniformly the representation (*what* information to convey) as well as the presentation (*how* to convey the information) in the different information domains. Furthermore, the interaction with both parts of the information space should also be uniform to enable users to access the information through a common interface.

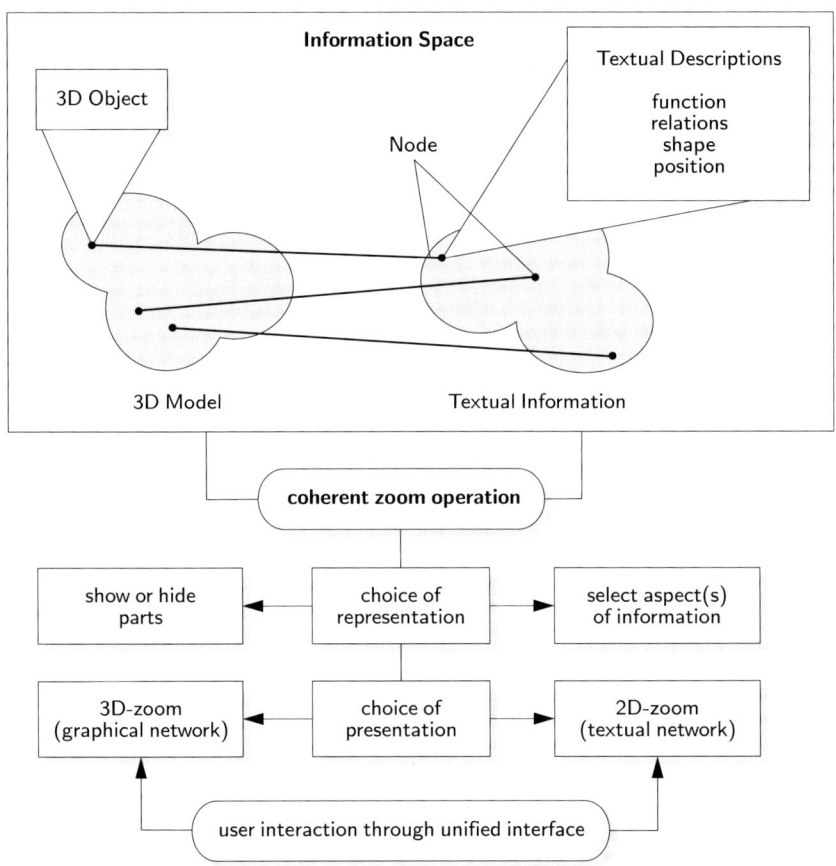

Figure 13.4: Coherent zooming in an integrated image-text illustration system

The application of fisheye views to graphical as well as to textual navigation helps to achieve these goals. User interaction based on zoom operations give comparable feedback if applied to the graphical or textual parts. We will refer to this point later.

As a prerequisite for the application of fisheye views we define a representation matrix for each category (recall Chap. 9 and [RPR96]). The choice of a representation can be approached by either explicit user interaction or the computation of what we call the aspect of interest, based on the interaction history and on the level of detail (LOD). By defining a representation matrix, the approach is adjustable to different domains. For each category there is a different set of representations. Each category, e.g., an organ system in anatomy, is characterized by aspects for which textual descriptions are provided.

In the ZOOMILLUSTRATOR the representations are as follows (see Fig. 13.5): all nodes have a label-representation. The more extended representations differ depending on the category. For instance, muscles have explanations as to their function, their nerve supply (innervation), and their shape, whereas bones simply have an explanation as to their location. Since the muscle category is an example with different aspects for one LOD, the system must decide whether the user is interested in the shape, the innervation, or the function. Based on the representation matrix, an appropriate representation is selected. The details of this process were given in Chap. 9 where the ZOOMILLUSTRATOR was described as an application of the Zoom Navigation paradigm.

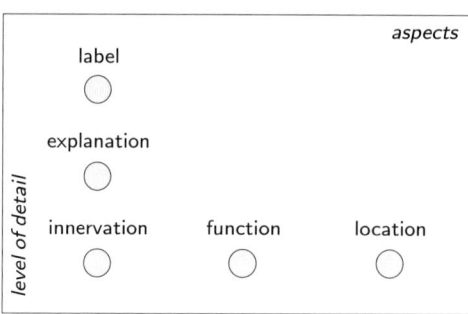

Figure 13.5: Representation matrix for one category in the ZOOMILLUSTRATOR

13.4.1 Zoom Techniques for Navigation in Textual Information

The distribution of the screen space available into areas for image and text display (recall Fig. 13.3) is only a starting point. Text networks and the 2D bounding box of the rendered image are parts of a top-level zoom network. When interaction occurs, the DOI of the two label networks and the graphics box change, which results in a varying size (from -10 to $+10$ percent compared to the original size). With this top-level zoom, a network can provide more space if several explanations are requested. Moreover, individual nodes are allowed to extend their width by 10 percent to accommodate more information.

Interacting with textual information is accomplished by scaling a rectangle which accommodates the information. The zoom component is invoked to redistribute the place for all rectangles of this network. The continuous zoom algorithm is adapted to take into account the legibility of textual information (as minimum size) and the space needed to display explanations (as maximum size). Figure 13.6 presents an example with two nodes explained after having been zoomed up continuously to accommodate an explanation.

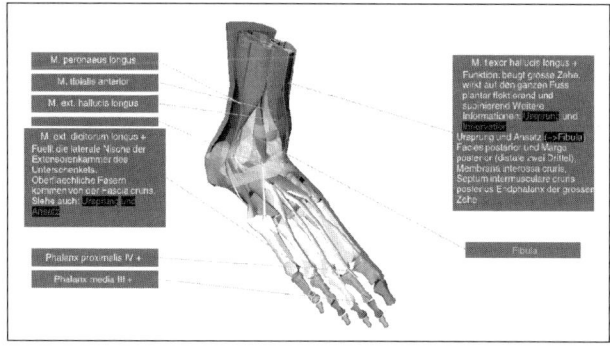

Figure 13.6: Integrating explanations in an illustration with zoom techniques

Interaction with the textual information causes currently explained objects to be automatically colored to be recognizable (corresponding Rule 2). The color of the explained object depends on its original color which will become more saturated when it is explained. However, the space available allows no more than one or two explanations to be displayed simultaneously. Therefore, explained objects can be colored without confusing the whole presentation.

Furthermore, the 3D model is transformed automatically if an object for which a user requested an explanation is not visible. For this purpose, objects which hide the object to be explained are rendered semi-transparent. If too many objects are in front of the interesting one, this technique does not ensure the recognizability of the hidden object. In this case the whole model is rotated (compare Chap. 3, where the same approach was used to emphasize objects in the model view after being selected in the view of the model's structure). For this adaptation the information about "optimal" viewing directions from the visibility information is exploited.

The size of the explaining text is limited to some 30 words per explanation. However, in most cases this is enough for describing spatial relations. Usually, the continuous zoom works independently in the left and right text areas to prevent irritating changes in one part due to interaction in the other. However, if one explanation is displayed which consumes all the space available on one side, one or two nodes are moved to the other side. This movement consists of a zoom step to provide the space in the target network and an animated movement. If users ask for an explanation, the corresponding node is zoomed up to accommodate the required amount of text. Other nodes are scaled down appropriately. If they become too small to display their label, only a rectangle with a reference line is displayed, so that interaction with this node is still possible. If the node becomes even smaller it is closed completely. We describe later how users can prevent nodes from being closed and how to get nodes back which were closed inadvertently.

13.4.2 Zoom Techniques for the Exploration of a 3D Model

In geometric models with a level of detail appropriate for explanation purposes there are many objects of very different sizes, leading to the problem of how small objects can be illustrated clearly. Furthermore, interactive illustrations should support learning goals directly derived from a graphical model such as (compare [RR96] and Chap. 9):

- recognizing relationships between several objects,
- recognizing the positions of objects in the model, and
- inspecting the shapes of (occluded) objects in the model.

As was shown in Chap. 9, these tasks can be accomplished with the 3D fisheye zoom. For the application in the ZOOMILLUSTRATOR it is important that an object can be scaled up while the overall model size remains constant. The constant model size is necessary to prevent labels and image hiding each other. Separate windows for images and text cause other problems, for example, they have to be placed in a location where they do not hide the current illustration window.

The advantages of integrating the 3D zoom in the ZOOMILLUSTRATOR are similar to those for the ZOOMSTRUCTOR (recall Chap. 3).

13.4.3 Adaptive Graphical Zoom

We still have to describe how we incorporate the graphical zoom in the user interface. At first glance it might be not convincing to zoom within the 3D model at all, because the study of topological relations is an important issue and these are distorted to a certain extent by the graphical zoom. However, adaptive scalings are employed in traditional teaching materials as we pointed out in Chap. 3 when we described the enrichment of geometric models with the ZOOMSTRUCTOR. The 3D zoom is used in very similar ways in both systems. The 3D zoom is only invoked by the system in a restricted way (for small objects with small scale factors) to prevent heavy distortions.

This feature is for the ZOOMILLUSTRATOR even more important than for the ZOOMSTRUCTOR because its users are not supposed to know the model very well (in contrast to the person who prepares the data). Figure 13.7 gives an example of an illustration with a muscle enlarged to support its verbal explanation (left side).

Users can reset the 3D zoom so that all changes as to relative sizes are undone. The 3D zoom enables us to emphasize graphical objects which are textually explained according to Rule 2.

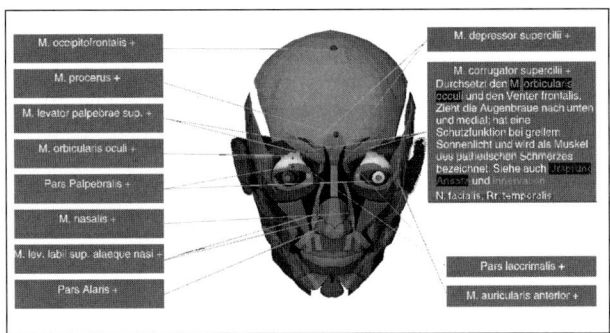

Figure 13.7: One muscle (above the eyes) has been enlarged to be explained, while others have been scaled down and moved away

13.4.4 Enhancing Navigation in Textual Information

One important question when applying zoom techniques concerns hiding nodes automatically. While the zoom algorithm generally produces comprehensible layouts, it might be irritating, especially for beginners, when a node disappears due to the size request of another node. Even when users understand what has happened they might not know what they are supposed to do to get a node back which has disappeared inadvertently. The method of getting the hidden node back by scaling down another node is not very intuitive and, moreover, a trial-and-error process. This raises two questions:

- How to prevent nodes from being closed (*preventive action*), and
- How to get nodes back which have been closed (*curative action*).

We present one possible solution for each question.

Prevent Nodes from Being Closed. To prevent nodes from being closed (preventive strategy), we introduce an additional network, a *pinwall*, as a container for some privileged nodes (up to four). These nodes are not exposed to the zoom and can therefore not be closed, but they can just as little be scaled up to show an explanation as long as they belong to the pinwall. This strategy is more natural than modifying the zoom algorithm itself.

The user can initiate an animated movement of a node to the pinwall (above the rendered image) where it remains at a fixed position (see Fig. 13.8). If there are already nodes at the pinwall, they are smoothly moved away to provide the space necessary for another node. The node is scaled so that just its label can be accommodated. The movement to the pinwall is followed by a zoom step to consume the space in the source network no longer needed. Nodes residing at the pinwall are still connected to the image via reference lines, which are updated as usual if the 3D model is rotated.

Selection of Hidden Nodes. While the movement to the pinwall prevents a node from being closed, we still need an intuitive way to get a node back once it has disappeared (curative strategy). Several approaches are possible:

- Selection of a label via picking the related graphical object, or
- Selection of a label from a container which holds all labels available.

We offer the first selection facility, as it is clearly useful to understand the image-text relation. Moreover, this approach is similar to the way students learn anatomical terms, which is by covering labels and trying to guess the correct name. However, this approach is restricted to visible objects which are large enough to be picked.

Therefore, a container for all nodes is also necessary because it allows a selection independent of the visibility and size of graphical objects. The straightforward idea to do this is to construct a hierarchical menu with layers, sublayers, and individual nodes. However, there is a clear cognitive gap between a menu (either a pop-up menu or a pull-down menu) and the illustration. Therefore, we designed a 3D widget we call a *rondell* which contains all labels grouped according to their category. The design of this 3D widget

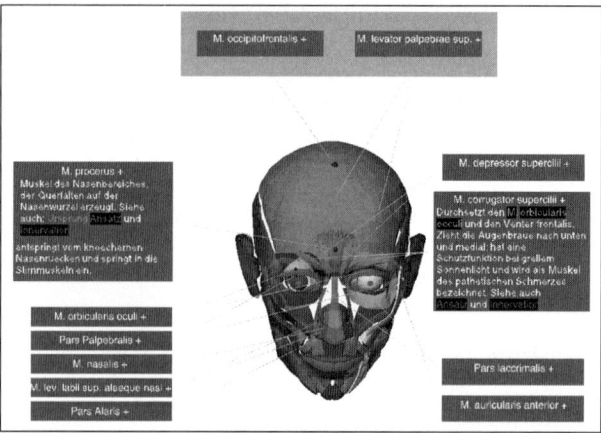

Figure 13.8: An illustration with two nodes residing at fixed positions at the pinwall (upper part)

is inspired by the work carried out at XEROX Parc on 3D interfaces (see MACKINLAY et al. in [MRC91]). Like the *perspective wall* and *cone trees*, the rondell is a 3D widget with an implicit fisheye view (in the terminology of NOIK, [Noi94]). The integration of detail (labels at the front) and context (labels at the side walls) is based on perspective transformations. It is designed for selection of non-hierarchical data.

The rondell can be rotated by clicking on the disks at the top and the bottom part, one for a rotation to the left and one for the rotation to the right. The color of the nodes that are closed is a saturated blue (instead of a weak gray for the nodes already presented) to encourage the user to invoke the node (see Fig. 13.9). The rondell is capable of displaying non-hierarchical data. Informal tests with medical students revealed that the ability of the rondell to browse to all textual information available is regarded as useful and justifies the screen space occupied.

The user can select a label on the rondell, which results in the display of the corresponding node with an additional highlighting to emphasize what has happened. The rondell can also be used for exploration of the 3D model. If a certain option is set, a simplified material editor is presented. This allows the user to show/hide the related graphics part and to change its color. Informal usability studies indicate that this freedom is useful. Users like to be able to hide objects occluding something essential. While users tend to recognize the rondell as an appropriate 3D widget and indicate they like it, it also has disadvantages:

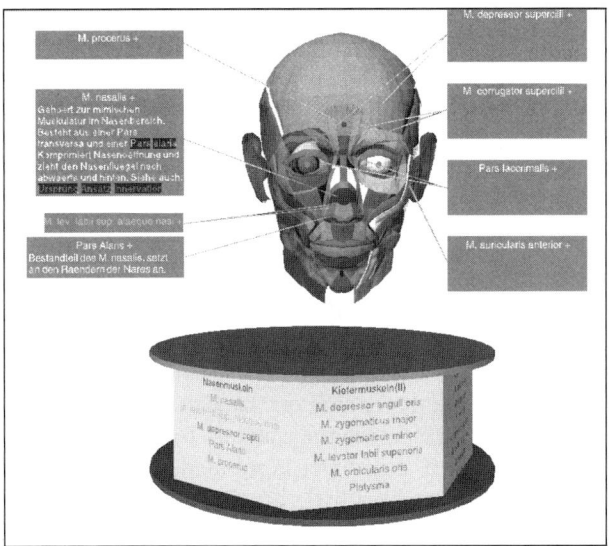

Figure 13.9: A label from the rondell was selected which is subsequently displayed in the illustration (left side)

- A rondell is less familiar than conventional menus.
- A 3D widget with 3D text requires considerable computing resources to render, which either slows down the system or requires a reduction in the quality (resolution) of the text presentation.

The selection of a hidden node – no matter whether the selection has been carried out by picking in the 3D model or via the rondell – leads to a zoom step which smoothly creates the space necessary for the selected label. Selection via the rondell is emphasized by coloring the rondell entry and the newly selected label with the same color.

Continuous Zooming Discrete Representations. Some problems when applying the continuous zoom for navigation in textual information are due to the fact that there are discrete representations for text which differ considerably in the space needed to display them. Each representation is hidden if the space does not suffice to display them entirely. This strategy is reasonable because fragments of a sentence the last words of which have been cut are not helpful. However, this can result in an ineffective usage of screen space with large rectangles which only display their label. Therefore, the result of the zoom algorithm is not directly mapped onto the presentation. Instead, the result is evaluated as to whether annoying effects would arise. If this is the case, a postprocess is carried out to improve the layout. Annoying effects and the postprocess to circumvent them are described in [PRS97].

13.5 Interactive Handling of Images and Text

The interaction facilities offered include navigation through textual information and transformation of an image. The reference lines which connect textual information with the image cannot be altered directly, but are updated automatically according to the position of the objects and textual information (according to Rule 1).

The zoom algorithm (recall Sect. 13.4.1) influences the size of the rectangles. While this is the main feature of the zoom, it is questionable whether additional modifications of the presentation are useful to emphasize the nodes which are explained (according to Rule 2).

Tests were carried out to discuss whether it is helpful to adapt other presentation variables, like the size of the font, the color of the rectangle, and the thickness of reference lines, depending on the size of the rectangles. The idea behind a color change is to increase the contrast between the rectangle's color and the background color if the object is zoomed up. Reference lines, which are originally very thin, become a little bit thicker if the corresponding label is zoomed up to make the correspondence between the textual information and the reference object clear. However, this technique is not applied when a label is zoomed up which has several reference lines because this would hopelessly overcrowd the image. Because the value of these adaptions turns out to be controversial, the features can be turned on and off interactively. If they are turned on, they influence the presentation after zooming a label and after rotating the model (in the case of a rotation the rectangle's size is adapted to the depth values of the reference objects). Figure 13.10 shows an example with all features turned on.

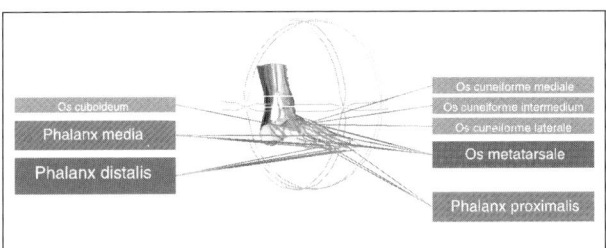

Figure 13.10: Color, font size, and line width are adapted to the size of the rectangles due to differing depth values after a rotation

13.5.1 Managing Consistency when Geometric Transformations Occur

Compared to traditional media, the great potential of interactive illustrations lies in the interactive handling of 3D models. To use this potential, an intuitive and direct approach for 3D interaction is required. For this purpose we exploit 3D widgets which allow the direct manipulative handling of 3D models (note that only 3D widgets can exploit the advantages of direct manipulation for 3D models). These widgets have separate handles to control the degrees of freedom inherent in 3D interaction. The virtual trackball (see Figs. 13.11 and 13.13) allows separate rotation around the x, y, and z axes. [HvDG94] gives an overview on problems of 3D interaction, while [Hou92] deals in detail with 3D object transformation. The correspondence between geometric transformations of the image and textual information with respect to the consistency rules defined in Sect. 13.2 is complex. While scaling leaves the relation between labels and image intact insofar as the same objects are visible and the relation of their sizes remains the same, rotation changes the visibility of objects. Experiments have shown that strictly applying Rule 3 (adaptations of objects to labels) is neither easy to achieve in real time nor useful for the student, because small rotations could lead to dramatic changes of the labels. Instead, precalculated visibility is employed to update the labels displayed only after major changes.

Another problem concerning rotation is that reference lines, which were originally well aligned, may cross each other after a rotation (violation of Rule 4). Furthermore, very long lines arise due to rotation if objects move from left to right while their labels remain in the same position. These effects

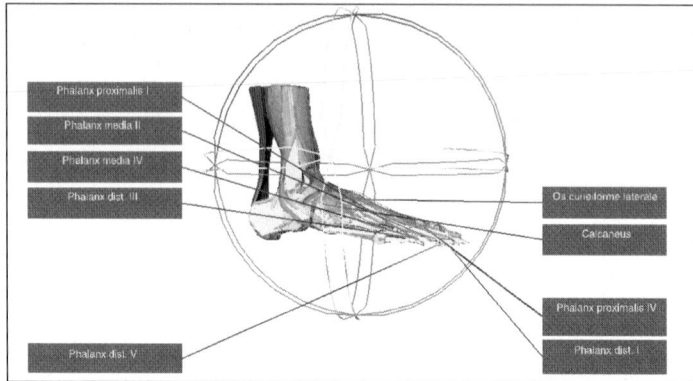

Figure 13.11: Bones of the foot after rotation with the virtual trackball. Due to the rotation very long reference lines from the labels on the right side to reference object in the left part of the image arise

are illustrated in Fig. 13.12. While studying the subject, the alert eye will find that the crossing lines are annoying. On the other hand, rearranging labels in real time would result in a permanent movement of both labels and reference lines, which is highly irritating. To provide both smooth transitions on the fly and well-balanced displays for carefully studying, rearranging labels to prevent crossing lines is initiated by a user only.

Whether the maintenance of Rule 5 (the adaption of the size of labels to the depth-value of the objects referred) is helpful or not depends to a large extent on the number of labels. While it allows an easy comparison of the positions of a few objects, it is irritating for several dozens of labels, the position of which cannot be recognized at a glance. To cope with this, a threshold value for the number of labels is taken into account.

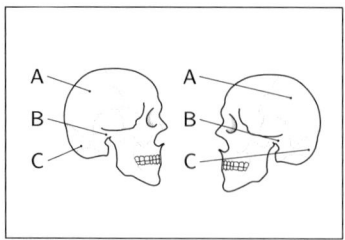
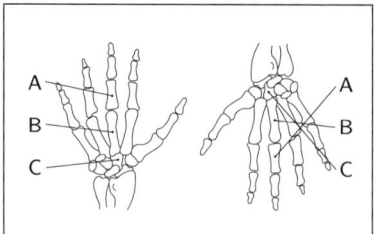

(a) The labels are near the reference points in the left image, but very long lines arise after rotation by 180°

(b) Reference lines which were well-aligned (left) cross each other after a rotation by 180° (right)

Figure 13.12: Problems with annotations after rotation

Besides allowing a user to manipulate a single image, a second image of the same subject can be added and transformed independently of the first. To present a subject from two different views is a common technique in anatomical atlases (see, e.g., [Sob88]) and very useful to develop a mental model of the spatial relations. The images are placed beside each other with labels on the left side of the left image and on the right side of the right image.

Those organ systems which are not in the focus are drawn even more transparent than in the case of one image, because the total amount of information has increased. This way a concentration on the parts of interest is supported. Figure 13.13 shows an illustration created this way.

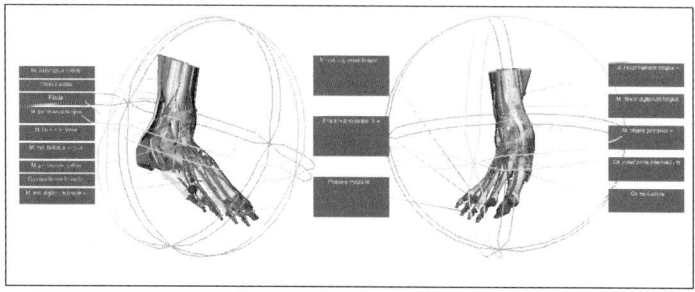

Figure 13.13: Two instances of a geometric model can be operated independently of each other with labels in the middle which refer to objects visible in both instances

In the case of two views of the same object, presented at the same time, the rearrangement of labels after rotation involves the determining which objects are visible in both images. The labels referring to these objects are placed between the images with reference lines to both to support the student in mentally integrating the two model views. See Fig. 13.13 for an example of this technique. When a second instance of the geometric model is created and one object is visible in both instances, it must be decided which of the two depth-values is judged to modify the font size of the label according to Rule 5. In the current implementation, the reference object nearest to the observer determines the size of the labels. With this decision, an object which is visible in both images is labeled large, and thereby emphasized, if it is near to the observer in at least one of the instances of the geometric model. This seems to be reasonable because objects visible in both images should have a higher priority than those parts which are only visible in one image.

13.5.2 Implementation Issues

A careful selection of quality–speed trade-offs is crucial for the acceptance of interactive illustrations. However, implementation issues are – by their very nature – very much dependent on a specific environment. Despite this, some aspects are relevant beyond the very specific environment in which the ZOOM-ILLUSTRATOR was developed. Quality is important when the illustration is "static", when no zoom operation or geometric transformation is carried out. By contrast, when the model is manipulated via a virtual manipulator it is essential that the system "answers" in a reasonable period of time. Quality is less important in this situation because the user has no time to look at the illustration carefully. Based on this consideration, several rendering parameters are worth considering:

- Antialiasing,
- Rendering transparent objects, and
- Resolution of implicitly defined objects.

Antialiasing, especially when applied to lines and to letters, improves the appearance of an illustration considerably. However, it is realized usually by rendering the whole model several times in *accumulation buffers*. This method is time-consuming and should be switched off if no hardware support is available.

There are several methods to render objects transparent. While high-quality methods sort all objects as to their depth-value and apply a blending method, better performance is achieved with stippling approaches which simulate transparency with textures at the cost of introducing visible artifacts.

While the 3D models to be illustrated (in our examples the foot and the face) are explicitly defined with the coordinates of their polygons, several objects in the illustration have no explicit representation, as there are spheres, cylinders (the rondell), and text. These implicitly defined objects are transformed into triangle strips before being rendered. This transformation can be realized with very different resolutions. To give you an idea how crucial this parameter is, the 3D text projected to the rondell is transformed into more than 100K triangles if the highest available quality is used, which is much more than the anatomic model being illustrated. Clearly, the rondell cannot be rotated in real time with this high-quality text presentation. Fortunately, the highest resolution is not necessary as the text cannot be read while the rondell is moving.

The decision which approach to take is of course strongly influenced by whether or not hardware support exists. The environment we choose for our development, the OPEN INVENTOR (see [Wer94]), supports a variety af hardware. In [PRS+95] implementation issues are described in more detail.

13.6 Figure Captions for Anatomical Illustrations

This section presents the application of dynamic figure captions as introduced in Sect. 12.3. These figure captions are directly related to the analysis of anatomical atlases as discussed in Sect. 12.1.1. This application provides insight into what is necessary to transform the conceptual architecture presented in Chap. 12 into a working prototype (recall Fig. 12.5).

13.6.1 Important Parameters of Visualizations

(1) Task Analysis. When anatomical illustrations are studied, it is important to be able to integrate the depicted content into a larger context. The user should be able to interpret what is shown from which direction. Furthermore, the location and topological relations of objects are of interest. In anatomy, visualizations are labeled. It is not clear for the user, however, whether all objects of a category are labeled or whether some of them are not, e.g., due to space restrictions (recall Sect. 12.1.1).

From this analysis we derive the important parameters of a visualization. These include parameters of the textual and the graphics display. The state of the textual information is represented by the set of objects which are labeled or textually explained. The state of the graphical display includes the number of instances (usually one or two placed next to each other) and the viewing directions for each instance. Other parameters describe the state of individual objects. Objects are often rendered in a semi-translucent manner, e.g., to expose an object otherwise occluded. Transparency is the most important presentation variable because it affects not only the object modified but also objects behind it.

(2) Analysis of the Visualization Algorithms. For interactive 3D illustrations the most important analysis concerns the visibility of objects after changing the viewing direction. The 3D model has to be analyzed concerning what objects are hidden by what objects and to what extent as well as to which objects are now visible. Because this analysis is computationally expensive, a preprocessing is employed. Another aspect of this step is the analysis of color contrasts (users may modify colors directly, which has side effects for contrasts).

(3) Event analysis. All events are represented as messages in the Context Expert (recall Fig. 13.1). An example for an event is

$$rotated(model[left], user, [40, 30, 40])$$

which records that the user has rotated the left instance of the model with the last parameter specifying the amount of the rotation. Thus all important information about the event and its range and initiation is preserved. The effect of the event, such as that objects become visible and other disappear are not recorded. To describe the visibility of objects, a visibility analysis is employed (rays from the camera into the model are traced and the sequence of objects hit by them is returned).

(4) Content Selection. In the content selection process, events are filtered as to whether they affect the global state or only single objects. Furthermore, it is analyzed whether visibility or "only" presentation variables change. The filtering process considers both the a priori importance of events and the user specification.

(5) Linguistic Realization.

(5a) Text Structure Analysis. The text structure analysis resulted in seven categories for which templates are required. The caption should start with a description of the model view which includes the name of the model, the viewing direction, and the aspects selected. Different templates are required, depending on, for example, whether one model view is presented or two are presented simultaneously. The second category of templates describes the filtering process of labels (whether all relevant labels could be displayed or not). Other categories include system decisions on how to emphasize objects, the description of rendering styles and attributes. As a result, these categories are arranged in a sequence which represents the order in which they are realized.

(5b) Sentence Structure Analysis. Template definition yielded 27 templates, representing a small yet sufficient set of phrases for the composition of figure captions. The first category includes all templates which describe the overall view. Let us give an example of the templates for the first category, where [model] represents the name of a model to illustrate, [direction] a viewing specification, and [aspect list] a set of important categories:

1. The [model] from [direction].
2. The [model] from [$direction_1$] and [$direction_2$].
3. The [model] from [$direction_1$] and [$direction_2$] – on the left [$aspect\ list_1$], on the right [$aspect\ list_2$].
4. The [model] from [direction] – on the left [$aspect\ list_1$], on the right [$aspect\ list_2$].

With this collection we have four templates, of which one is selected by the system as the first sentence of the figure caption. If only one instance of the 3D model is depicted, the first template is chosen. If there is a left and a right instance of the 3D model, one of the templates 2, 3, or 4 is chosen.

(5c) Lexical Realization of Template Variables. We need phrases to name colors, transparency values, and viewing directions. The naming of viewing directions considers conventions of the medical domain. In medical images, the frontal view, for example, is referred to as *ventral*, which is more exact because ventral means "from the stomach". Thus a reference point of the human body is used to name a viewing direction. By analogy, other viewing directions are named accordingly with reference to the human body.

13.6.2 Examples

We start with an initial view of the system immediately after the user has specified which model he or she wants to look at and which aspects he or she is interested in. The system produces an initial view of this model. From this user specification, the system decides from which direction the model should be presented and which objects to label. The figure captions (see Fig. 13.14) describe this and inform the user that all objects relevant to the specification of interesting objects are labeled.[1]

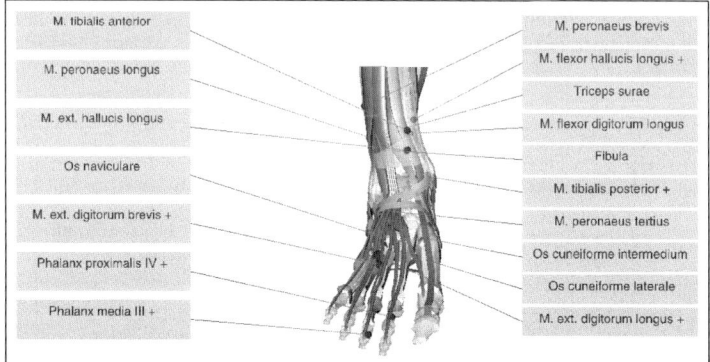

Figure 13.14: The ZOOMILLUSTRATOR has produced an initial view described by an appropriate figure caption (the layout corresponds to the sketch in Fig. 12.1).

Let us look at another example, using the model of a face for illustration. The user has manipulated the presentation so that the left and the right parts of the model look different. The figure caption includes a phrase indicating that the objects near the surface have been rendered semi-translucent in the right part of the model (see Fig. 13.15).

The next image shows again the model of a foot. The user has requested an explanation for a very small muscle. The system has automatically enlarged this muscle to emphasize it. This side effect is reflected in the figure caption (see Fig. 13.16).

Finally, let us have a look at a situation with two instances of a 3D model and its description in Fig. 13.17.

---

1 The captions are slightly enlarged. The bold parts result from the templates, while the words in plain text result from the substitution of variables. The sensitive parts are surrounded by a rectangle.

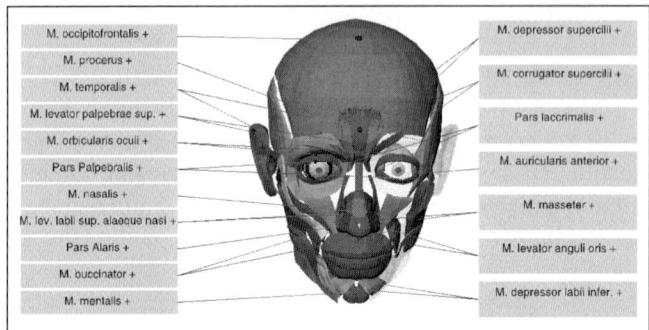

Figure 13.15: Different parameters were used in both halves of a symmetric model

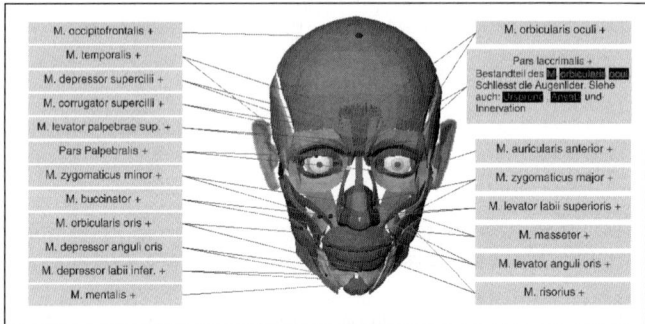

Figure 13.16: The figure caption includes comments on how the sizes have changed to explain an object

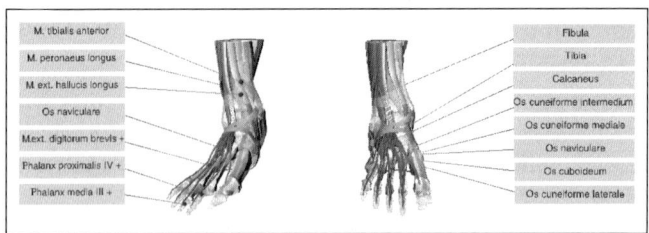

Figure 13.17: The caption for two instances of a 3D model consists of the similarities of both instances followed by the peculiarities of the left and right image

13.7 Concluding Remarks

Interactive illustration systems require facilities to explore text and graphics while maintaining a close relation between these basic media. We presented the ZOOMILLUSTRATOR, a system to illustrate complex models. Our system combines the direct manipulative handling of geometric models with the interaction facilities of a hypertext system. We investigated the relation between rendered image and textual information referring to it, and defined rules for *consistency* between images and text.

While it was relatively easy to derive rules for a consistent static presentation, it turns out that conflicts between these rules and the temporal coherence of successive images arise. It becomes apparent that these conflicts must be tackled carefully with dedicated strategies which differ in the amount of user involvement.

While the straightforward mechanisms which guide the generation of an initial illustration are sufficient, subtle presentation techniques are necessary to combine powerful interaction with an automatic placement of entities. To accomplish this, fisheye techniques are employed. They integrate different levels of detail in *one* window. This contrasts with many systems that allow the user to navigate in a large information space for the price of organizing lots of windows on the screen. The ZOOMILLUSTRATOR can incorporate small explanations as found in anatomical atlases (recall [Sob88] which has been used as a source for the explanations).

Coherent Zooming. We have applied fisheye techniques for the exploration of a 3D model and related text. We refer to this uniform interaction as *coherent zooming*. While it may seem natural to use fisheye views for navigating in textual information, our contribution is that we make it work uniformly on 3D models and in hierarchically organized textual information spaces. Although tested exclusively for anatomical examples, the strategies presented should be easily generalizable for illustrations of other complex 3D phenomena, for example in biology or in engineering. To transform the system to another area of application, a careful segmentation of the information space is necessary.

High-Level Support. The ZOOMILLUSTRATOR has been developed to enable users to directly manipulate an illustration with rendered images and text. But users also benefit from high-level support. The overall layout with separate areas for images and text (pinwall, rondell) is synthesized automatically. Labels and reference lines are calculated and placed by the system. The most important support our system offers has to do with managing a close relation between images and text. It is especially helpful that the system performs automatic transformations and material changes to show an object the user is interacting with. Although these transformations do not provide optimal results in every case, they help users to locate objects. This help is appreciated if objects are involved which are small or difficult to access.

Enriching and Exploring Geometric Models. Many similarities exist between the ZOOMILLUSTRATOR described in this chapter and the ZOOMSTRUCTOR to prepare the necessary data as described in Chap. 3. These similarities are not surprising at second glance. Both the student as the end-user and the person who prepares the data must understand a complex 3D model and the relations between its parts. Both benefit from navigation facilities which integrate detail and context, as fisheye techniques do. Furthermore, an integration of symbolic and graphical information is necessary in both applications. While structure and context information in the ZOOMSTRUCTOR have been presented in different windows, textual descriptions for an end-user are integrated in one window together with the image. While the ZOOMILLUSTRATOR enables the presentation to be tailored to certain categories, the ZOOMSTRUCTOR cannot offer this feature because the categorization has not taken place.

Figure Captions. It is useful for an interactive system to produce figure captions to assist users in orienting themselves in the information space. Helpful captions can be generated using the internal representation of the modifications made on the 3D model. Adaptive scalings caused by the 3D zoom and the use of semi-transparency are graphical means which "deserve" to be mentioned in a figure caption. Furthermore, figure captions can describe the current viewing direction and important objects which are hidden.

Usability Evaluation. The development of our system has been accompanied by informal tests with medical students and colleagues. However, a more systematic usability study is necessary to evaluate the interaction facilities offered. This study should help to find out whether the visualization techniques are adequate and sufficiently flexible. A lot of assumptions have been made, e.g., about the appropriateness of the effect of transparency, which must be validated.

Contributor of Chap. 13: Bernhard PREIM

Part V

Abstraction in Time

Up to now in this book, the emphasis has been on methods and tools for abstraction to produce still images, or key frames. Animation has been used primarily to provide for a smooth transition between such key frames so as to enhance the user's ability to understand what has happened. In this part, we turn to abstraction in animation as a means of expression.

In Chap. 14, Maic MASUCH and Frank GODENSCHWEGER take up the topic of animating non-photorealistic graphics. The main problem they discuss is how to achieve frame-to-frame coherence. Their emphasis is on line drawings where shadows and shading are carried out with cross-hatching.

There are situations in which what is sought are not the key frames, but a process of abstraction to be applied to the transitions themselves. In Chap. 15, Ralf HELBING and Bernhard PREIM study examples where the key frames are "normal" views of objects, but some aspect of the transition between these frames should be highlighted, hence the movements of objects are modified as a means of expression. Along the way, the authors survey how film techniques can be formalized and used by animations systems to generate interesting and informative inbetweening. They give examples both from anatomy as well as technical documentation.

This part only scratches the surface of the topic of abstraction in time, and considerable thought should ultimately be put into other aspects of abstraction in time. For example, what happens to labels when objects are moved? Can figure captions, or more appropriately, animation commentaries, be used to describe what is happening to a viewer?

Chapter 14

Animating Non-photorealistic Computer Graphics

This chapter deals with the creation of 3D non-photorealistic computer animations. It reviews the basic concepts for traditional and computer-generated animation with an emphasis on non-photorealistic animation which, when examined closely, covers more than just the mere rendering of a number of subsequent images. This chapter will not discuss new techniques for object deformation or motion specification but concentrates on the visualization of moving non-photorealistic images. As we will see, this requires new rendering methods for "drawing" a picture.

After a brief introduction to the basics of traditional and computer animation, including main concepts such as keyframes and inbetweening, principles of animation are reviewed. Then we will address the main issue of this chapter, techniques for creating non-photorealistic computer animation. This leads us to the problems of "frame-to-frame coherence" and the "shower-door effect" in non-photorealistic computer animation. We introduce two systems for non-photorealistic computer animation, with a detailed review on animated line drawings, and investigate the behavior of shape, contour, and hatching lines over time.

14.1 A Brief Introduction

Animation has its origin in the word *animare* which means "to bring to life", but one of the most intriguing definitions can be found in [Mea92]: "Computer animation is the heady mixture of visual poetry and mathematics".

An animation creates the illusion of movement by exploiting the inability of the human eye to differentiate very fast subsequent visual impressions into a single image. If the images are displayed with a certain speed, the human visual system integrates the images to create the illusion of continuous movement. The rate at which the displayed image stops flickering depends on the brightness of the image and is at about 25 fps (frames per second). Feature films at the cinema are shown at 24 fps, while common frame rates on TV are 25 fps (European PAL system) and 30 fps (USA) resulting in a refresh rate of approximately 50 Hz, respectively 60 Hz, by the use of half images.

Although animation is always considered to be the motion of objects and cameras, the term animation covers all visual changes of a depicted scene. This includes shape, color, material properties, changes of lighting, camera properties, and even rendering techniques.

Today we find 3D computer animation in many areas of application, like science, business, education, and entertainment. Ranging from the latest eye-popping special effect for a feature film to scientific visualization of meteorological phenonema, computer animation has developed to a powerful tool of visualization.

14.1.1 Traditional Animation

As the production process of a traditional animation is pretty much the same as in computer animation, this section will introduce techniques for creating an animation. The traditional production process will be explained in more detail, because non-photorealistic computer graphics has – to a certain extent – more in common with the natural way of hand-drawing than with modern photorealistic rendering techniques. As stated in Chap. 4, if we want to create a photorealistic image, we should simulate the photographic process, whereas if we want to render non-photorealistic images we should investigate methods that simulate painting and drawing.

Traditional animation has a long history reaching back into the early days of moving images. It spans a wide range from the first animated sequence *Humorous phases of funny faces* by J. STUART BLACKTON (1906) and *Gertie the Dinosaur* by WINSOR MCCAY (1914) to the first cartoon with synchronized sound, *Steamboat Willie*, by WALT DISNEY (1928). This development reached its first height with the production of the first full-length feature film, DISNEY's masterpiece *Snow White and the Seven Dwarfs* (1937).

Like all creative projects, the production process starts with an idea from which the story is developed. Then a screenplay is written, providing a description of every single detail that is depicted in a shot, the dialog of acting characters, and further production notes. This screenplay is subject to many changes throughout the production. In the next step the screenplay is translated into a storyboard, which can be seen as the visual adaption of the screenplay. It consists of frames from all shots of the animation. A refined version of the storyboard is used as basis for the *keyframes*. These are a number of images from the animation (e.g., every 10th frame) that show acting characters or objects in certain *keypositions*, e.g., a very characteristic facial expression. Keyframes are – literally speaking – the framework of the animation and are drawn by skilled senior animators. The images that lie between the keyframes can be drawn by less experienced animators who are guided by the appearance of the keyframes. This process is called *inbetweening* (see Fig. 14.1).

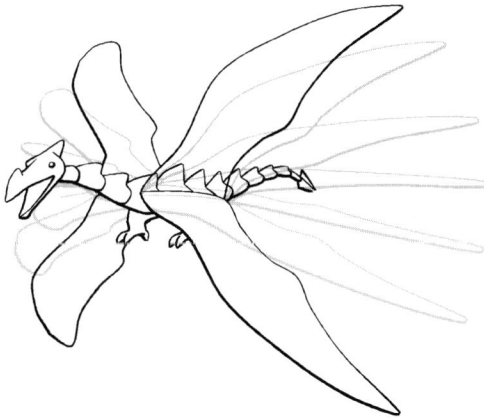

Figure 14.1: The process of inbetweening: The dark outlines show the wing in the highest and lowest position, the keyframes for the wing movement of the dragon, the gray outlines depict interpolated wing positions

In the next step all drawings are transferred to *cels* (special transparent layers that allow the objects to show through) which are colored with opaque paint.[1] These cels hold the entire scene: one cel contains the background, on the top of this cel other cels are placed which contain parts of the scene. The topmost cel, which is almost empty, contains the main character. These cels result in one frame of the animation. The frame is recorded and the cels are replaced by subsequent ones, showing the character in a slightly different position. In order to spare work, it is common to split not only the scene, but also a character into various parts, and draw them separately on different cels. A very good insight into the complete production process of professional animation is given by CULHANE in [Cul90].

All in all, this production process is highly iterative and time-consuming, and includes a lot of hand-crafting. Imagine that for the Disney feature film *Snow White and the Seven Dwarfs* – a landmark in traditional animation – about 1.2 million drawings were made! Finally, about 130 000 made it into the movie.

---

[1] As even transparent cels are not absolutely transparent, painting equally colored objects on different cel layers requires a color adaption, because the object behind four or five cels will appear slightly darker than the one on the first cel, and must therefore be painted in a brighter color.

14.1.2 Computer Animation

While the production process for a computer animation is similar to traditional cel animation, the generation of a single frame is quite different. As mentioned before, it is based on computer simulation of the photographic process. Here characters, objects, and their environment are designed, using techniques ranging from 3D scanning to 3D modeling. Then a material is applied to each surface, lighting, cameras, and atmosphere are set up, and a rendering technique is determined. After that, scene components can be animated by specifying their motion using various animation techniques like:

- Keyframe interpolation
- Hierarchical animation
- Inverse kinematics
- Procedural animation
- Morphing
- Motion capture

For a description of these techniques the reader is referred to WATT and WATT [WW92] or O'ROURKE [O'R95].

After the final rendering of all frames a number of post-production techniques like digital compositing or mixing with live action can be applied. In the end the final images are either recorded on film or video, or they are combined to a digital animation encoded in *MPEG*, *AVI*, or *Quicktime* format, depending on the platform and purpose of the animation.

Computer animation is still relatively young in comparison to traditional animation. It started in the late 1970s after computer technology became more practical and usable at all. Visual milestones include (among others, of course) *Voyager 2* (1980), the feature film *TRON* (1982), *Luxo jr.* (1985), the feature films *The Abyss* and *Terminator II* (1993), and finally *Toy Story* (1995) as the first full-length digital feature film. A more detailed overview of the history of computer animation can be found in KERLOW [Ker96].

14.1.3 Principles of Animation

Over the last decades animators have developed several fundamental principles concerning how characters and objects in motion should behave to create a convincing and thus entertaining illusion. These methods have been developed and perfected mainly at DISNEY studios and became the fundamental principles of motion. Everyone who is not going for simulation of physical laws should know them.

An excellent and most entertaining illustration of the following principles of animation is given in the book *Disney Animation: The Illusion of Life* [TJ81] written by THOMAS and JOHNSTON.[2]

---

2 Sometimes, this work is also called "The Animation Bible" due to its size and the value of its content.

- *Squash and stretch*
  Every object that is not extremely rigid changes its shape like the bouncing ball in Fig. 14.2. It squashes when hitting another object and stretches when moving away. During these actions the volume of the ball is preserved.
- *Anticipation*
  Prepare the audience for the next movement by preceding each major action with a specific movement that anticipates what is to come.
- *Slow in and slow out*
  Every object needs a certain amount of time to reach a certain speed. It is important to consider the time spent for the acceleration.
- *Secondary action*
  Enrich the liveliness of characters by adding subsidiary actions that support the primary action, e.g., a sad figure wipes a tear as it turns away.
- *Exaggeration*
  Actions do not have to be exactly naturalistic, they have to be *convincing*.
- *Appeal*
  Create characters that are fun to watch, not necessarily cuddly bunnies but appealing characters that have character and charm.

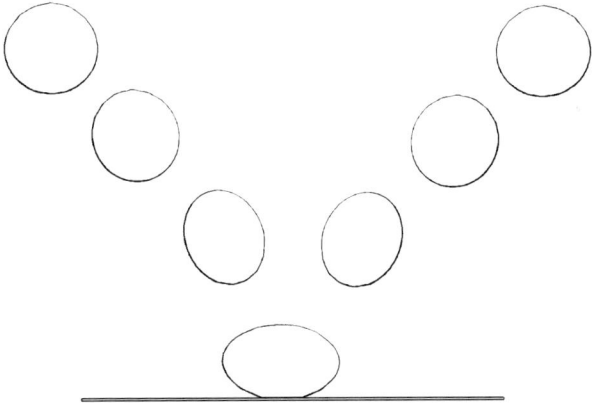

Figure 14.2: Squash and stretch

Although there are more principles (like *Staging, Straight ahead action and pose to pose, Follow through and overlapping action, Arcs,* and *Timing*) to consider, these are the most important. Despite the fact that these principles have been developed for traditional animation, they can be adapted to computer animation. JOHN LASSITER applied these principles very successfully in his short animation *Luxo jr.* [Las87]. Many of the animation techniques mentioned in Sect. 14.1.2 have been developed to support these fundamental principles.

14.2 Non-photorealistic Computer Animation

In the following sections, the usability of existing methods and new approaches for the generation of non-photorealistic computer animation are presented. With the new approach the images are created using 3D models and a modified animation pipeline to generate subsequent images of line drawings.

14.2.1 Why Use Non-photorealistic Computer Animation?

Even lifelike high-end computer animations have to face the criticism that they are somehow cold and hyperrealistic, because they show a world consisting of mathematically perfectly shaped objects without scratches or dirt. Computer animations have to face this criticism more than still images. As a consequence, a lot of effort in designing realistic-looking animations is made to meet these demands. To make them become more realistic, dirt, bumps, and scratches are applied to surfaces, mathematically correct shapes are deformed, and instead of computer modelled objects, 3D-scanned objects are used.

Today, computer graphics concentrates almost exclusively on photorealistic images, although traditionally created drawings have an artistic quality that computer-generated images lack. However, up to now only very few approaches deal with the creation of non-photorealistic animation in 3D. This is in part because the focus of most 3D rendering research lies on creating photorealistic images and also due to historical reasons and the development of 2D animation. Although in recent animated movies nearly all production steps involve the use of computers, the depicted characters remain flat shaded and the animation process is based on (digital) layers.

The abstraction of a depicted scene can have essential advantages. The artist can simplify a picture by leaving out unnecessary and distorting details, and can focus the viewer's attention on important features. Then the artist can stress the importance of certain parts of a depicted scene through variation of the drawing style, e.g., less important regions may be painted with light, fading lines, while relevant parts may be depicted with strong, bold lines. The resulting image is still somehow realistic, but it may differ from a photorealistic representation in shape, color, or texture, and even leave out lights and shadows. Despite – or just because of – these deviations, non-photorealistic images are common in the fields of scientific illustration and classical arts.

When creating non-photorealistic images on a computer, one soon thinks of combining successive pictures into an animation that also benefits from abstraction and simplification. Due to the temporal nature of moving pictures, the viewer always has less time to decode the presented information, so it is of utmost importance not to distract the viewer's attention with unnecessary detail.

14.2.2 Problems Using Existing Concepts

First, we should investigate existing methods for creating a non-photorealistic animation to see if they can be applied simply. All in all, the reviewed concepts can be subdivided into two types:

- 2D animation systems
- 3D non-photorealistic imaging systems

All 2D computer animation systems, like TIC-TAC-TOON [FBCT95], for example, are strongly related to traditional animation. They are designed to create images that look like their traditional equivalents and are therefore based on two-dimensional drawings. These, however, lack exact shading and correct perspective for the characters and objects depicted. In addition, this approach turns out to be futile, if we want to render animations using three-dimensional models to cope with these deficits.

In Chap. 4 several approaches for the generation of line drawings from 3D models were introduced. Another approach is quite straight forward: One could use 2D image processing methods like edge enhancement, Gaussian noise, color particle placement, etc., on the single images of a photorealistically rendered animation to create non-photorealistic images. However, all these systems concentrate on the creation of single images and are based on user interaction, which makes them unsuitable for the generation of animations, but this is just a minor hindrance. When applying one of these approaches, the user confronts two major difficulties: a lack of *frame-to-frame coherence* and the *shower-door effect*.

The Lack of Frame-to-Frame Coherence

The main difficulty in applying existing (still) image creation methods for animations result from the usage of stochastic processes to achieve a hand-crafted look. These methods are non-deterministic, i.e., no two successive frames of an animation look the same. Even if there is no motion at all, there is a disturbing distortion due to the random changes in the appearance of the depicted scene elements as no two strokes (or their digital equivalents) are drawn at exactly the same position. This absence of frame-to-frame coherence results in an unintended disturbance of the animation.

The Shower-Door Effect

If a 2D image is postprocessed for an animation using operations like those mentioned above on successive images, the user has the impression that the strokes and color particles effectively stick to the viewplane and not to the object. The depicted scene looks like it is being viewed through structured glass, comparable to the effect encountered by someone looking out of a shower through the waterdrop-covered glass door. This effect results from the fact that all postprocessing methods are indeed 2D (pixel-based) operations.

As all depth information is lost after projecting a 3D scene onto a 2D image plane, this information cannot be encoded in, for example, the size of strokes or color particles. So all areas of an image are treated equally and this causes the strokes and color particles to stick to the viewplane and not to the object.

14.2.3 Rendering Non-photorealistic Computer Animation

Recalling the rendering pipelines introduced in Chap. 4, we can derive a pipeline for rendering an animation (see Fig. 14.3). After designing the scene and the motion paths these settings have to be parsed.[3] An animation engine evaluates the motion specifications from this data and calculates the corresponding transformations. This description is passed to the rendering pipeline (see Sect. 4.3), which generates a still image. The image is written to a storage medium and the calculations are performed for the next frame until the last frame is written.

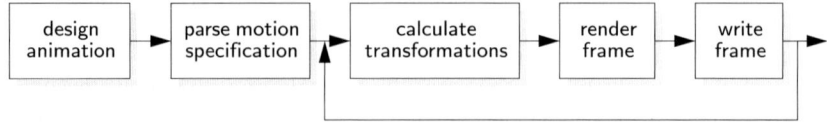

Figure 14.3: An animation pipeline

Let us summarize the requirements for a basic animation system capable of generating non-photorealistic animations. The system should

- render non-photorealistic images from a 3D model,
- render subsequent frames according to some kind of motion specification,
- maintain frame-to-frame coherence, and
- avoid the shower-door effect.

If we want to meet the special demands summarized above, we have to use a rendering pipeline for the image creation process that is capable of drawing an image using deterministic line styles.

14.3 Animating Paintings

A system for rendering animations in a painterly style is presented by MEIER in [Mei96]. There, the problem of random changes in the frame appearance is solved by placing particles directly on a 3D model. These particles are transformed to screenspace and sorted by a painter algorithm [FvDFH90] on the basis of their perspective depth. Each particle represents a brush stroke,

---

[3] For the sake of simplicity we concentrate on the motion of objects, although there are other animatable parameters.

which is a small monochrome texture image with alpha information.[4] This is used to represent the characteristic structure of a stroke. The appearance of a single brush stroke is determined by taking position, size, orientation, and color information into account. The color information is calculated with the aid of lighting information from a separately rendered reference picture. The attributes for a particle are looked up at the same position in the reference picture. The resulting animation preserves to a certain extent the frame-to-frame coherence and resembles oil paintings from impressionistic painters.

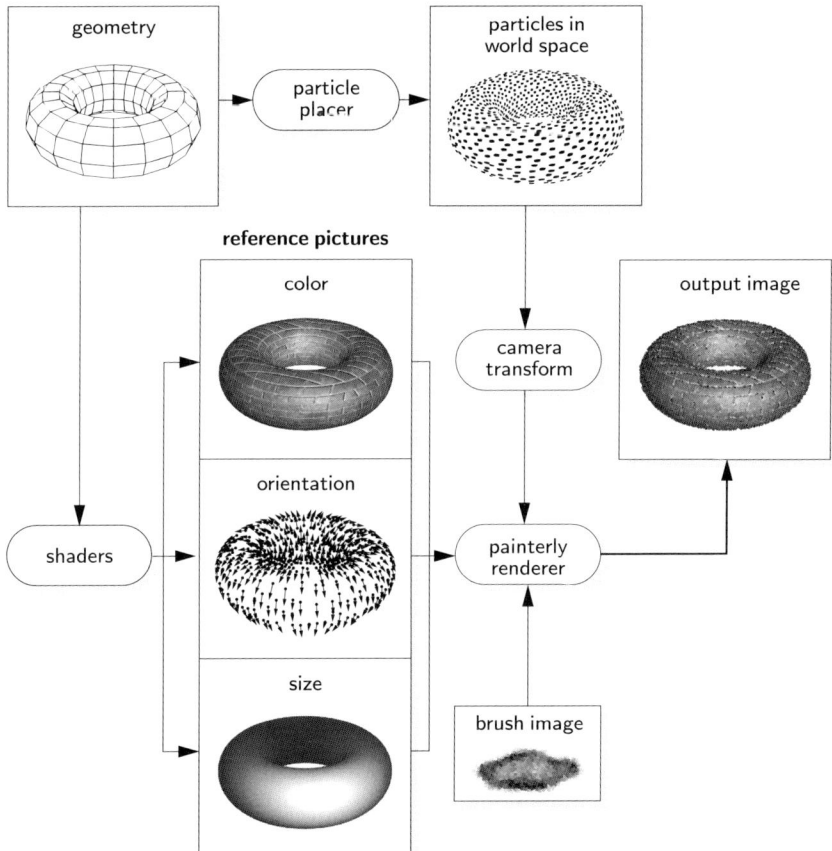

Figure 14.4: The rendering process for generating a single frame simulating the color placement process of an artist

This system shows its strength in simulating the process of painting an image by placing color strokes on the output medium and is therefore well-

---

4 The alpha channel is used in compositing operations to define the degree of blending between two images (see [Ker96]).

suited to create painterly animations that resemble oil or pastel paintings. However, this approach seems unsuitable for use in the fields of scientific illustration. In order to extend the means of (computer) graphical expression in visualization tasks to these fields, we should investigate methods for the animation of line drawings.

14.4 Animating Line Drawings

In this section a new approach for the generation of animated line drawings based on a polygonal model and on freeform surfaces is presented. The frame generation is performed using the standard rendering pipeline for line drawings (see also Sect. 4.3) with an enriched 3D model as input. The polygonal rendering engine provides an analytical description of the image as output, which, in contrast to comparable approaches, is deterministic. The animation engine is based on keyframes and modifies the given scene for subsequent frames.

In general, the animation engine has to perform two main tasks:
- to determine the object movements according to the given keyframe data, and
- to supply the render engine with new scene information.

14.4.1 Animating Polygonal Models

As mentioned in the introduction to this chapter, we concentrate on the visualization of moving non-photorealistic images. We use a standard animation program (3D Studio) for creating and setting up an animation. It is important to benefit from the power of an existing modeling and animation tool as we concentrate on the visualization of the rendered images. Therefore, the data for the animation is read by an input filter, the parser, which acts as input processor for the animation engine.

The animation engine receives the following different types of data:
- The 3D geometry of scene objects (in a polygonal description, including information about lights and cameras),
- additional information (hierarchy, importance, line styles, etc.), and
- the animation data, which can be separated into
  - animation settings (number of frames, image size, etc.) and
  - the movement of all objects described with keyframes.

One part of the input for the animation engine is the 3D geometry model and possibly corresponding additional information about importance and line styles used in the rendition. The other part is a set of keyframes that describe the movement of the objects and general animation settings. An object can be of any 3D shape, it may be a light source or a camera. The animation engine can therefore be seen as a filter that provides the render engine with the

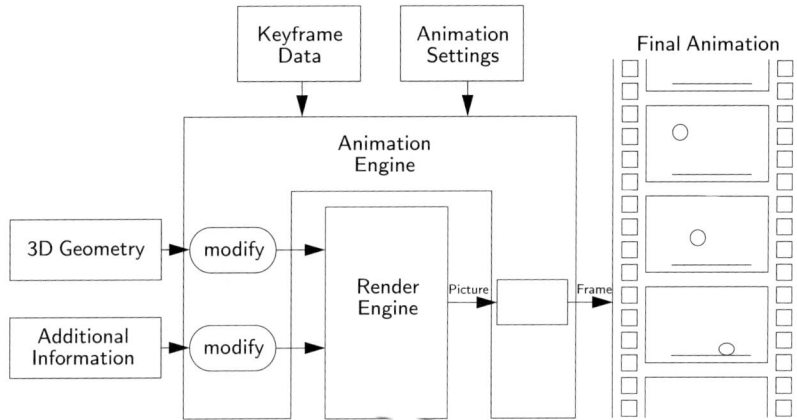

Figure 14.5: The system design for an animation system capable of rendering animated line drawings

necessary animation data combined with the additional information, which consists of the number of frames and settings concerning the line styles. In order to generate a sequence of images for each object, its transformations are calculated. For the given keyframes, this calculation can be done directly, whereas for the intermediate frames, the object movements have to be interpolated. As a linear interpolation would lead to discontinuities that result in jerky and unsmooth object movements, the use of splines is common. In order to achieve smooth motion, these splines have to satisfy the condition of second-derivative continuity. Furthermore, a high degree of locality is desirable in order to keep the implications for a designed motion path as small as possible when making adjustments to the animation. Here, a development due to KOCHANEK is important. In [Koc84] he introduced a spline class that satisfies the demands mentioned above, using the control parameters *tension*, *continuity*, and *bias* to specify the shape of the spline. The tension parameter controls the bending of the curve that represents the motion path. The continuity influences the "velocity" of the object passing through a key, i.e., the number of frames that locate the object "near" the keyframe, and the bias can shift the number of frames toward a keyframe or away from it.

One can think of a scene as a collection of objects. These objects may have common and distinctive features. It is possible to model common features only once and allow these features to be inherited by child objects. For instance, every scene object – no matter if a 3D geometry object, a camera, or a light source – can be moved. Consequently, this movement can be inherited by child objects. Thus the mechanisms implemented in the animation engine can be applied to every object in the scene. Another attribute that can be inherited is an object-specific line style. This allows the user to draw objects

– or subobjects – with different line styles and to change the line style only for selected objects.

The scene is rendered by performing the line rendering pipeline and passing an analytical description (technically speaking: a collection of lines) back to the animation engine, which paints the vector-oriented frame representation on an abstract image. After that, a special output device writes subsequent frames into a predefined directory. Currently, our system supports *PostScript* as a resolution-independent output format and *TIFF*, *BMP*, *GIF*, and *AnimatedGIF* as resolution-dependent output formats. Finally, the series of images can be combined into an animation using standard *MPEG* or *Quicktime* encoders. However, we discovered that for animations consisting of black and white images the *FLIC* format is most useful.

14.4.2 Animating Curved Surfaces

In "complex" movements of objects, like clothes or flags waving in the wind, or when soft objects are pressed or strained, the objects undergo mostly smooth deformation. In order to simulate such behavior in an animation, the representation used should guarantee ways to easily deform surfaces, and here the polygonal representation fails. With freeform surfaces, where the surfaces are controlled by control points and the movement of those control points results in a smooth deformation of the surface, such problems of complex movement can be resolved. Chapter 5 deals thoroughly with curved surfaces and introduces a technique for producing line drawings. In this section we combine these rendering techniques and the animation techniques described in the previous section in order to render animated curved surfaces.

The animation engine explained in the previous section is extended to use curved surfaces and supplies the renderer with the information for localization and deformation of all objects in each frame. The data for the deformation is gained by the explained keyframe interpolation with distinct interpolation functions, such as linear, exponential, smooth in and out, fast in and out, etc. The transformation in time, which includes localization and deformation, is applied either to whole surfaces or to a collection of control points of surfaces, which makes the controlling of parts of surfaces in time possible. This collection of control points is called a *cluster* and the deformation process *cluster deformation*. A cluster is driven as a separate object in our system; it can include control points from more than one surface and the control points can overlap further clusters.

Figure 14.6 shows a bowling pin with two declared clusters, where the control points above the throat are chosen for the first cluster and the remaining control points for the second cluster. A deformation applied to the first cluster (rotation and scaling) results in a different, but still smooth surface. A line rendering with a brush-like line style simulates a painted graphic on the right of the figure.

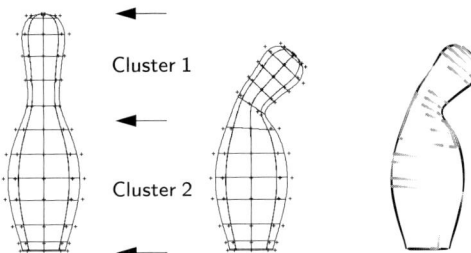

Figure 14.6: A bowling pin, where two declared clusters split the control points in two regions (left). A rotation and scaling applied to Cluster1 deforms the pin with resulting smooth surface (middle). The line rendering with brush-like line style simulates a hand drawing (right)

The application of these techniques to create an animation can be seen in Fig. 14.7. In this animation, three bowling pins move out of the way of a bowling ball. The figure shows a couple of frames of the sequence in which two pins are jumping over the ball and one pin is moving sideways. This example nicely illustrates the deformation of curved surfaces to create the "squash and stretch" effect mentioned earlier.

The movement of the pins is controlled with keyframes and the steps between them are smoothly interpolated. The keyframes refer to the defined positions of the surface control points. Unfortunately, the few frames illustrated in the figure do not show the harmonious transition of the deformation of the pins as the animation does. In this scene the bowling pins are displayed with horizontal hatching texture, the ball is stippled and the shadow is drawn with vertical lines.

14.4.3 Animating Line Styles

If we are able to specify the line styles for an animation, it is possible to keyframe the parameters of a line style and perform an *inbetweening for line styles*. This means that a line style or certain attributes of a line style are transformed into another style. This feature allows, for instance, an object to change its importance over the time in a line drawing animation. Among other attributes, changing the brightness of a stroke is a very useful way to depict a change of importance.

Figure 14.8 depicts three frames from a sequence that shows the bending of the toes of a footbone. The importance of a certain bone is altered by gradually changing the line style of all other (unimportant) bones from dark to light gray. In contrast to the first frame, the bone in the third frame is striking by its different drawing style. The emphasized bone can be distinguished clearly and remains in its spatial relationship. Other parameters that can be animated include the width of a line, the line style, and the deviation a line. These effects can be used primarily in educational or visualization environments.

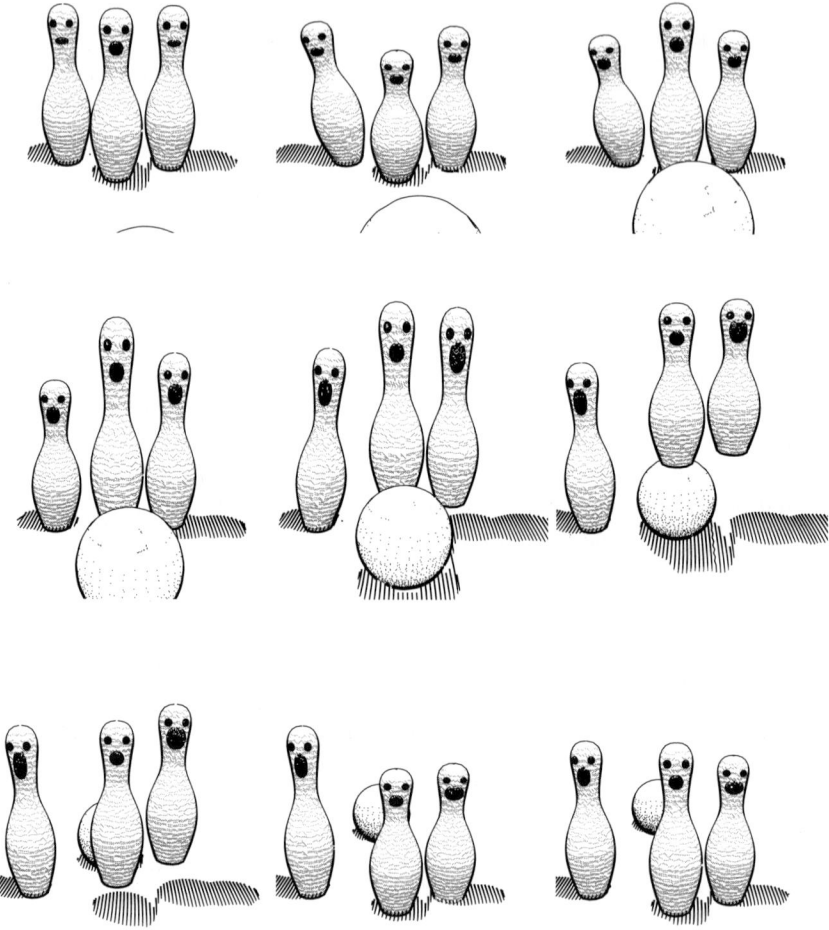

Figure 14.7: Some frames of the bowling pin animation showing deformations of freeform surfaces displayed as line drawings

14.5 Future Work

In this chapter we introduced two basic animation systems representing current work, and although these systems are capable of rendering basic non-photorealistic animations, there is still a lot of undiscovered country ahead. For instance, we would like to implement a refined hatching method for texturing different surfaces with different line styles. The behavior of these lines during a surface deformation should be comparable to conventional texture mapping. Animating these lines could result in a completely new way to express surface deformations, e.g., to simulate wrinkles on a face. In addition, as the rendering in our polygonal renderer is done entirely analytically, the generation of shadows raises some new problems that could easily be solved

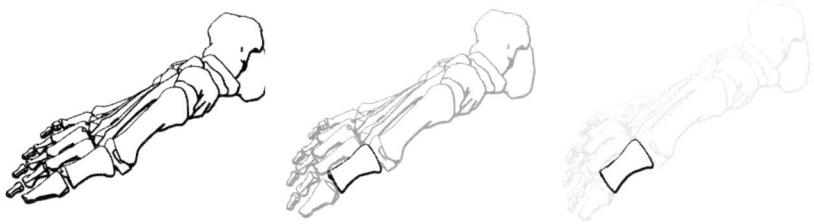

Figure 14.8: Gradually emphasizing an object in a scene while maintaining its spatial relationship to other objects and deemphasizing the surrounding objects

in a photorealistic context. This will be one of our tasks for the near future. The painterly renderer experiences difficulties with adapting brush strokes to the size of an object if this size changes. Furthermore, the particle placement is unsuitable for rendering curved surfaces as there are no long, deformable strokes. We experience similar problems when drawing lines resulting from cluster deformations.

Finally, we think it can be promising to develop new techniques for the representation of many objects, e.g., leaves on a tree or clouds. In the past, artists developed some powerful techniques to depict these kinds of objects, e.g., painting a tree, with a few characteristic strokes rather than painting every single leaf. But this task seems difficult to accomplish, as the human artist – due to his massive parallel perception – experiences a tree as a whole object, not as a collection consisting of n million leaves and m thousand wooden substructures. It might be promising to transform a polygonal representation consisting of several hundred thousand polygons into a simplified, yet characteristic shape. A more interesting approach might be to turn away from a polygonal representation of such objects and attribute them with structure information like "has leaves" or "is cloudy" that evokes a special drawing technique. It is still open how this would look in an animation.

Contributors of Chap. 14: Maic MASUCH and Frank GODENSCHWEGER

in the MIT Artificial Intelligence Laboratory in the late 1970s, entitled *Creation of Animations from Story Descriptions* [Kah79]. It was the first attempt to fully translate a high-level description into a set of frames. Later, ZELTZER [Zel90] described the generation of computer animations from high-level scripts and defined some important terms:

- *Task-level specification* – the specification of communicative intent. With this terminology, emphasis is placed on the fact that this is the level on which the designer of an animation thinks. Examples for task-level specifications are *show-object, show-action,* or *show-relation.*
- *Decomposition rules* – describe how task-level specifications are translated into low-level commands an animator can execute. This translation process can be rather complex and involve several levels resulting in a hierarchical *decomposition tree*. The decomposition process is often not straightforward but includes back-tracking. Decomposition rules, for example, describe in which steps a 3D model or a virtual camera must be transformed to show an object. To show an action, decomposition rules state which movements are necessary to communicate how a depicted entity in a 3D model can be handled.
- *Elementary sequences* – form the result of the decomposition process at a level an animator can handle. In other words, exact time and positional parameters are available for each movement. Elementary sequences can either be executed immediately, or (if they are independent of a specific description language) they can be translated straight into an executable sequence. An example of an elementary sequence is the description of a transformation (e.g., a translation) with the exact timing specification and exact coordinates where the transformation starts and ends.

We will use ZELTZER's terminology within this chapter because it allows to compare intent-based animation systems based on their use of task-level specifications and decomposition rules.

One of the most difficult problems in specifying animations is to plan the path of a virtual camera, e.g., when it should be moved through a complex environment. DRUCKER and ZELTZER [DZ94] describe how this complex task can be solved automatically. The *intelligent* camera control thus achieved is an important example of intent-based animation design.

Our work was inspired by KARP and FEINER [KF93], who describe a knowledge-based approach to using scene structuring techniques for computer generated animations. They are focused on animations that demonstrate or explain objects and actions, which is close to our focus. Their ESPLANADE (Expert System for PLanning of ANimation DEsign) system exploits a sophisticated planning scheme to fulfill communicative intents. The design of ESPLANADE is guided by the assumption of a hierarchical structure of traditional films with sequences, scenes and individual shots. This structure is mapped to a decomposition tree. From the ESPLANADE project we learned that decomposition rules (how to achieve an effect) can (and maybe should) be borrowed from the film medium.

In a similar way, BUTZ [But94, But97] applied film techniques to automatically generate animations that describe the handling of technical devices. His CATHI system is integrated in the multi-media presentation system PPP [AMR96] which also includes modules for presentation planning and text generation. In the animations generated, a variety of advanced computer graphics techniques (e.g., depth-cueing, directing a spotlight towards certain locations) are applied to shift the *visual focus*. CATHI also animates exploded views, which is very effective because a viewer can see the actual movement from an undistorted view to an exploded one (see Fig. 15.1 for an example).

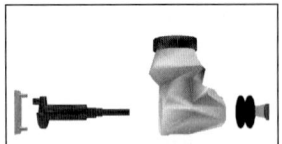 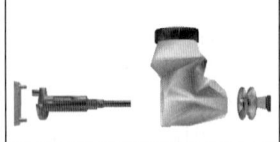 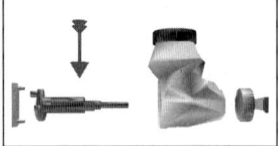

Figure 15.1: Example sequence generated by CATHI to explain a construction group: after animating an exploded view, arrows and changes of object's material are used to highlight important objects (courtesy of Andreas BUTZ)

One thing which is of special interest in the context of this book is that CATHI automatically adapts the level of detail in the animation (see BUTZ and KRÜGER [BK96]). In contrast to other systems, they strive to simplify the shapes that are not in the viewer's focus in order to enhance his or her perception.

Comparing the communicative goals supported by these systems leads to an interesting observation: The goals themselves (*show-object, show-action*) are very similar across the systems described above but the ways in which they are realized differ considerably. These differences comprise not only the techniques applied but also the effort required to carry out the calculations. Moreover, the systems differ in the flexibility of the generation process, which can be affected by several constraints. The CATHI system, for example, can handle constraints regarding the graphics hardware available and constraints from the presentation planning process.

Most of the work done so far concentrated on the automatic generation of animations based on high-level specifications. For this purpose, large knowledge bases are required which incorporate knowledge on how to realize communicative intents. Furthermore, a large number of very domain-specific assumptions are incorporated in the knowledge bases.

15.2 Creating Animations from High-Level Specifications

Although useful, automatic generation alone may not be sufficient to entirely capture the creative process of designing an animation, even for rather rational domains such as technical and educational animation. We assume that automatic generation can lead to a meaningful "suggestion" on how to convey information but that further refinement is necessary. Therefore, we focus on the *creation* of an animation rather than on fully automatic *generation*. By creation we refer to an iterative process in which a first prototype of an animation is generated in the computer. The user is then encouraged to refine this prototype in an interactive fine-tuning process.

Manual editing of the animation specification, however, necessitates a file format or even a scripting language since the author must be able to store and retrieve his or her work for later editing. This language must reflect the internal data structures in a meaningful way, especially if the author is expected to carry out modifications directly in the script. Therefore, we need scripting languages that support the specification of communicative intents as well as the specification of animation techniques with their parameters. With this approach we aim at an integration of automated generation with interaction facilities.

15.3 Theoretical Foundations

To achieve a higher impact of computer animation, we borrow ideas from the domain of film-making, which, in its one hundred years' history, has developed a number of structuring techniques that convey information and emotions in a very specific way not possible in other media [Mon95]. However, the application of these techniques in the rather rational and objective domains of technical and educational animation contrasts with applictaion in commercial films that require a much greater emotional involvement. In a technical animation, we cannot look into a character's eyes and see how he or she feels, but this does not mean there is nothing to learn from film-making techniques.

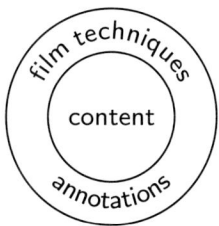

Figure 15.2: Relation between content and augmenting techniques

These techniques form another communication channel in addition to the actual displayed scenery and action. Using film and annotation techniques in a presentation layer above the underlying graphics model and animation techniques (see Fig. 15.2), one can exploit the understanding people have developed for the film language. In addition, we take some liberties with the scene content. On the scene level, we emphasize important objects by taking into account their visibility and recognizability. For this purpose we employ two strategies:

- *Direct emphasis*
  The attributes of an object and the lighting specification are modified to emphasize it. Objects are accentuated using a different color or texture to direct the viewer's attention. A unique color or color flashing while explaining the object are variants of this technique. An appropriate lighting specification can also contribute to the emphasis on an object, for instance spotlights can be very effective in directing the user toward parts of a 3D model.
- *Indirect emphasis*
  To emphasize an object, the attributes of other objects may be modified. Direct emphasis fails if the object to be emphasized is not visible or hard to differentiate (despite highlighting) from surrounding objects. In this case, direct emphasis should be complemented by a simultaneous deaccentuation of other objects. We refer to this as *indirect emphasis*. Moreover, the lighting specification is adapted so as *not* to highlight other objects. Besides assigning another color to less important objects, visibility has to be taken into account. This is accomplished by clipping or removing objects. Objects can also be rendered translucent to show things that would be occluded otherwise. While this sounds simple, it can take some time to find the occluding objects as they depend on the current viewing direction.

More specialized emphasis methods are given below in the detailed discussion of our illustration system. These methods have in common that they modify the scene. However, an important design criterion for these techniques is that they must not alter the scene or its objects beyond recognition, as this would certainly interfere with the educational intent behind their creation.

In the case of technical animation, such arbitrary alterations are not desirable, as the animation reflects a simulated process. Since this simulation is done before the presentation in another application, it could use, e.g., the same coloring techniques for other reasons so as to indicate an object status. In order not to interfere with the original content, we must choose the emphasis techniques carefully. For technical animation, we thus focus on techniques at the presentation level only:

- *Camera position and direction* (perspective)
  In a film, the camera position is never chosen only with visibility in mind. Instead, the perspective adds meaning, e.g., by choosing a certain ele-

vation that makes people and things look either small and insignificant or big and troublesome. This can be used to achieve very subtle effects that are rarely perceived as an effect of the use of camera perspective. Outside of films, however, the camera perspective is usually chosen to provide a clear and unobstructed view of objects that must be visible in the situation at hand.

In small-scale models such as those used for medical illustrations, the change of perspective is usually accomplished using another paradigm: instead of maneuvering a virtual camera through the scene, the object itself is rotated and moved while the camera remains fixed. This has essentially the same effect, but reflects a different relation between the user and the real object.

- *Camera motion*

  A change of perspective generally follows or prepares for a change of action. A moving camera makes this transition gradually and therefore comprehensible for the viewer. The camera following a moving object makes a clear statement that this object is the center of focus and thus indicates a high relevance. Even if the object does not move, the camera can convey the same information by approaching the object. Likewise, backing away from a previous focus prepares the viewer for another communicative intent.

  One more property of camera movements makes them particularly interesting for computer animations. Monoscopic images often give too few depth cues to support the viewing of complex scenes. Our human three-dimensional vision is achieved using multiple "cameras" (and hence, perspectives) at the same time. Now, a single moving camera can compensate the missing camera by slowly altering its perspective. Thus, a moving camera supports and improves three-dimensional vision.

- *Shots and cuts*

  Cuts divide a film into shots. Like a camera movement, a cut changes the perspective, since the camera usually points somewhere else after the cut (see *multi-angularity*, Sect. 15.5.1).

  A very important difference, however, is that cuts can also consume time. That suggests the use of cuts whenever uninteresting actions should be skipped to keep the presentation reasonably short. Long animations that show a simulation spanning many weeks of real time, for example, cannot be animated for that long. It is also impossible to increase the time scale until it fits in a time short enough, since details would be lost or become indiscernible. Cuts are therefore a necessary element in complex animations. Fortunately, they also enable a number of interesting methods to convey information and aid the viewer's comprehension.

  Film makers use various forms of scene structuring techniques that group shots and put them in a context to each other. The structure of a sequence adds meaning above what is provided in the shots themselves, e.g., alternating shots indicate a strong connection between the two views. Some popular techniques are described in SHARFF [Sha82] and MONACO [Mon95]. These techniques are elements of a *film language* that viewers learn from watching movies.

As mentioned before, for a real application these concepts must be taken out of their kinesthetic origin and adapted to a specific domain. The next two sections show examples of implemented systems that apply these techniques in educational and technical contexts.

15.4 Animation for Educational Purposes

Educational videos play an important role in the explanation of spatial phenomena. Compared to textbooks with their two-dimensional images, videos do a better job in explaining spatial relations. In particular, continuous transitions between different camera positions are valuable for building a mental model of spatial relations.

We are especially interested in animations for anatomy teaching. Anatomy with its highly irregular and complex shapes is an interesting area for developing animation techniques. Besides camera (or object) movements, pointers are used to direct the student to certain parts of the image. Computer animations in this field can learn from these techniques. However, with computer animations other effects can be achieved which are hard to accomplish with conventional videos. While for videos the model to explain is colored once (to ensure high contrasts), a computer can easily adapt the color and thus emphasize whatever is important in a specific context.

Based on these observations, we developed the animation component of the ZOOMILLUSTRATOR to combine techniques from traditional media with the flexibility of a computer system. Our system generates animations which are tailored to what is currently being explained.

In this section we describe the script language that controls the animation. The interpretation of a script results in commands to present text and to accentuate parts of the underlying 3D model. To enhance comprehension, smooth transitions for both the display of textual information and changes of the graphics are realized.

The animations generated are especially useful for beginners who work with prepared film sequences, whereas the advanced student will switch more to the interactive exploration of geometric models.

15.4.1 Design of Animation Techniques

With the animation component described here we enable the author of an animation to specify what should be explained in how much detail. In particular, we implement the following task-level specifications:

explain <*anObject*>
explain <*aGroup*>

The development of decomposition rules and animation techniques is guided by educational videos for anatomy teaching. These videos show in great detail the shape and location of complicated objects. In addition to the techniques described in the last section, two specialized methods are used to demonstrate complex shapes, such as blood vessels and muscles:

- *Clarify shape*
  Pointing devices follow the contour of the object to be explained. In order to accomplish this, a path on the object's surface is interactively specified or extracted from a topological analysis. This method is very well suited for branching structures.
- *Separate*
  The object is taken out of its context and shown alone in a separate window. This way the object can be manipulated in a different context.

These techniques are implemented in the ZOOMILLUSTRATOR. They are dedicated to the explanation of highly irregular shapes, as they occur in natural phenomena. For the explanation of regular shapes, conventional techniques like a close-up are more appropriate.

15.4.2 Data Structures

In this section we shall describe which prerequisites and data structures are necessary to implement the techniques described above.

First, a careful segmentation of a 3D model into objects is required. Furthermore, it is necessary that objects are meaningfully classified. In anatomy, the membership of an object in an organ system (e.g., bones, muscles, blood vessels or nerves) is crucial; therefore, objects are categorized according to this criterion. On the basis of this classification default animation techniques can be assigned. Hence, for example, the topological structure of bones is usually very easy to understand. Nerves and blood vessels, however, require more sophisticated strategies to be explained. The categorization and the assignment of default animation techniques is summarized in the *structure information*.

Besides a well-organized scene graph, additional data structures are necessary especially to handle the occlusion tests without unacceptable delays. Also, the automatic viewing transformations require some knowledge about the "optimal" viewing direction and the size and position of the projected object. Together we call these data *visibility information*. In our implementation, 26 pre-calculated viewing directions are realized (eight steps along the azimuth and declination axis, respectively).

The off-line model analysis is performed by casting rays into the scene and recording the order in which objects are hit. Each object o has a visibility value expressed as the ratio of the number of rays that hit o first to the number of those that hit *o* together. In addition, the system also stores how often an object *p* occludes another object *o*, so that the relative degree of occlusion can be used to decide how the deaccentuation will be performed. Small occlusions are handled by clipping against the bounding box of the occluded object, while large occlusions result in transparency or removal of the occluding object.

15.4.3 Script Language

The application of the animation techniques described so far requires a formal language in which the techniques can be specified and parameterized. It is important that meaningful default values exist so as to minimize the effort to specify an animation.

Important questions when designing a formal language are *what* should be expressed and *who* should use it. We call the person who writes a script the author (see above). The author is assumed to be familiar with the content. The script language makes it possible to specify easily what should be explained in how much detail.

For this purpose, the author does not need to know which data structures are used and relies on the information organized by a content provider. The role of the author is similar to that of a lecturer who uses a textbook someone else has written.

Our experience with interactive illustrations is that the connection between rendered images and related text is crucial for comprehension (see Chap. 13). From this experience we hypothesize that a coupling of these media is also essential for the efficiency of educational animations. This hypothesis is also supported by the fact that animated movements in educational videos are carefully accompanied by textual comments. Therefore, we provide constructs to state that changes on the graphical part are accompanied by simultaneous changes of text presentations. Smooth transitions are required for changes both on the textual part and on the graphical part. For smooth changes of text presentations, fisheye techniques DILL et al. [DBHH94] are exploited. This is the same approach as employed in the interactive ZOOM-ILLUSTRATOR (recall Chap. 13).

The heart of the script language is the *explain* statement. It specifies which named object should be explained. An optional parameter list specifies the timing and the techniques (see above) to apply. An *explain* statement may be complemented by an *emphasize* statement to specify which techniques should be used. This incorporates techniques to emphasize an object directly or indirectly (Sect. 15.4.1). An optional *while* statement defines what should happen on the textual part when certain transformations take place on the graphical side. The language is described in more detail in PREIM et al. [PRS96]. The statements can either be defined explicitly or (at least partly) generated by a teach-in mode, in which the system records interactive movements and translates them into the Script Language.

15.4.4 Architecture

The ZOOMILLUSTRATOR reads a *scene description*, containing a polygonal model, and related *textual information* derived from a medical textbook [Sob88]. The structure of the *scene description* corresponds to that of the *textual information*. Furthermore, the *visibility information* and the *structure information* (see Sect. 15.4.2) are read in. From these sources an *internal representation* is constructed which guides the execution of the *animation script*. Figure 15.3 shows the relation between these components.

15.4.5 Implementation and Examples

We have developed and tested our animations with polygonal models, some from anatomy and one technical model to verify that our concepts are valid not only for anatomical objects. Because models with the level of detail required for illustration purposes are difficult to create, we rely on models which are commercially available [Dat96]. These models differ in their complexity from some 6K polygons to some 110K polygons.

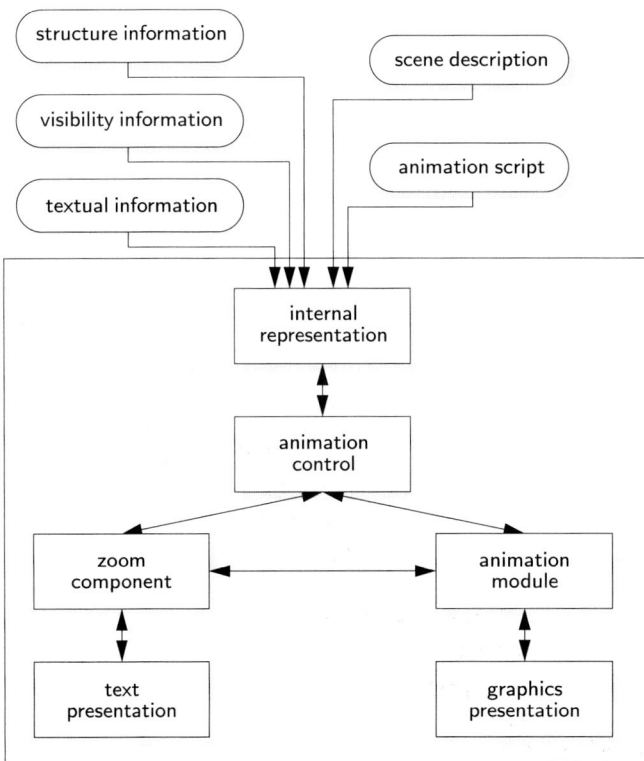

Figure 15.3: Architecture of the ZOOMILLUSTRATOR with the Animation

The animation is implemented using OPEN INVENTOR [Wer94] and C++. Special engine classes support the interpolation between initial and final states. Several changes can be specified to happen at the same time. This mechanism is employed for geometric transformations as well as for changes of material properties.

Path Specification. In Sect. 15.4.1 we did not consider how the path to show an object's shape is defined. We developed an interactive tool in which the object to be explained is handled separately. The author marks the starting point, branching points and endpoints resulting in a tree structure of the path to show (see Fig. 15.4). The path contains world space 3D points and is therefore independent of the viewing direction. Additional points are derived from the coordinates of that object, so that the interactive specification is used as a starting point for an automated process.

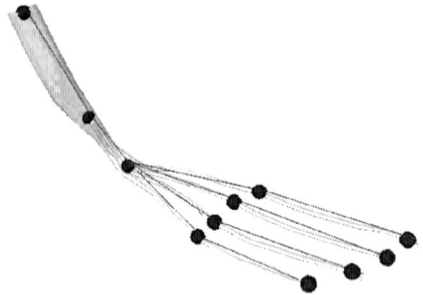

Figure 15.4: Path specification

Selection of Pointing Devices. Path specification is not the only interesting detail in the demonstration of an object's shape. Other important issues are: Which pointers are appropriate? How is the pointer moved along the path? On the basis of our observations, we modeled objects used in videos for anatomy teaching to point at something. These include tweezers, scissors, and ballpoints. In addition to these "real-life" objects, we modeled some 3D arrows. They are very useful because their size can be flexibly adjusted to the size of the objects to be explained. Note that "real-life" objects cannot be scaled arbitrarily because we "know" the relation of the sizes between a ballpoint and some anatomical structures. When the shape of an object is to be explained, pointing devices are selected automatically; however, this behavior can be overridden by a manual specification of a pointer.

The movement of a pointer is guided by the current surface normal, that is, the pointer is always chosen to be perpendicular to the path. The tip of the pointer touches the surface directly. This is in contrast to human pointing gestures, where a gap between the pointer and the object to be explained remains. We believe that this gap is due to concern not to damage the object and is therefore not necessary for our virtual objects.

Examples. Figure 15.5 shows on the left the start of an animation, while the right image shows modifications to explain a muscle.

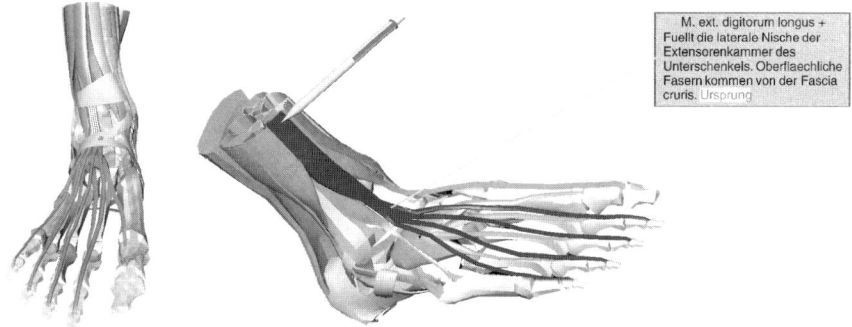

Figure 15.5: Original position (left), modifications to the original image prepare the explanation of the shape: the camera position has been adjusted and a ballpoint is directed toward the origin of the emphasized muscle (right)

Figure 15.6 shows in the upper part how the animation continued. The course is explained with arrows, while the ballpoint remains unchanged. An explanation is displayed, which describes the course. Structure information is used to display the labels of related nodes.

Finally, the lower image in Fig. 15.6, arrows reach the lower parts of the muscle. As a consequence, on the textual side, other nodes appear which are related to the muscle's lower part.

The techniques developed for educational animations are inspired by videos for anatomy teaching but are not limited to this domain. At the end of this chapter a film sequence is shown to describe a complex situation in a technical model.

15.5 Film Techniques in Technical Animation

This section describes the use of film-making heuristics in a technical animation system, ANIPLUS [LH95]. ANIPLUS is a 3D real-time animation system designed for the visualization of simulation runs. This application differs from the ZOOMILLUSTRATOR in a fundamental way: the content (the scene and the animation actions) is predefined and cannot be altered. The remaining degrees of freedom are therefore limited to the camera control and the assembly of shots into sequences.

Since the simulation itself is a strong abstraction of a real system, it is often hard to comprehend, especially for non-technical audiences. Computer

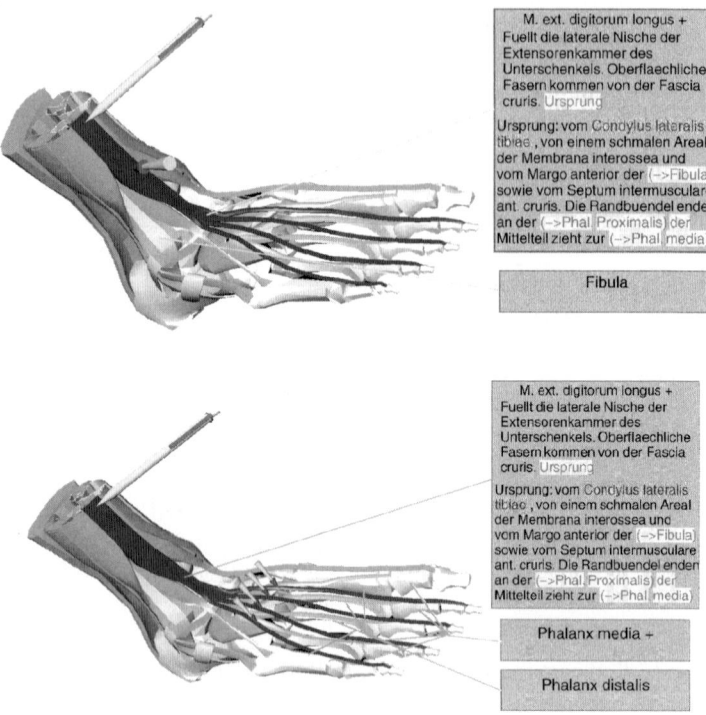

Figure 15.6: A large arrow demonstrates the upper part of the shape and moves downward (top). After reaching a branching point, the arrow splits into several small arrows. As the motion continues, the label of the bone where the muscle starts disappears while others become visible (bottom)

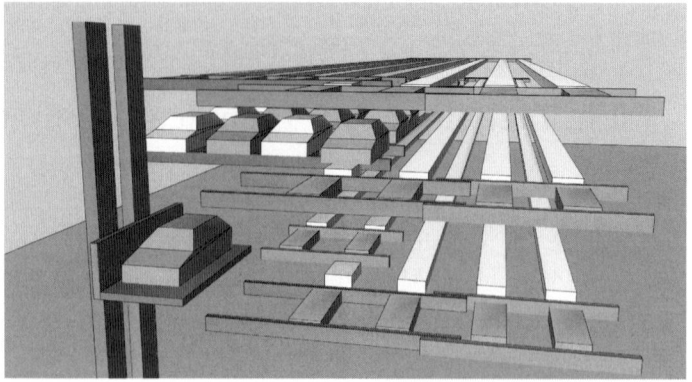

Figure 15.7: AniPLuS scene

15.5 Film Techniques in Technical Animation

graphics, especially animations (for an example see Fig. 15.7), help to bridge the gap between abstract simulation models and the real system. By watching the animation, the simulation expert can spot problems that are not easily detected in a statistical report.

However, with the increasing complexity of the simulated worlds (and hence, their visual presentation), mental abilities must be taken into account when designing the presentation. Today's tools allow both the creation of complex scenes and long detailed animations. This creates problems for the end-user: a large and complex scene is not explored at a glance and simulations covering weeks of real time cannot be animated for that long. Besides complexity, there are other issues that call for better presentation design, among these aesthetics is surely important although usually neglected.

15.5.1 Design of Animation Techniques for Technical Animation

Design of animation techniques makes planning of the presentation necessary, which results in a number of communicative goals that are to be expressed one after another. The techniques listed in Sect. 15.3 can help to establish these points.

In ANIPLUS, there is one shot sequence for each communicative intent. These shots are created using a number of structuring techniques [Sha82].

- *Separation*
  Used often in dialog scenes, alternates between two shots showing the speakers. Separation makes the viewer part of the scene and creates a much greater emotional involvement. It conveys the sense of a strong correspondence between the two alternating shots and can be used in technical animation to link two separate, but related processes (see Fig. 15.8).

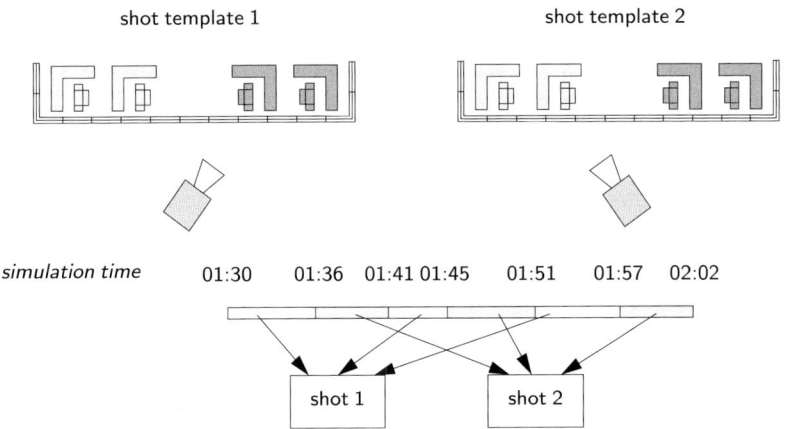

Figure 15.8: Shots and time settings in a separation

- *Parallel action*
  Similar to separation in that there are at least two locations involved, but here, showing them in a single shot is not an option. Parallel action is better suited for long-running animations where the action has some time to develop.
- *Master shot sequence*
  A master shot introduces the scene. Close-up and medium shots – with occasional returns to the master shot – tell the story.
- *Multi-angularity*
  Show the same spot from a different perspective. This technique is often used after cuts that consume time and skip irrelevant actions. Leaving the camera at the same position would create a disturbing jolt.
- *Camera movement*
  The most important reason for camera movements was already explained in Sect. 15.3. There are, of course, other situations where they are useful. When not forced by the need to follow a moving object, the camera movements can also be used (e.g., in an introductory pan) to provide a better feel for the scene and to assist the viewer's orientation.

15.5.2 Creating Animation Sequences

This section gives a brief overview of how ANIPLUS supports the creation of enhanced animation sequences from simple animation files.

Figure 15.9 outlines the basic work flow with ANIPLUS. First, an animation model complete with a scene description and animation actions must be opened. In this model, the author can walk around interactively in both space and time. This includes jumping to arbitrary points in time as well as playback with any speed (*time factor*). The author can thus thoroughly explore the model and derive the communicative goals that are to be expressed with this animation. These goals form the conceptual basis for the rest of the work.

To build a sequence, the user must first specify the communicative intent that this sequence should support. This includes a goal type, a verbal description and the time frame that the whole sequence should fill. The verbal description is not really used by the program, but it serves as a useful reminder as to what was intended and allows a user to validate the resulting sequence later with respect to the original goal.

Next, a film technique must be chosen that generates the actual shots for the sequence. Not all of the techniques generate multiple shots. For *camera movements*, only one shot must be specified. For the other techniques, two or more shots serve as templates for the actual shots that make up the sequence. These template shots are specified before generating the sequence by interactively placing the camera (as when exploring the scene) and associating a fixed position, a path, or a graphics object with the camera position and/or viewpoint.

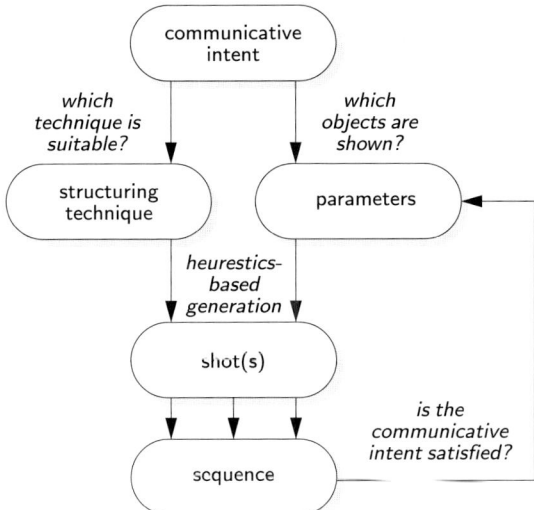

Figure 15.9: Workflow in the design process

Generating the shots then creates instances of the templates in a series defined by one of the structuring techniques, e.g., alternating between two templates in a *separation*. Each of the techniques has a different parameter set that controls the initial setup of the shot sequence. One could say this step adds the *time parameters* to the *positional parameters* of a shot.

For example, when using the multi-angularity technique, the user first defines the perspectives for the shots as mentioned above. Then, the timing parameters are derived from the previously defined overall length of the sequence, divided by the number of shots (three or four).

The system generates the shots so that there are no gaps between them. Whenever the start of the sequence is moved to another time, all shots are updated accordingly. If a cut is to consume time, its starting time can be set manually. The system supports time settings by interactive manipulation of a time slider. When the user finds the right time, it is entered automatically in the dialog form. To prevent overlapping when the start or the length of one shot has been changed, the following shots are delayed, if necessary, to make sure they start after the end of the previous shot. If that is not desired, these shots can also be edited.

Similar to the time settings, the camera positions can also be changed for each shot. All settings are initialized during the creation of a sequence. Since the heuristics employed are only rules of thumb, it is very important to give the user a chance to override them, if necessary.

Figure 15.10 shows a dialog box for editing a single shot. On the top, there is a timeline for the whole film where the current shot is highlighted.

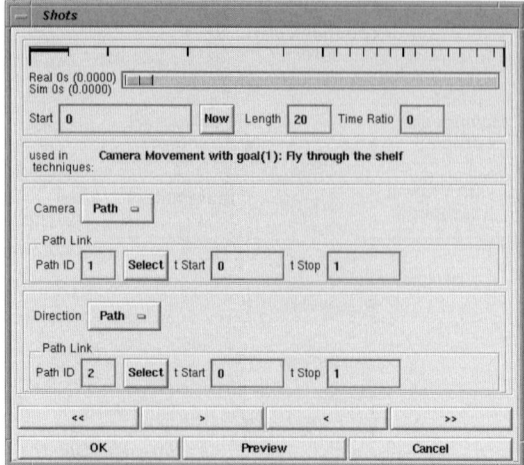

Figure 15.10: Dialog box for shot editing

The slider allows the user to adjust the current time within the shot. Since in each shot the camera position and/or viewpoint can be bound to a fixed position, a path, or an object, this helps to evaluate the camera movements. Below the top, the start of the shot, its length, and its time factor can be edited. Their initial values are set when the shot is generated as one of a certain sequence. The comment states which sequence the shot belongs to and what communicative goal is to be satisfied with this sequence. The next two boxes control the camera bindings (position and viewpoint). In this shot, the camera position remains fixed while the viewpoint follows a scene object. Object bindings can be specified by selecting the target object in the 3D scene and adjusting the camera. The system will then maintain the relative camera position and/or viewpoint with respect to the target object. Using the buttons below, a shot can be placed on the start or end of the film or switch places with the previous or next shot. The preview button allows the user to verify the settings for this shot.

15.6 Concluding Remarks

We have presented a concept for creating animations on the basis of the intents specified. Intent-based animations help to minimize the effort required to specify an animation. Animated movements are generated based on high-level statements on the level of communicative goals. The processing of high-level statements requires decomposition rules to break them down to low-level commands for an animator. These decomposition rules can be derived from film-making heuristics. Besides very general film-making techniques, dedicated knowledge about the application area is highly useful. This includes, for example, an analysis of videos for educational purposes.

15.6 Concluding Remarks 277

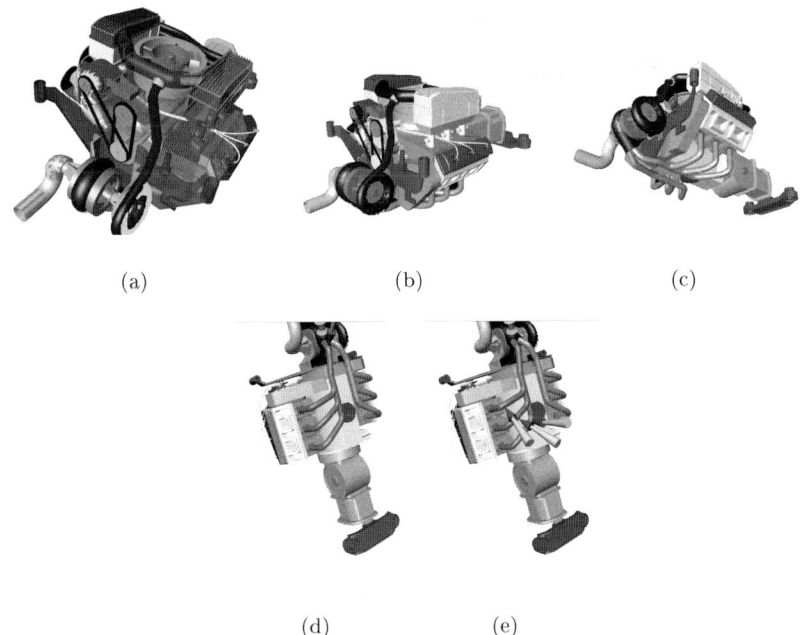

Figure 15.11: (a) Explanation of an engine's exhaust pipe: Original situation, (b) After an automatic rotation to recognize the exhaust pipe, (c) Rotation continued, (d) Arrows clarify the shape ..., (e) ...and structure of the exhaust pipe

Script languages for intent-based animation design support the specification of high-level statements directly. However, high-level statements should be added by more specific commands which allow a fine-grained control. Intent-based animations require a comfortable script language but can also benefit from facilities to interactively specify animations (or at least parts thereof). The integration of high-level specifications and interaction facilities for fine-tuning provides a comfortable way to create animations.

In particular, a teach-in facility which records the movements (e.g., object transformations, camera control) an author has performed is a useful add-on for intent-based animation design because it allows a fine-grained control over an animation.

Future work should concentrate on the validation of the concepts developed. For this purpose, a usability study which includes potential authors as well as viewers is required.

Contributors of Chap. 15: Ralf HELBING and Bernhard PREIM

Part VI

Abstractions in Interactive Systems

The methods and tools for abstraction in graphics described in the preceding five parts of this book can be applied selectively to a variety of different areas. In the chapters of this part, the methods of abstraction are explored primarily in connection with line drawings. The resultant images lend themselves well to emphasizing certain important features of the underlying model, while other details can be deemphasized without adversely affecting the overall impression. Each application draws on some aspect of the general concepts of abstraction introduced thus far, putting them to a test. However, each also brings with it its own specific challenges to be met.

First, Michael RÜGER, Kornelia ULLRICH, and Ian PITT show in Chap. 16 how the concepts of zooming can be applied to graphical user interfaces. In particular, they show how screen space can be saved by enabling the user to enlarge windows of interest while in response, the system makes other windows smaller to make them all fit in the screen space available. The concept of the aspect-of-interest (AOI) introduced earlier in Chap. 10 is put to use in deciding on the specific visualization of each window based on both its size and its context of use. The authors report on a user study comparing zoom navigation to the pan-and-zoom method of interaction. The results show that the new method of zoom navigation is an attractive alternative.

As pointed out earlier in this book, medical illustration, which Stefan SCHLECHTWEG and Hubert WAGENER take up in Chap. 17, relies heavily on methods of abstraction. The authors discuss how abstraction can be used in an interactive, text-driven illustration system for anatomical models. In particular, they address the following problem: Given a marked up medical text describing an organ, produce an illustration which highlights the relevant parts and which can be explored interactively by the user. The result is a toolbox for managing the mapping of features of the text to be illustrated onto graphical means of expression. The prototypical system called TEXTILLUSTRATOR which the authors describe is but the tip of the iceberg in this field of application.

Chapter 18 by Frank GODENSCHWEGER also deals with the human body, but from a more macroscopic point of view. He applies the concepts of abstraction to produce animations of gestures as they are used in sign language for deaf people. Up to now, systems for producing sign language have concentrated on shaded images, even though printed handbooks use line drawings almost exclusively for explaining signs. Indeed, using such simpler, abstract graphics allows the viewer to concentrate on the essential features of the presentation. To date there are no systems that can produce really natural-looking photorealistic animations of moving hands, but the author's goal is to produce convincing line drawings in which the graphical features do not distract the viewer from the intended message.

While thus far we have concentrated on rendering geometric models, Ralf HELBING looks in Chap. 19 at animating models of processes. The work is motivated by the observation that a given process can be simulated but then visualized in many different ways. In particular, abstraction is a prerequisite for the visualization because not all the available data could possibly be encoded in a single image or a sequence of images. The author develops the notion of plugins for modeling visualization and applies these to simulation and visualization of material flow in factories.

Chapter 16

Zoom Navigation in User Interfaces

Many authors have observed the impact of the increased cognitive load users are confronted with when using today's high-functionality computer systems. Graphical (direct manipulation) interfaces tend to use the notion of infinite working sheets. Yet existing screen real-estate is finite, partly due to current technological restrictions but mainly because of the limitations imposed by the human perceptual system.

In real-life complex situations, people rely on global context while exploring local detail, a perceptual ability imposing no conscious cognitive load. FURNAS' generalized fisheye view [Fur86] exploits this ability for the computer screen by displaying several levels of detail simultaneously. This technique has been used in a wide range of applications, as surveyed and classified by Noik [Noi94]. Fisheye techniques are also discussed in Chaps. 2, 9, and 10 of this book.

Reducing the organizational and navigational overhead, however, is only one part of the story. Active user support also aims at helping the user to deal with the applications at hand. There seems to be a trend to modeless interfaces as, for instance, the graphical Smalltalk-80 environment [Tes81] and direct manipulation [Shn92]. Relatively unobtrusive support mechanisms like command expansions and navigation by defaults are gone in such modeless interfaces.

Furthermore, active task support has become extremely complex due to the degrees of freedom offered by today's graphical user interfaces.

GENTNER and NIELSEN [GN96] propose what they call an *Anti-Mac-Interface* to overcome the restrictions of the WIMP (windows, icons, menus, pointer) interface. They emphasize the computer's role in cooperating with the user by providing support for the user's interaction. According to the

Table 16.1: Some Mac and Anti-Mac characteristics

Mac	Anti-Mac
WYSIWYG	Represent meaning
User control	Shared control
Modelessness	Richer cues

authors' proposal, this can be achieved by breaking with the paradigm of complete user control and allowing the computer to actively participate in presentation and interaction issues. Three of the Anti-Mac interface characteristics (see Table 16.1) in particular match the design rationale behind a new interaction technique called zoom navigation (as introduced in [RPR96], see also Chap. 10).

In addition to the degree of interest (DOI), whose computation is based on the geometric and conceptual distance to the current focus point, an aspect of interest (AOI) is introduced based on the history of the user's interest in aspects of the information space. Zoom navigation interprets a user's navigational actions as shifts in his or her point(s) of interest (DOI and AOI). Like NORMAN [Nor90] who uses the term *affordance* to characterize the way real-world objects supply usage cues, we introduce the term *navigational affordance*. In terms of the Anti-Mac interface characteristics, zoom navigation helps in adjusting the navigational affordance (supply richer cues) as well as choosing an appropriate representation (represent meaning) according to the user's estimated information needs (shared control). In addition, zoom navigation is application (domain) independent.

16.1 Prior and Related Work

Research on reducing the interaction effort when navigating in large information spaces has utilized FURNAS' generalized fisheye view in a variety of techniques. "Classical" fisheye viewers as described in SARKAR and BROWN [SB94] make use of cartesian or polar transformations to enlarge the view at the point of interest (focus). In PAD++, BEDERSON et al. [BH94] apply a similar technique to navigation and visualization by supplying a special widget set supporting zooming. Though not a fisheye technique, it also relies on detail and context.

In DILL et al. [DBHH94] the variable zoom technique is introduced, which allows more than one point of interest to be handled in an efficient and intuitive manner. This technique is combined with a rather sophisticated reasoning process to give "contextual assistance" by using agents to guide switching of representations. The authors call their technique "intelligent zoom".

Strategies for automatically placing windows according to domain-specific assumptions have been developed for a calendar visualizer [MRD94] and a hypertext system [BH94]. A more generic technique is presented in [LE95] and describes an algorithm based on the concept of simulated annealing to produce an optimal screen layout. Computational costs associated with this method seem to be too high, however, taking approximately four seconds for the optimal layout of twenty nodes (=windows) on a high-end workstation.

Reducing the number of windows by performing editing in place is accomplished by a number of methods. The concept of visual editing realized in Microsoft's OLE2 enables applications to invoke other applications to let the user edit some foreign document part in place without navigational effort. Within OpenDoc this becomes the basic interaction paradigm so the user does not need to switch between application windows.

16.2 The Zoom Navigator

The concept of zoom navigation was used to implement the zoom navigator within the CREATE! simulation development environment. The CREATE! system provides a number of tools for building and running discrete event simulation models as well as tools for modifying the environment itself [RB95]. Zoom navigation was integrated into the two-dimensional graphical model editor. Model elements are mapped onto nodes in the pluggable zoom structure and the interval bounds are computed based on the bounds of the current graphical representation (see Fig. 16.1).

The ZOOMNAVIGATOR enhances interaction in several ways. The zoom with its fisheye properties directly allows for a better navigation in large and especially hierarchical models as already reported by SCHAFFER et al.

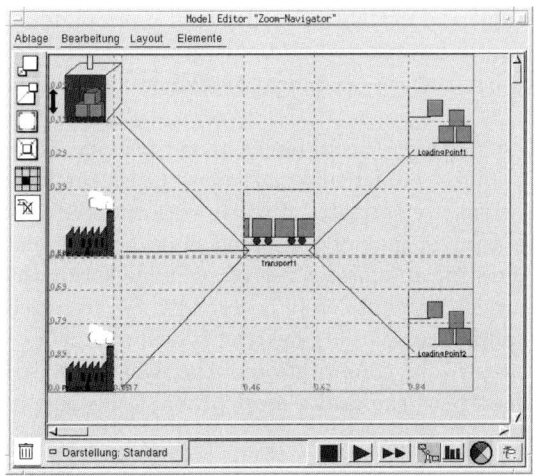

Figure 16.1: ZOOMNAVIGATOR: the graphical model editor with the interval structure overlaid

[SZB+93]. Although quite unusual, pan-and-zoom interaction is not disabled, as can be seen by the scroll bars and zoom icons remaining on the screen (see Fig. 16.1). When working on large models, users often prefer to zoom into a certain part of the model, and then use the fisheye zoom within this area.

We encountered several problems when using zoom techniques in this environment. One of them was mixing pan-and-zoom techniques with fisheye techniques. When working on very large models, users preferred to use pan-and-zoom to zoom into a certain part of the model, and work with the fisheye zoom within this area. Since the zoom algorithm affects all nodes, zooming up a node can force other nodes out of the field of view. There is currently no solution to this problem, although one possible idea would be to restrict the zoom to the actual visible subset of nodes.

Aspects or information categories for model elements are the graphical appearance in the layout (icon), parameter values, program code, and the textual or graphical results from a simulation run. Figure 16.2 illustrates the different aspects associated with model elements at different levels of detail. The level of detail here corresponds directly to the node size in the graphical model editor.

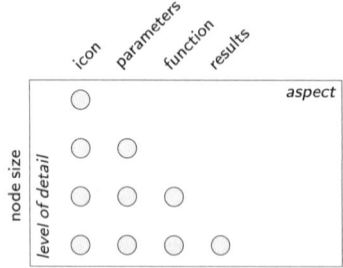

Figure 16.2: ZoomNavigator representation matrix

Working with simulation models usually implies a number of iteration cycles between modeling, simulation, and evaluation. Advanced users building and testing new elements frequently have to switch between tools in the development part of the environment and the graphical modeling, simulation, and evaluation part.

Zoom navigation smoothly integrates the different tools into the main working context, namely the graphical model editor. Depending on the level of detail (node size), representations are activated directly within the graphical model. Figure 16.3 shows a screenshot of a zoomed node with its parameter dialog activated. To allow for an efficient use of available space, the node's graphical representation (icon) is completely covered by the activated dialog. As the dialog background is transparent, the user is still able to recognize the overall graphical context. The computation of the AOI estimated the editing or viewing of parameters as the user's most probable interest in the current interaction context.

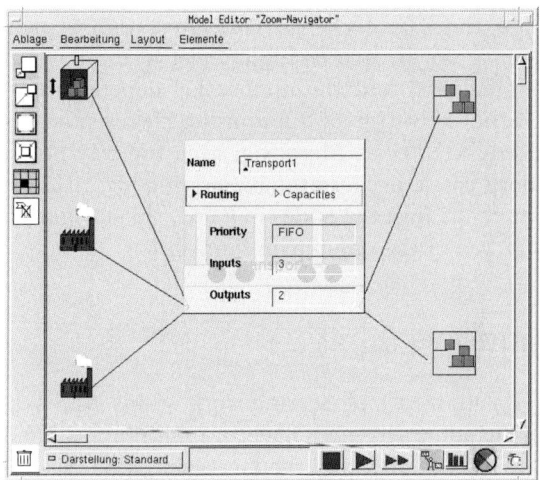

Figure 16.3: Result of zooming the center element in Fig. 16.1: zoomed element has the parameter dialog activated

With the progress of work in the simulation model, the user's interest shifts from editing tasks to validation and evaluation tasks. This involves repeated comparison and changing of parameters as well as evaluating and displaying results of simulation runs.

Advanced users typically extend the predefined set of simulation elements by making use of the integrated development environment. Zoom navigation supports viewing the component's code or parameter definitions (see Fig. 16.4) while iterating through development and debugging cycles from within the graphical model. Nodes of interest can be zoomed up and easily revised.

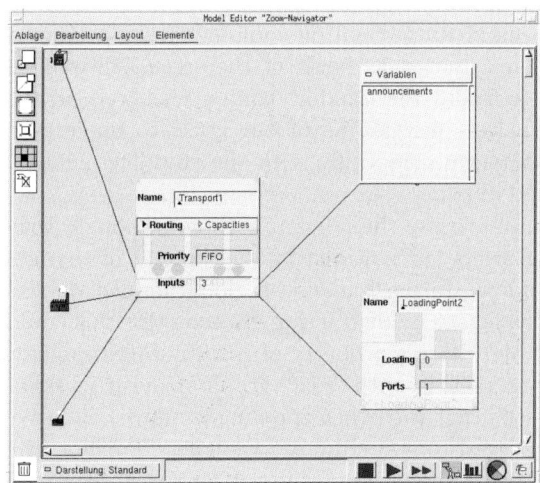

Figure 16.4: Zoomed elements with different dialogs activated

If we analyze interaction in the ZOOMNAVIGATOR, navigation is performed as in the one-dimensional case: by expressing interest in items, item groups (by selecting multiple elements) and the application-dependent aspects. The system reacts with the activation of appropriate representations in the same way as in the ZOOMCALENDAR. Moreover, even the way nodes grow or shrink is uniform in both cases, because the underlying algorithm is exactly the same. If a user were to arrange the nodes in a line, the navigation behavior would be exactly as it was in the one-dimensional case.

16.3 Zooming Windows

It has been a long way from ENGELBART's pioneering work on his NLS system [EE68] to modern multiple-window systems. Their graphical appeal and flexibility serves as a basis for dealing with an ever increasing amount and complexity of information. By using separate windows for different tasks, users can handle several applications and documents simultaneously and switch back and forth.

There are several drawbacks, though. As screen space is a limited resource, only a limited number of windows can be used. Movable overlapping windows compensate this by reusing screen space in a third (or more correctly second-and-a-half) dimension. The housekeeping task associated with this, however, binds increasing resources in terms of user interaction and cognitive effort. Some multiple window strategies like tiling or stacking [Shn92] try to reduce or avoid this overhead, but provide only partial solutions or sacrifice flexibility.

As the amount of housekeeping effort is directly related to the number of windows, there are two ways of tackling this problem: supporting users in managing multiple windows or reducing the number of windows necessary to accomplish their goals. Using zoom navigation combines these methods. Windows and their contents are treated as parts of the same hierarchical structure, allowing the user to zoom the window contents as well as the windows themselves. Nevertheless, it was one of our goals to make sure that window zooming would integrate smoothly with the standard window management actions mentioned above.

Our first approach was simply to use the pluggable zoom. Though early results looked quite promising, users felt irritated by the number of changes going on when zooming a window. In particular, the global impact on size and position of all windows was felt to be distracting. Reasons for this could be traced back mainly to the algorithm's property of maintaining topology. Although appreciated when interacting with "real" graph structures, strict topological correctness is not seen that way when zooming windows. Relative positions of windows were preferred to stay "almost" the same, but not in a strict topological sense. In order to enhance the results of window zooming we analyzed the degrees of freedom in the original variable zoom algorithm and

16.3 Zooming Windows

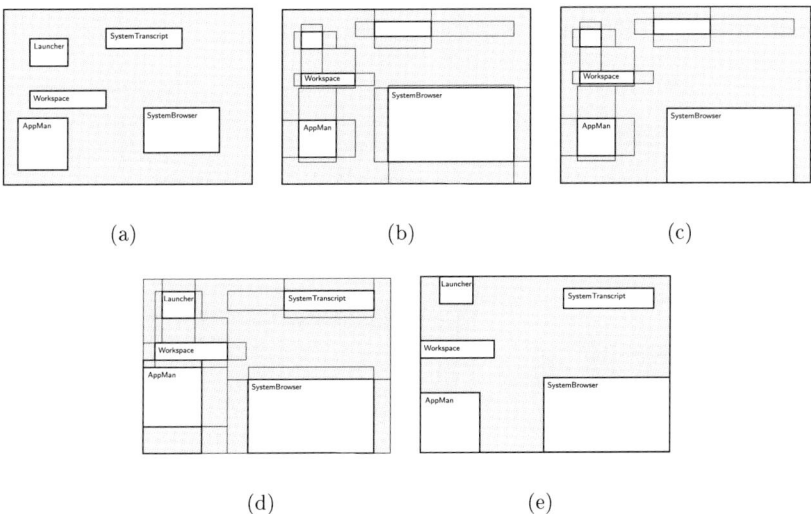

Figure 16.5: Window zooming: (a) the initial layout, (b) after zooming, (c) the first iteration, (d) the second iteration, (e) the final layout

decided to explore relaxation of the fixed properties topological correctness, ratio, and overlap.

As shown in Fig. 16.5(a), we select the rectangles formed by the window borders and the adjacent empty intervals already existing in the variable zoom instead of computing optimal growing areas. Each window then determines which of the four resulting areas to use. The order in which windows have the right to choose depends on a grow demand factor computed from several window-dependent factors like size, distance from original position, and ratio.

A gravity parameter describes the preferred direction of growing and shrinking windows with size limitations (min, max) within a larger area. Capturing and losing space in alternate directions caused windows to wander around. Size and position constraints of one window do not prevent others from growing, so this can lead to overlaps. Nevertheless, windows will never be completely covered due to the inherent properties of the variable zoom algorithm and our postprocessing steps.

All postprocessing steps cause a violation of topological correctness and render the internal data structures of the variable zoom obsolete. One property of the pluggable zoom, however, is its ability to re-setup its internal state at any time, which we make use of here. Smooth integration with existing window management functions was one major goal in our application of the pluggable zoom to window management. Closing simply removes it, moving is treated as deletion and insertion, resizing initializes the zoom structure.

Opening a window either inserts an empty area which is zoomed to make room, or adds to the top of a stack (see Fig. 16.6).

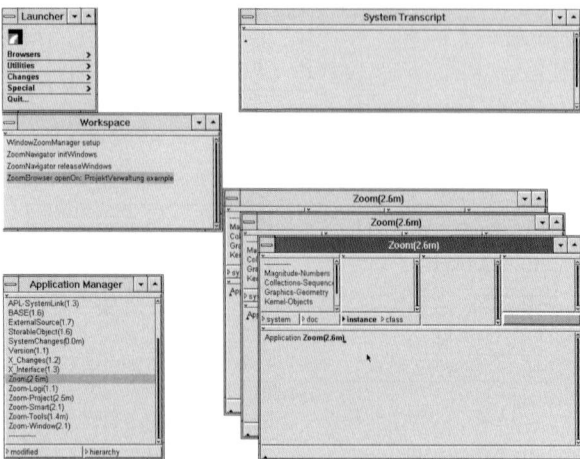

Figure 16.6: Opening windows on a stack

16.4 User Study

In order to evaluate the impact of zoom navigation, we carried out a user study involving both standard pan and zoom techniques as well as zoom navigation. The ZOOMNAVIGATOR was used in this study, because both the ZOOMCALENDAR and ZOOMVIZ are still prototypes and allowed only some informal observations to be collected.

16.4.1 General Setting

Because the ZOOMNAVIGATOR is part of a large simulation development environment providing a rich set of tools, it requires rather extensive domain-specific knowledge to operate. In order to allow a sufficient number of subjects to successfully complete the tasks, we had to isolate some characteristic work situations and emulate these without having to rely on domain-specific knowledge.

16.4.2 Hypotheses

Based on the experiences with the CREATE! system, we formulated a set of hypotheses to compare typical tasks from the different phases in the simulation lifecycle with and without use of zoom navigation.

We applied a technique similar to that used in [LBT96] by measuring motor and nonmotor times and used the nonmotor times as an indirect measure for the user's cognitive load.

Hypothesis 1
The total time required to complete a task will be less using zoom navigation than that using pan-and-zoom.

Hypothesis 2
Less nonmotor time will be required relative to the total time needed to complete a task using zoom navigation than by using pan-and-zoom.

16.4.3 Variables

The independent variable in this experiment was the interaction technique used first (pan-and-zoom, fisheye). Subjects were assigned randomly to either of the two groups.

The dependent variables consist of two components, the total time needed to accomplish a task and the amount of nonmotor time in relation to the total time.

16.4.4 Subjects

A total of six subjects, all computer science students or researchers, participated in the study.

All had worked with graphical simulation systems before, but only three of them with the CREATE! system used in this study. However, the experiment was designed to abstract from CREATE!-specific interactions and rely instead on tasks found in most graphical simulation systems. Three had worked briefly with fisheye zoom systems before.

Each participant was briefly introduced to the purpose of the experiment and the goals of the different tasks.

16.4.5 Overall Experiment Structure

Experiments took between 30 and 40 minutes followed by an interview of approximately 20 minutes. The steps in the experiment were as follows:

Step 1 (Interaction exercises)
Through the initial exercises we made sure that subjects achieved sufficient competence with the basic interaction techniques.

Step 2 (Measurement of motor times)
The tasks within this group were aimed at measuring the times taken for drawing connections under varying circumstances like different node sizes

and the number of intermediate points. No extra navigation steps or recognition efforts were needed to identify the source and destination elements. The values measured allowed us to isolate the nonmotor times in the more complex connection experiments. The times were collected by recording all user interactions into a logfile.

Step 3 (Allow subjects to perform tasks)
After the initial recordings were made, subjects carried out the main three tasks using pan-and-zoom and, after completion of all tasks, using zoom navigation. Half of the subjects performed the tasks in reversed order to compensate for learning effects.

16.4.6 Experiment Tasks

Graphical models in the CREATE! environment consist of elements representing simulation entities and connections between these elements denoting the flow of information (recall Fig. 16.1). Typical interaction tasks vary depending on the project state. Within the construction phase, placing elements, drawing connections, and specifying parameters are the dominant tasks. Throughout the validation and experimentation phase, comparing and changing of parameters as well as understanding dynamic relationships dictate the user's interaction. We therefore designed tasks to reflect these typical interaction structures.

Task 1 (Validating connections)
Simulation studies typically involve a lot of work on validation. In the CREATE! environment this almost always requires a consistency check of the existing connections. The first task was a simulation of validating an existing model by finding out the names of connected nodes.

Task 2 (Connecting nodes)
The second task was the simulation of building a new model. In CREATE! a major part consists of connecting simulation elements at connectors (small areas in the nodes). The model was large enough either to require several zoom operations or to point at very small areas.

Task 3 (Connecting by name)
A typical situation in different phases of simulation development in CREATE! involves the identification of several nodes and, afterwards, to connect some of these. In the third task, subjects were given a list of names (of already existing elements in a model) to connect.

16.4.7 Collection of Data

The data were collected by automatically logging each user interaction to a task-specific logfile. Each log entry contained a time stamp and information about the interaction type (button press, drag) and the position or distance of the operation.

16.4.8 Results

Motor times for drawing connections consist of a mouse click at the starting point and a drag operation. Each intermediate point adds an extra drag operation. From a total of 90 connections we measured a mean value of 3.0 seconds. For the task of connecting some small elements a mean time of 11.0 seconds was measured, caused by the difficulty of pointing at small areas.

Table 16.2: Comparison of mean task completion times

| Task | Mean times to carry out tasks | | Improvement |
	pan-and-zoom	zoom navigation	to pan-and-zoom
1	29.3 s	27.4 s	6.9%
2	39.3 s	28.2 s	39.4%
3	200.2 s	86.4 s	131.7%

Hypothesis 1
The comparison of task completion times between the interaction techniques (Table 16.2) showed a general advantage for zoom navigation. To determine if any of the differences were significant, the results were analyzed using a WILCOXON test. The times obtained for each task using pan-and-zoom were compared to those from using zoom navigation.

The difference for the task of validating existing connections (task 1) showed only a small difference (6.9%), as pan-and-zoom allows for a fast navigation to the endpoints of connections (repeated overview and zoom-in).

Connecting small elements (task 2) was significantly faster (39.4%) using zoom navigation, although additional zoom operations were required. The difference in motor times when connecting small versus larger sized elements made up for this effect.

For tasks 1 and 2 no statistically significant difference was found.

The largest percentage improvement of zoom navigation over pan-and-zoom (131.7%) was detected in the task of connecting by name list (task 3). The total time using zoom navigation was found to be significantly lower ($p \leq 0.025$) than that using pan-and-zoom. We think the ability of the zoom navigation to display additional information within the overall context explains this result.

Hypothesis 2
The motor times made for 19% of the total time needed with pan-and-zoom and 60% for zoom navigation. We found this difference to be statistically

significant ($p \leq 0.025$). As the nonmotor times indicate periods where the user is engaged in mental activity, the relatively low portion of nonmotor times in the pan-and-zoom case indicates a much higher overhead resulting from the extra effort required to identify elements by zooming in and out.

For task 3 we found empirical support for both hypotheses. Zoom navigation not only enabled the users to perform the task in less time but also reduced the cognitive load significantly.

16.4.9 Interview

The interview directly following each experiment aimed at collecting users' impressions and suggestions for changing or improving the ZOOMNAVIGATOR. There were another three subjects performing the tasks whose logs were not used in the statistical analysis for various technical reasons. However, the data taken from the interviews are included here, too.

Table 16.3: Subjects' overall ratings for the techniques

	Excellent	Good	Not so good
pan-and-zoom	0%	33%	66%
ZOOMNAVIGATOR	55%	44%	0%

Most users were surprised that "it really worked"; although some users already had experience with fisheye zoom techniques, the activation of representations within the surrounding (graphical) context was felt to be a real improvement. Most users rated the ZOOMNAVIGATOR higher than the pan-and-zoom interaction (Table 16.3).

In general, reactions to zoom navigation were positive (see Table 16.4). Most users preferred zoom navigation over pan-and-zoom and rated it more user friendly.

Table 16.4: Comparison of user judgements on pan-and-zoom and zoom navigation (ZN) as the main interaction paradigm

	Agreed	Not agreed
prefer ZN	88%	11%
ZN more user friendly	88%	11%
ZN worked as expected	77%	22%

Arguments supporting this opinion were the ability to select multiple focus points, reduce uninteresting details, and activate representations. Some users mentioned that zoom navigation was "simply fun". The main argument (44% of all mentioned) concerned the underlying zoom with its detail-and-context view. Of the suggestions brought forward, some dealt with basic interaction techniques not directly related to zoom navigation like drawing connections. Those regarding the ZOOMNAVIGATOR suggested a finer control over zoom speed, either by the user and the system or by replacing the constant speed by an automatic zoom to the next available representation.

16.5 Conclusion and Future Work

The ZOOMNAVIGATOR is a realization of the concept of zoom navigation in an existing complex application environment. This demonstrated the feasibility of the pluggable zoom as an object-oriented, reusable software component.

We introduced the notion of navigational affordance, borrowing from ideas advanced by NORMAN By providing clues about contents and using an estimation of user interests by computation of the *DOI* and *AOI* values, the computer is able to assist in interaction within complex systems.

Work is still to be done in making better use of the information gathered throughout the interaction. Last but not least, user interaction with the system is a reflection of his or her way to a problem's solution for which SCHOEN [Sch82] coined the term *reflection in action*.

Contributors of Chap. 16: Michael RÜGER, Kornelia ULLRICH, and Ian PITT

Chapter 17

Interactive Medical Illustrations

In anatomy, and even more in surgery, the viewer's expectation of a good illustration is to get reliable information about form, structure, and sometimes also texture of the depicted objects. Within printed illustrations this can be achieved by using different kinds of drawings or even photographs. Here structure can be depicted by color coding, texture by "shading" the surface differently. The general presentation goals, as stated in Chap. 4, also apply here. Besides that, medical illustrations include an artistic handling of the subject and thus a medical illustration can be regarded as a fusion of science and the graphic image.

Although computer graphics today has a major influence in many areas, medical illustrations are still almost exclusively done by hand. This has at least two reasons. First, producing a scientific or medical illustration requires a lot of training and knowledge about the subject as well as the drawing technique. This knowledge can hardly be represented by algorithms or data structures. Second, today's computer graphics tools are not designed for the purpose of these illustrations and are thus only marginally applicable.

With the tools and methods described so far in this book, we can now open the field of scientific and medical illustration to computer graphics. There are basically three possible ways:

1. Creating strictly two-dimensional drawings and other images by using painting and drawing tools which are already available.
2. Creating images from a 3D geometry model by specific rendering methods. Here also special "shading" methods must be developed to meet the requirements in the area of medical illustration.
3. Designing tools for interactive creation and manipulation of medical illustrations. Here it is essential to cater for interaction facilities as well as

for new ways of conceptually integrating textual (symbolic) and graphical information.

Special rendering techniques for the creation of illustrative images from 3D models have already been discussed in Chap. 4. The main focus of this chapter will be on the last of the three points: designing tools for interactive creation and manipulation of medical illustrations. Thus this chapter goes along with Chap. 13 in the sense that here also techniques for combining textual and graphical information in illustrations are examined.

The chapter is organized as follows: In Sect. 17.1 we make some observations on illustrations in traditional media and derive a new concept for interactive illustration systems. This approach is further examined in Sect. 17.2. Within the field of interactive illustration systems, other approaches have also been developed. Some examples of other systems are presented in Sect. 17.3 and compared with the text-driven techniques. Finally, Sect. 17.4 poses some interesting questions regarding future application and development of interactive illustration systems.

17.1 Interactive Medical Illustration

Looking at anatomy reference material, two big categories of books can be found: textbooks (e.g., [WM92]) and atlases [Sob88]. Textbooks – as the name implies – focus primarily on a verbal description of the subject matter at hand. The images used here have to be chosen and designed carefully since their function cannot be understood without the surrounding text. However, even textbooks require extensive use of images since the underlying problems and subjects must be visualized. We will give a short overview of the relations between images and text:

- *Text illustration*
  Images accompany and illustrate the *text* rather than the *subject*. This means that they do not cover the whole bandwidth of facts which might be interesting for a given subject but depict selected items in great detail, whereas all other parts are shown to give the viewer a certain orientation. For example, an illustration belonging to a paragraph dealing with the muscles which move the eyeball may show other parts of the eye as well (e.g., the optic nerve, the lens, ...), but the focus is on the muscles. Thus they are shown in great detail and everything else is visually thrust into the background.
- *Abstraction*
  Besides elements of the text at hand, images also show abstract information like the direction of blood flow or the degrees of freedom in joint movement. This is achieved by placing arrows or other abstract graphical symbols in the picture. This information is described verbally in the surrounding text.

- *Labeling*
  The labeling of the images is sparser than in anatomic atlases. In most cases, only labels with a reference in the text are shown.

Since images used in textbooks only focus on special parts, the number of images needed to illustrate a subject to any degree of completeness is rather high. In certain situations one fact has to be illustrated by several images, since some information can only be gained by looking at an object from different directions. But this means that illustrations may be spread over several pages, aggravating problems associated with the mental integration of all the information.

In contrast to this, an anatomy atlas contains almost no text at all. The images illustrate the *subject* and hence contain much more information in each individual image. Images used in atlases are in most cases larger and thus more detailed than in textbooks. Labels are shown in overwhelming numbers (up to 80 labels per image can be found). Those labels have to be mentally integrated and – much more important – sorted out by the viewer to get the information he or she wants. Additional information is given within the figure caption or, somewhat more rarely, in accompanying texts or tables. In this context it is also important to show a subject from more than one viewpoint to build up a 3D mental impression of the depicted objects.

Although the categories – textbook and atlas – seem to be different, they have many features in common. First, there is the need to incorporate several images illustrating one subject into one mental model. Second, the relationship between image and text is essential – either as correlation between labels and objects, or as assignment of images to a piece of text. Third, all images have to possess the qualities already mentioned above – clear recognizability of objects and the structures and relationships between them as well as esthetic appeal.

For interactive illustration systems which resemble, up to a certain point, those traditionally known media, we can also identify two big groups of systems with those differences. We will call systems which mainly focus on the graphics (and thus are similar to atlases) *graphics-driven*, and those which concentrate primarily on textual information (like textbooks) *text-driven*. Either way, to develop an illustration system a number of important points have to be considered:

- *Provide integration of text and images*
  An interactive illustration system should incorporate both textual and graphical information in such a way that the relationship between text and image becomes immediately clear to the user.
- *Facilitate interaction*
  Interaction facilities with the illustration (i.e., with the graphical part) should at least support change of viewpoint and zooming.
- *Provide multiple access to information*
  Access to information should not be restricted to one particular inter-

action method; instead, many possible ways should be offered to get a specific piece of information.
- *Provide flexible levels of detail*
  The amount of information (especially textual information) provided to the user should be controllable by the user, though in certain situations the system itself may decide that more or less detailed information will be presented.

In the following we will present the TEXTILLUSTRATOR, an example of a text-driven system.

17.2 A Text-Driven Illustration System

In medical textbooks, the primary information is encoded in the text. As already stated, illustrations help the reader to understand the text, they focus on special aspects, and their contents is closely related to the text. An interactive text-driven illustration system should therefore place the text at the center of interest and create images corresponding either to the contents of the visible portion of the text or to user interaction with the text. The following remarks are based on the implemented system TEXTILLUSTRATOR; a screen shot is shown in Fig. 17.1.

The display is divided into two areas. The graphical view on the left contains the illustration, which is generated from a three-dimensional geometric model. The text pane on the right contains the text for which the illustrations are generated. After starting up the application, the user selects a text and the corresponding 3D model, and an initial screen layout is generated. Within the graphics view all standard interaction techniques (i.e., rotation, translation, zooming) can be used to manipulate the graphics. Due to its length, the text does not fit entirely in the window, thus a scrollbar helps to choose the appropriate region.

With this system the user interacts by navigating through the text with the scrollbar. The point of the system is that while one does this the graphics automatically adapt to the contents of the text by changing the viewpoint or the presentation of objects (color, level of detail, transparent or opaque, etc.). While the user is building up a mental connection between the text and the illustration this reduces the effort needed to search for the parts of the image described in the currently visible portion of the text. Only the objects of interest are highlighted, and all other objects are visually thrust into the background, for instance by coloring them in different shades of gray. In this way the user creates an animation which always reflects the contents of the currently visible part of the text and thus also the reading history.

Furthermore, additional interaction facilities are provided to give a more detailed connection between graphics and text. Clicking on a name in the text highlights the corresponding graphical object. This enables the user to explicitly look up items described in the text and avoids the need to search

17.2 A Text-Driven Illustration System

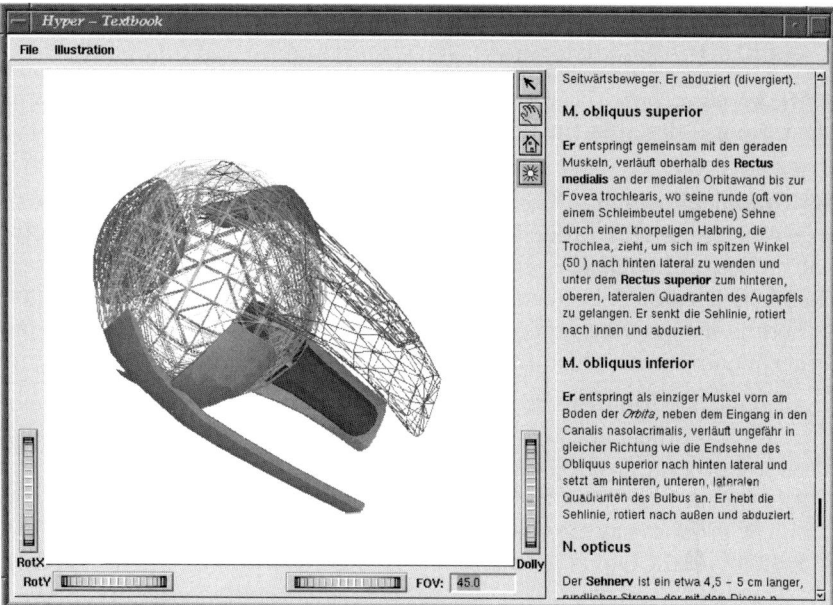

Figure 17.1: Screen shot of TEXTILLUSTRATOR, a text-driven system: the text pane on the right includes special interaction facilities, the graphics on the left is created from a 3D model based on the contents of the visible text portion (for easier reproduction on paper the selected parts are shaded, whereas all other parts are displayed as wireframe)

through a long list of labels. Also, the other way round is possible. Selecting an object in the graphics causes the text to scroll so that an appropriate description for the selected object is displayed. The selection of the part of the text to be displayed is either based on the document structure (i.e., the object's name appears in a title of a section or chapter) or the first occurrence of the object is chosen.

The interaction facilities provided in the TEXTILLUSTRATOR help the user to better navigate through a longer text by creating illustrations which always reflect the current reading position and which provide further possibilities to explore the contents of the text. The following sections describe the requirements and techniques behind text-driven illustrations.

17.2.1 The Information Space

The interaction facilities provided as well as the visualizations of graphics and text are built based on the information space which basically consists of three parts:

- the three-dimensional geometric model holding all necessary data to create the illustration,

- the text to display, and
- additional structures connecting graphical and textual information.

Before we show how the connections between graphics and text are established, we will describe the underlying models.

The Graphical Model. The 3D geometry model which is the basis for the generation of the illustration is rather simple. We concentrate here on polygonal model, although this choice is arbitrary; any geometric model (e.g., voxel models or models constructed from free-form surfaces) will do as long as there is a rendering component which can handle it. We impose some further requirements which can easily be satisfied:

- All objects within the geometric model have to be clearly differentiable from each other, i.e., the whole geometric model has to be divided into several objects (see Fig. 17.2).
- All objects have to be identifiable by a unique identification key. Also, object groups may be assigned such a key. This requires a structured model (recall Chap. 3 for additional structures within geometric models).

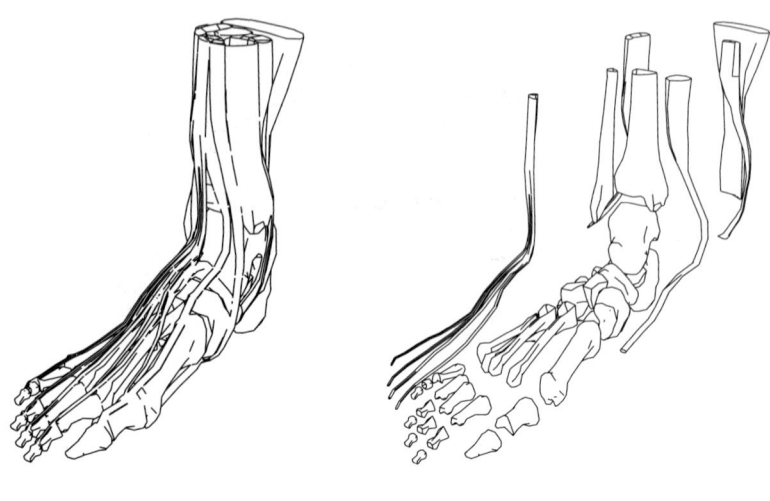

(a) The model as a whole   (b) The model divided in parts

Figure 17.2: Construction of the geometric model from individual parts

As data source we use file formats like 3DS (Autodesk 3D-Studio), or Inventor. Besides the pure geometry, color and transparency information as well as the object identifiers are used.

For display, the geometry model is rendered using OpenGL and presented to the user in a special viewer which is also responsible for all interactions on the graphics side.

17.2 A Text-Driven Illustration System

The Text Model. Since we are dealing with a text-driven system, the model for the text plays an important role and thus has to incorporate several kinds of information besides the given verbal description. At present, text formatting instructions as well as relations between parts of the text (i.e., text entities) and graphical objects are stored. A special text representation based on SGML was developed to build an internal representation which holds all necessary data and can be extended easily. This *TaggedText* contains for each character:

- the ASCII value,
- formatting instructions (boldface, italic, font size, etc.), and
- an array of tags which themselves hold arbitrary references (pointers).

This data structure is implemented very efficiently, i.e., for each character the data are not stored directly (which would lead to many redundancies) but are easily accessible. By using the TaggedText we are able to determine all additional information for each character position.

Within the parsing process of the given SGML file, markups which result in a formatting attribute are converted into the corresponding attribute and all other markups (as long as they are interpreted by the parser) are converted into tags which, in turn, are assigned to the text (see Fig. 17.3). These tags include, for instance,

- references (similar to hyperlinks) with their destinations,
- associations between different text parts with the positions of the associated parts,
- object names,
- the number of appearance of an object, and
- an importance value for an appearing object (e.g., objects appearing within the title of a chapter or a section are more important than those appearing within the normal text).

Some of the tags created this way are just placeholders for tags which have a direct connection to the graphics model. They are replaced by the actual data within the startup phase of the application.

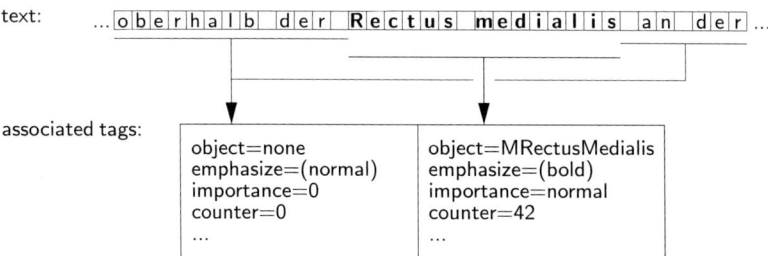

Figure 17.3: Within the TaggedText for each character, formatting instructions as well as other attributes are stored

Since the text is the most sensitive part within text-driven illustration systems, the preparation of a given text is crucial. However, a simple keyword search already suffices in most cases. The most important point is to establish connections between text entities and objects in the graphical model. In the medical domain, in which we are working, this can easily be done by searching for the Latin names of anatomic objects. Also, relations between several objects can be found within medical texts without a sophisticated linguistic analysis. One reason for this is that in the medical domain there exists a "pleasantly standardized" terminology. It is our belief that without including linguistic methods we can keep the approach as general as possible. In addition to keyword search, an interactive tool for text preparation serves the purpose well.

Besides pure text and graphics oriented information (as can be seen in Fig. 17.4) additional, so-called *context information* is used for both graphics and text. Here a possible model structure as well as other data influencing the graphical representation (e.g., color and transparency) of model parts are incorporated into the model and evaluated accordingly (see Chap. 3 for more information on the enrichment of geometric model with context information).

17.2.2 Coupling of Graphics and Text

The connection between the illustration and the verbal description is of great importance, especially in text-driven systems where the text cannot be displayed within the graphics (e.g., as labels). For the techniques used here, the following considerations are required:

- *Bi-directionality of connections*
  Connections between text and graphics have to be bi-directional so that interactions on either one trigger actions on the other side.
- *Loose coupling*
  Text and graphics should be loosely coupled. This allows easy registration of new interaction facilities as well as the enabling/disabling of existing ones.
- *Standard interaction facilities*
  Standard interaction facilities on the graphics as well as on the text are to be supported to provide a familiar environment to the user.

The text-graphics mediator[1] (see Fig. 17.4) as implemented in TEXTILLUSTRATOR fulfills exactly those requirements. It builds the connection between the text and the view which displays the model. Furthermore, it keeps a list of registered special mediators which, in turn, are responsible for special interaction scenarios. During the setup process of the application, the text-graphics mediator gets the geometric data as well as the enriched text. As

---

[1] The term mediator is used with reference to the design pattern "Mediator" (see [GHJV95]) although it is not entirely the same.

a next step, a table for all registered special mediators is created and initialized. Special registration functions for adding entries are provided. The following three entries in this table are always present:

1. A "picking mediator" which supports selections based on picking actions in the text.
2. A "scrolling mediator" which triggers reactions on a change of the visible portion of text (which happens when the user scrolls through the text).
3. A "selection mediator" which triggers reactions on the selection of a graphical object within the illustration leading to a change within the displayed text.

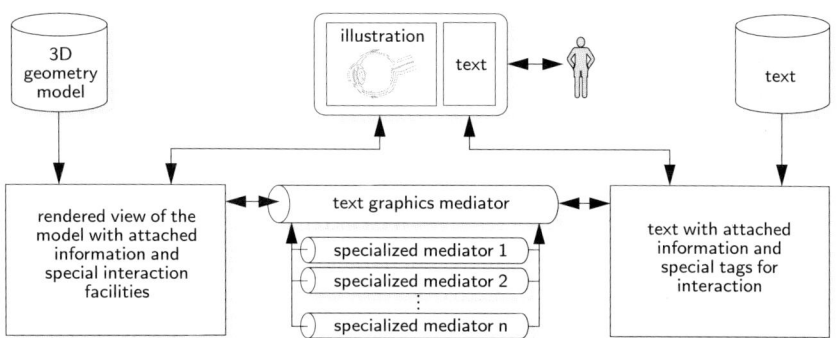

Figure 17.4: TEXTILLUSTRATOR system overview (the arrows to/from the text-graphics mediator symbolize that the information flow here is bi-directional)

17.2.3 Interaction Support

Whereas the general text-graphics mediator keeps the link between objects and text locations referring to them, the registered mediators are responsible for interaction. Each of them keeps track of special events occurring in one of the two items connected by the mediator (graphical object or text entity) and triggers appropriate actions on the other side. For interaction events on the text, the mediator gets a list of all the tags assigned to the portion of text involved (be it a single word or a longer paragraph). Based on these tags, the objects involved and parameters for a special action are chosen. On the other hand, interactions on the graphics result mainly in search actions within the text's tags to find certain positions or regions.

The concept of registering objects which are responsible for triggering actions when interaction events occur has many advantages:

- For each event type, a different reaction can be implemented and used. Even different actions for one particular event are possible.
- New interaction facilities can be added easily.

- A specific interaction scenario can be put together by selecting appropriate mediators.
- Text and graphics remain relatively independent from each other, i.e., they do not form a single monolithic model. This allows the use of a new model (during runtime) if the one currently used is no longer appropriate (for instance switching to a more detailed geometric model for the illustration).

Some examples illustrate the general concept (see Table 17.1). This list may be continued with more elaborate methods.

Table 17.1: Events and appropriate reactions in a text-driven illustration system

Interaction event	Reaction
Selecting a word (preferably a medical term) in the text	The corresponding object in the graphics is displayed either in a different color or with more detail (textured).
Selecting a word in the text where the corresponding object is currently invisible in the graphics	The graphics is transformed (e.g., rotated and translated) to ensure the object is visible.
Selecting a word in the text	If information about relationships of this particular object to other objects is available, they are visualized in an appropriate way (e.g., objects which are connected to a selected muscle may blink, objects which are supplied with blood by a selected vein may change color).
Scrolling through the text	All objects currently mentioned in the visible portion of the text are displayed using appropriate colors, whereas all other objects remain gray.
Scrolling through the text	All objects contained in the visible portion of the text are labeled in the illustration.
Picking an object in the illustration	The text is scrolled automatically to the position of the first (or most important) reference to the object.

Interaction events may also show reactions in the same representation, i.e., interaction on the text changes the text and interaction on the graphics changes the graphics. This leads to the already known behavior of graphics applications where the model can be rotated, translated, and scaled at the user's command. This is very important in the context observed here, since users can orient themselves within the graphics to better understand changes initiated by the system as reactions to the interaction. Transformations within the graphics can be carried out at any time without affecting the other interaction facilities. So the user can explore the image by zooming and rotating it, while the text-driven animation always continues with the state of the image in which the user leaves it.

On the textual side, we gain some hypertext functionality, where by selecting a particular part of the text either hyperlink behavior is simulated and leads the user to a different text location, or more information is displayed at this point in the text or in the image. Within the text we take advantage of the given document structure, so that in a first step only an overview of the document (similar to a table of contents) is shown to the user which can be explored further by requesting the next level of the structure until all text is displayed.[2] However, we do not aim to integrate a typical hypertext system on the textual side, since the risks involved (getting "lost in hyperspace") are too high and may disrupt the advantages gained by the interaction facilities provided.

17.3 Comparison to Other Approaches

So far we have described the general techniques behind a text-driven illustration system. In Sect. 17.1 we have seen that there is at least one other big category of systems which are built upon a different approach – graphics-driven systems. In this section we will compare our text-driven approach with graphics-driven systems as well as with a third group: knowledge-based illustration systems.

A text-driven system creates illustrative images based on a given textual description. This is done by analyzing the contents of the description. The connections to the graphics have to be on a global level. This means that a complete text is connected to a three-dimensional model, while local references exist between smaller text parts and single graphical objects. This global link allows interaction on different levels, i.e., single words, paragraphs, or even a complete text. The text itself can be processed for use in a system without having much additional information. The only data necessary are definitions of links between words in the text (i.e., names) and graphical objects (i.e., identifiers). For medical texts with a standardized terminology (Latin names), these links can be created even *without* any user interaction and for texts in different languages.

In graphics-driven systems, where the textual elements are included together with the graphical model within one model, more preparation time (and effort) for the textual descriptions is needed. They have to be provided in a form which matches the requirements for their use. For different pre-

---

[2] This behavior is well known from so-called "folding editors" where the contents of a paragraph are hidden behind the headline and selecting the headline brings up the paragraph.

sentations – as label or more detailed description – different models have to be given which are then used accordingly. Also the model for the graphical illustration has to be processed in advance in terms of adding structure and specific information (recall Chap. 3). Generally, the connection between text and graphics here is more local. A particular scene object has references to one or more textual descriptions (labels). This allows interaction on a per-object basis, but prevents interaction on a more global level which includes more than one object. Nevertheless, the graphics-driven approach is well suited for reference materials, where unequivocal connections exist between graphical objects and pieces of text.

The two approaches seem to be contradictory, but it should be possible to integrate them in one system yielding a rich set of possibilities to create illustrations which:

1. are closely related to a paragraph of text,
2. show graphical information from different viewpoints and with different levels of detail,
3. incorporate graphical information in texts by creating illustrations which reflect the information within a specific part of the text,
4. incorporate textual information in the graphics as labels with more or less information displayed, and
5. are easily to handle in terms of interactively changing the contents as well as the appearance.

The following examples give an overview of some applications which belong to the field of graphics-driven systems. We will emphasize some of the properties of those systems and compare them with our text-driven approach.

17.3.1 The Zoom Illustrator

The ZOOMILLUSTRATOR is presented in Chap. 13. The system fits into the group of graphics-driven applications. The user interacts with the graphics, which are extensively annotated with labels. The labels give not only the name of a specific object but also further information. The limited space *within* the graphics makes it necessary to select the most important points for display. However, by applying zoom methods (see Chaps. 9 and 10) on the labels the space actually needed for the presentation of the text is distributed among the labels based on certain given conditions. Interaction facilities provided include transformations of the graphics (rotation, translation, scaling) and picking where the respective text-graphics connections are affected. Here interaction is possible not only directly in the graphics but also with the textual labels, yielding changes in both text and graphics.

As the simplified system overview in Fig. 17.5 shows, the information space is built upon the graphical model (scenegraph). All textual information, i.e., labels as well as further descriptions, are directly attached to the graphical objects leading to a rather tight coupling of graphics and text. This offers potential for interaction only on a local level. Also, due to the limited screen space for labels, the information gained through the text is limited.

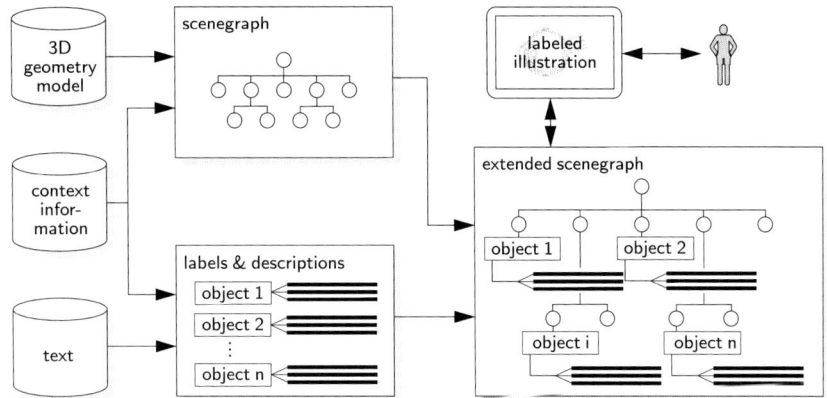

Figure 17.5: ZOOMILLUSTRATOR simplified system overview: the user interacts with the labeled illustration which is created from an internal representation containing graphical objects with attached textual information

However, compared to a printed anatomy atlas, the ZOOMILLUSTRATOR has many advantages. First, there is the possibility to freely transform the image in order to view it from different directions. Second, the close relation between objects in the illustration and the referring labels – even while interaction with the graphics takes place – helps users to orient themselves within the illustration and to get the information they want.

17.3.2 VoxelMan

The VOXELMAN developed by HÖHNE et al. [HPR+94] can be regarded as state of the art in medical visualization. Here volume models are used for generating the illustration, other images (e.g., CT, MRT, or x-ray images) are included. The user has numerous possibilities for interaction including queries for different types of information. The basis for the system is an extensively structured information space which is created upon the graphical model. Here not only labels and short explanations but also all kinds of anatomic and physiological detail are included. The user can even simulate different examination procedures like x-ray or tomography. The visualization is done within a single illustration. This makes orientation easier and also helps to interpret the examination results within the context of the three-dimensional anatomic structures.

Longer textual explanations are included but without any connection to the graphics. However, the philosophy of the system is that all information can be obtained by interacting with the graphics.

17.3.3 Other Graphics-Driven Systems

There are many other systems which deal with medical illustrations, but not all of them can be called "illustration systems". Nevertheless, some of the features they use are of interest here.

One of the standard anatomy atlases, *Sobotta: Atlas of Human Anatomy* [Sob88, German version] is available on CD-ROM as an interactive system. Here the user cannot modify the illustrations, and digitized images are used. An interesting feature is the connection between regions in the image (i.e., objects) and labels or tables with describing facts. A bi-directional link ensures that the object belonging to a particular label and vice versa can be found easily. This system shows all the properties of an anatomy atlas – many extensively labeled images and almost no text. The main drawback is the lack of interactivity for the graphics. As in a regular atlas, many images have to be mentally integrated to get the "big picture". The images used within the system are the same as in the standard paper edition so that the electronic version still profits from the extraordinary quality of those illustrations.

Systems based on three-dimensional models allow flexible interaction with the graphics, but they often lack descriptive texts. Silicon Graphics offers an Internet-based system called CYBERANATOMY. Here the user navigates through a VRML model of the human body and can call up a more detailed explanation of an object by selecting this object. The use of VRML enhances the interaction facilities with the graphics and enables the use of this application via a network. The explanations here are also limited to small images with attached labels. There is no direct link between images and text. However, the network based approach makes this system interesting for future use.

17.3.4 Knowledge-Based Systems

Systems built upon knowledge-based methods are a third direction which has not been examined yet. As far as we know, they have not been used within the medical domain so far. These systems are often used to generate step-by-step instructions for a given action. Illustrations accompanying those instructions can be generated automatically. At the German Research Center for Artificial Intelligence the systems WIP [WAF+93] and PPP [AMR96] are developed to generate not only illustrations but also multimedia presentations. S. FEINER et al. use similar techniques in connection with sophisticated visualization methods. Their systems IBIS and APEX [SF91b] use transparency or the combination of more than one image to depict the information. The use of texts in this context is rudimentary, however, and problems of transforming the graphics according to the presentation goal also arise.

Although not used within the medical domain so far, knowledge-based illustration methods are an interesting alternative for the future. Given a knowledge base of anatomical and physiological information, this approach can be used for the creation of illustrations for such different purposes as reference (as in atlases and textbooks), step-by-step instructions (for preparation of surgeries and reports), and presentations (animations). If we directly compare the knowledge-based and the text-driven approach, similar problems in the area of visualization have to be solved. In both cases there is a presentation goal (either directly derived from a knowledge base or given in a verbal description) which has to be fulfilled by transforming the graphics appropriately or by other visualization techniques. Thus, the visualization techniques described in this book can be applied in both cases.

17.4 The Road Ahead

In this chapter we have presented a new technique for interactive illustration systems. From the comparison to other approaches in Sect. 17.3 one can see that a wide variety of techniques for interactive medical illustration – based on different types of data – are in development.

The text-driven technique as presented here opens up a new avenue for text illustration by providing two key conceptual advances over previous approaches. First, the user can choose a geometric model for the illustration of a given text in SGML. This allows more flexibility in creating illustrations for different purposes and with different levels of detail. The choice of the model being used may depend not only on the illustration task to be fulfilled but also on the contents of the given text. It is even possible to switch the models during runtime so that a user may start with a rather simple model in order to get a first overview of the facts being described in the text and later switch to a more detailed model for a deeper insight.

Second, the user can interrupt the text-driven animation and explore the image by zooming and rotating it, while the text-driven animation always continues with the state of the image as the user leaves it. This combines the properties of an anatomy textbook and an atlas. Exploring the illustration by transforming the graphics and viewing the objects from different sides helps in recognizing topological relations. On the other hand, all information contained in the text for which the illustration is created influence the graphics. Thus, selective information retrieval becomes possible.

Putting it all together, the text-driven approach combines features known from textbooks and atlases. Compared with the typical scenario for learning in anatomy where different books are used to acquire information and where even within one book information is spread out over different pages, this improves the learning process. However, there are still some concerns. The most important is the use of rather long texts in connection with online applications. Here a system displaying long texts has to incorporate methods for navigating through the text by either giving the user an overview of the text structure or providing hints on how the current reading position is related to the document structure. The second point is easily accomplished with a dynamic illustration created from the contents of the text. The technical concepts described in this chapter also allow one to encode a "reading history" in the illustration or animation by evaluating which part has already been displayed. A visual clue in the generated animation might be to "age" an already discussed part by applying a color different to the color used for new objects.

Looking into the future of interactive medical illustration, there are a few key items to consider. An interactive system should outrun the possibilities of traditional media (like books). Here the systems already available have added a new dimension to medical reference and teaching by different methods of connecting different kinds of information as well as by the ability to interactively explore the information.

Furthermore, network-based information systems will increase their relevance for everyday work. Surfing the World Wide Web, most of the pages one can find there look as if they were "taken from a textbook". Selecting a link referring to an illustration generally opens up a new page and thus may disrupt the reading. (Here we have the same effect as when flipping pages in a book.) Adding interactive features to the WWW which go beyond what one might expect today from Java or VRML would also open up a new arena for medical illustration systems. The following points are of special interest here:

- The client-server architecture prevents the user from storing all required data locally. So 3D models as well as texts could be stored on special servers. The user's client is then responsible for interaction with those models.
- The quality of models will increase, since the latest research results can be incorporated much more easily in a model held on a global server than in thousands of models stored on thousands of local machines.
- Networks offer a corporate environment for many users. For effective communication between several persons, techniques have to be provided for expressing their ideas not only in textual form but also as illustrations and by interaction with illustrations.

The success of interactive illustration systems as presented here depends mainly on two key points: the text to illustrate and the 3D model the illustrations are created from. Medical texts are available from different sources, such as publishing companies, hired authors, or practitioners. The availability of 3D geometric models – either as surface or voxel models – has been increasing within the last few years. With the "Visible Human Project" [SASW96] a huge database is available for the creation of very detailed models. However, the capabilities of today's graphics hardware have to be taken into consideration. For interactivity we need real-time responses from the system. Thinking of models with 250 000 polygons and more (voxel models are even more complex) either a high-end graphics system is needed or the model has to simplified. Nevertheless, technological progress in the field of graphics hardware as well as rendering algorithms will allow the interactive handling of these models in the near future. Thus it is our belief that interactive illustration systems will become more important, and not only in the field of medical illustration. In this chapter we have presented some tools that will help to pave the "road ahead" so that it will be easier to drive on.

Contributors of Chap. 17: Stefan SCHLECHTWEG and Hubert WAGENER

Chapter 18

Rendering Gestural Expressions

In this chapter, computer generated illustrations and animation sequences of hand gestures are discussed. The animation of gestures is very useful in the teaching of sign language.

We propose algorithms for rendering 3D models of hands as line drawings and for designing animations of line drawn gestures. Presentations of gestures as line drawings as opposed to photorealistic representations have several advantages. Most importantly, the abstract nature of line drawings emphasizes the essential information a picture is to express and thus supports easier cognition. In addition, when line drawings are rendered from simple 3D models (of human parts), they can be esthetically more pleasing than photorealistic renderings of the same model. This leads us to the assumption that simpler geometry in 3D models suffices for line drawn illustrations and animations of gestures, which in consequence eases the 3D modeling task and speeds up the rendering. Other advantages of line drawings include fast transmission over networks, such as the Internet, and the wide scale independence they exhibit.

We built an application for designing and animating hand gestures in order to illustrate sign language as line drawings. An interactive animating module controls sequences of gestural expression, which allows easy repetition of misunderstood sequences of sign gestures. Furthermore, the underlying 3D representation makes it possible to view the gesture sequences from arbitrary directions for a more rigorous inspection of illustrated words and phrases in the sign language.

18.1 The Problem of Visualizing Human Bodies

Modeling and rendering human bodies or parts thereof is a well-known problem that has attracted the attention of many research groups. It seems that our perception of humans is very sensitive to many fine details: the cell structure of the tissue (wrinkles, etc.), the hairs, and in animations the exact movement of muscles that press and stretch the tissue. Various approaches have been developed to deal with these problems and to incorporate other details, but at the moment no esthetically fully satisfying solution exists to produce presentations that look realistically human.

In the field of facial animation, for example, PARKE proposed in his pioneering work [Par82] a parameterized model for facial animation. He identifies for each facial expression a set of parameter values such that an appropriate change of these values results in distinct facial expressions. TERZOPULOS and WATERS [TW90] developed a hierarchical trilayer as a physically based 3D model of the human face in order to simulate bones, muscles, and tissue. The appearance of the tissue is approximated in their model by a simulation which takes into account elastic forces between different parts of their model. These and similar approaches can be adapted for rendering illustrations and animations of hand gestures. But the models required are extremely complex and the rendering times are very high. At least for interactive applications, these problems are prohibitive.

When designing a teaching system for sign language, interactive speed is more important than esthetically acceptable graphics. GEITZ, HANSON, and MAHER [GHM96] followed this route by providing such a teaching system for use over the Internet. The 3D VRML models they use for representing the human hand are very coarse. This allows fast rendering of graphics and the system can be used interactively. Currently, single static signs of the manual alphabet can be viewed from arbitrary directions by rotating the model online. A disadvantage of such crude models of human body parts, especially when rendered in a photorealistic style, is the tendency of viewers to pay at least part of their attention to criticizing the esthetic shortcomings of the presentation [Bru95]. It has been observed that viewers of line drawings are less concerned with criticizing the crudity of the underlying model, and the focus of concentration is directed instead towards the information conveyed. This leads us to the assumption that graphical presentation of hand signs may be more appropriately done as line drawings. Indeed, books dedicated to the task of teaching sign language usually present the signs as line drawings instead of using photos, mainly because line drawings ignore irrelevant details and thus force the focus onto the essentials (for example [SCC76]).

The main problem in employing line drawings as a presentation style arises from the fact that rendering engines (and hardware support) for producing line drawings are quite rare. Furthermore, animation of line drawings poses additional problems with respect to the selection of characteristic lines as well as frame-to-frame coherence.

18.2 Drawing Optimization for Gestures

In our application, gestures are represented within the computer as geometric 3D models of hands. But before we go into detail on this representation, it is useful to classify the gestures we have to present. Here we follow a classification scheme given by HARLING and EDWARDS [HE96]. In this classification, a distinction between hand posture and hand location is made, where hand posture refers to the positions of individual fingers relative to the hand. In performing a gesture, hand posture as well as hand location may be either static or dynamic. This leads to four different classes of gestures. For example, the gesture representing the letter "J" in the manual alphabet consists of a static hand posture and a dynamic hand location, while the letter "A" is static in posture and location.

The following parts of this section describe the representation of finger and hand movements for forming a chosen gesture.

18.2.1 Representing the Hand and Its Movement

The 3D model of the hand we use in our application is composed of freeform surfaces which have been modeled with Alias|*wavefront*. Using freeform surfaces for deformations, such as performed in hand movements, gives the advantage of a more realistic shape but is harder to control. This is why many systems which deal with hand and finger movements use rough representations; for example, the phalanxes of a finger often consist only of cylinders.

In our application, each finger (including the nail) is modeled by two patches, plus one additional patch each for the palm and the lower arm. Besides this freeform surface modeling of the tissue of a hand, we supply a skeleton structure that approximately mimics the natural skeleton of the hand. This simplified skeleton is illustrated in Fig. 18.1 (middle).

The movements of joints in this skeleton structure have different degrees of freedom that are chosen to match those of real hands. LEE and KUNII [LK95] studied exhaustively the constraints of hand movements and finger flexions. They defined constraint functions for the hand and each phalanx of the finger. In our application, we only include the constraint for single joints so that, for example, a finger cannot rotate backwards. Including constraints concerning the combination of rotations is intended as future work.

In our system, a posture can be applied to the freeform surface which models the tissue of the hand by a technique called cluster-based deformation, which is a well-known feature in computer animation systems. When defining a posture of the skeleton, a set of rotation angles for the different joints is

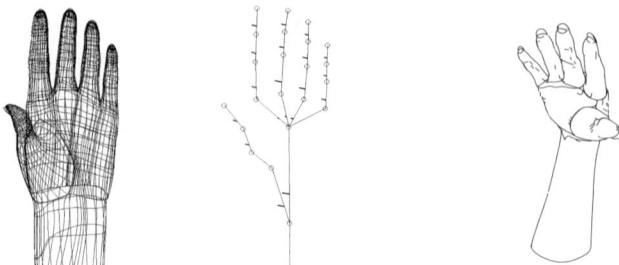

Figure 18.1: Deformation model of the hand: the freeform surfaces of the hand (left) are supplemented with a skeleton (middle), and inverse hierachy is used to perform deformations; (right) an example as a line drawing

specified. Using the principles of inverse hierarchy, a posture of the hand is computed by a set of rotations.

In order to specify a gesture, it suffices to give the rotation of all joints. In practice, the designer of static gestures in our system has to be careful, since no collision detection for the resulting model is performed. This means that although all rotation parameters lie in their appropriate constraint range, auto-penetrations in the resulting model may occur. We consider this deficiency to be negligible, because in a resulting line graphic the areas of penetration are very small. Indeed, this tolerance in the perception of line graphics supports our preference for this presentation style.

18.2.2 Temporal Control

Many gestures, especially those accompanying speech, consist of many hand movements, i.e., they are inherently dynamic. Such gestures are best illustrated by animations. Our general approach for generating such animation consists of specifying a sequence of static gestures that constitute the keyframes of the animation. The transition between consecutive keyframes is obtained by an interpolation that can be chosen from different interpolation schemes.

A meaningful animation of a series of gestures requires appropriate timing. For example, when a human spells a word in sign language, the signer makes fast movements between the gestures representing single letters (he or she *throws* a letter), and then remains in this position for a few milliseconds. This gives a viewer time to recognize the letter in the case of a static gesture. If a dynamic gesture is performed (e.g., letter "J" or "Z"), the movement of hand and fingers follows a quite controlled timing.

The timing specification incorporated into our system is currently quite rudimentary, but easy to use. For each specified keyframe (i.e., static gesture), a preceding period and a following period are specified. The time spent to move from a keyframe K_i to a keyframe K_{i+1} is given by the sum of the following period specified for K_i and the preceding period for K_{i+1}.

Up to now this timing scheme is not fully validated. An easy, alternative scheme that allows for finer time-tunings consists of simply defining the transition time between any pair of gestures. The disadvantage of this is that the effort required to integrate new gestures grows with the number of gestures available in the system. Moreover, the size of the timing specification grows quadratically relative to the number of gestures as opposed to a linear growth in the former scheme.

The time-tuning values as well as the parameter sets for the joint rotation which represent each gesture will be taken from a library and are thoroughly described in the next section.

18.3 Animation of Gestures for the Manual Alphabet

The gestures available in our system are contained in a library, which can be extended by end-users in a quite convenient way. This gesture library consists of a table with an entry for each individual gesture. Within this table, the geometry of the gesture is encoded and timing specifications as described above are recorded. The geometric information for a given static gesture simply consists of the rotations at skeleton joints necessary to form the hand posture and location. In case of dynamic gestures, a sequence of key-frames and an interpolation method is stored, where key-frames in turn are specified as static gestures. The following two sections describe the user interface for building and expanding the library.

18.3.1 Interactive Dialogs for Library Maintenance

Entering the timing values for a gesture into the library is a trivial task. The interactive dialog window for adding and editing timing values is shown in Fig. 18.2.

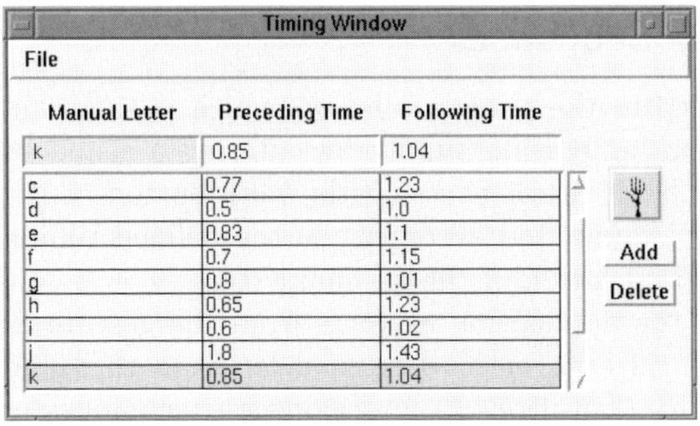

Manual Letter	Preceding Time	Following Time
k	0.85	1.04
c	0.77	1.23
d	0.5	1.0
e	0.83	1.1
f	0.7	1.15
g	0.8	1.01
h	0.65	1.23
i	0.6	1.02
j	1.8	1.43
k	0.85	1.04

Figure 18.2: Dialog window for adding and editing preceding and following time periods of each manual sign

After choosing a gesture in the list, values for the preceding period and following period can be entered or edited. Each gesture has a reference to its geometric specification. Clicking the "skeleton button" opens a dialog called gesture builder that allows inspection and redefinition of this specification. The dialog window for defining and modifying the geometry of static hand gestures is shown in Fig. 18.3.

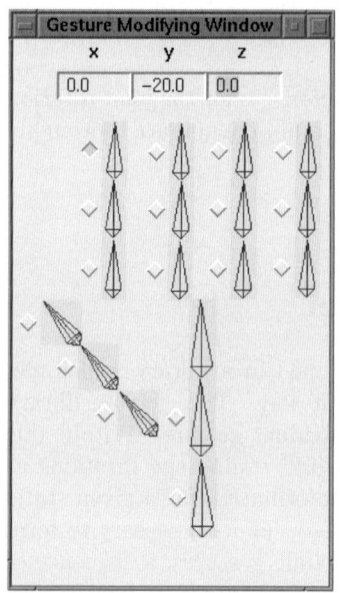

Figure 18.3: Dialog window for performing and modifying hand gestures. In the schematic illustration of the skeleton the different joints can be selected by radio buttons. The rotation for the selected joint is entered in edit boxes

Each individual joint can be selected and a rotation can be assigned. The user has to be aware that only basic constraints for the degrees of freedom are known to the system. In particular, constraints concerning combinations of rotations are missing. This means that a user can specify an unrealistic gesture without obtaining a warning from the system. But an associated window displaying a graphic of the defined gesture is immediately updated when a parameter is redefined. In this way we can ensure instant graphical inspection of the definition process which has proved useful in gesture design.

18.3.2 Building Gesture Sequences

Gesture sequences are controlled in the trigger window, which is shown in Fig. 18.4. A user can trigger an animation simply by entering a sequence of manual letters in the input field. After pressing the play button of the control panel the hand gesture is animated according to the defined timing schedule and the geometrical specification of the manual letters.

To perform the animation, the application extracts from the gesture library the geometric description of each entered manual letter in turn and produces specifications of gesture transitions by interpolation techniques in

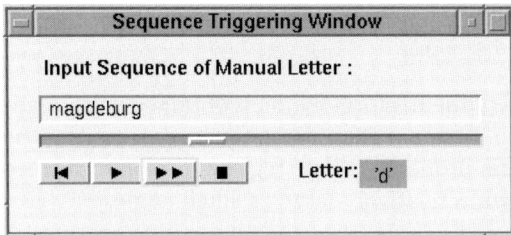

Figure 18.4: Trigger window for controlling animations of gestures

accordance with the defined timing constraints. The resulting composition of the gesture sequence is shown as a line drawing in the render window where an arbitrary view of this animation can be chosen.

The process of composing the manual letters into an animation takes more time when the sequence is played for the first time. In this case, for each frame of the animation a full rendering is performed which incorporates a special polygonal description of the hand model after deformation is carried out. We will discuss the rendering process in the next section. But when the animation is played for the second or a subsequent time, a special polygonal description, which is necessary for calculating the line drawing, is recalled from the memory of the computer, where we put it during the first calculation. If such a chosen gesture sequence is required more often, these calculated polygonal descriptions of an animation can be stored on the hard disk.

18.4 Generating Line Drawings of Freeform Surfaces

The specification of a hand gesture as described in Sect. 18.2 is transferred to the geometric hand model. Therefore, the first step consists of deforming the given hand model according to the joint rotation specifying that gesture and yielding an explicit 3D model for the gesture. After this, the second step consists of choosing an adequate drawing style of outlines and textures in order to obtain esthetically pleasing line drawing of hand gestures. These two steps are the content of the following subsections.

18.4.1 The Rendering Process

We refer to our work in Chap. 5 for a more rigorous description of presenting line drawing of freeform surfaces. In brief, we perform the following tasks in turn:

1. The freeform surface is transformed into a special polygonal mesh. During this transformation, we carry out the following process:
    a. reparameterization of the patch, so that a nearly natural parameterization of patches is obtained, and

b. approximation of the freeform patches by a polygonal mesh which is evenly spread in parametric space.

   In this way a polygonal mesh of the freeform model is obtained with quadrangles more evenly spread in 3D space than with standard isoparametric meshes. A consequence of this property is that regions of high curvature exhibit edges whose faces span a relatively large or small angle.
2. Analytic rendering is performed to give a vector-oriented description of visible parts. With this description, we are able to apply different line styles for contours as well as edges.
3. The contour lines are identified and inner edges are classified with respect to angles of adjacent faces. This classification is used to control the level of detail in the resulting drawing.
4. Chains of contour lines and inner edges of given classifications are approximated by cubic splines which can be drawn in different line styles.

This rendering process is designed to allow an interactive tuning of the desired line drawing. Changing the density of the polygon mesh, which actually consists of adjusting the number of faces in the mesh, results in a finer or coarser approximation of the freeform model.

A very prominent reason for employing 3D models of hand gestures is the arbitrary adjustment of the viewing direction. After changing the viewing direction, redrawing the hand includes only steps 2–4 of the rendering process for a fast update.

A readjustment of the level of detail does not require redoing all steps, but only step 4 of the rendering process, which results in a very fast update. The following variations of drawing styles are included in our application:

1. All lines, such as contour lines and edge lines, can be drawn in different linewidth and brightness. This makes it possible to emphasize patches of the model (e.g., focusing on a finger).
2. Drawing certain inner edge lines with a desired level of detail. The revealing of the edges depends on the angle between adjacent faces and therefore corresponds to the curvature. A minimal level of detail reveals only the edges with a high angle of the adjacent faces, which actually depict the parts of high curvature. The level of desired detail can be adjusted in a nearly continuous range. At the maximal level of detail the underlying polygonal mesh is drawn (a result that usually is unwanted).
3. Computing shading by drawing simple hatching lines, cross-hatching, and stippling.

Users should avoid high levels of detail, since these show the artifacts of a crude 3D model more clearly and thus annull in particular the cognitive benefits of line drawings over photorealistic presentations.

A short demonstration of these different styles is given in the next subsection.

18.4.2 Demonstration of Drawing Styles

We are now in the position to demonstrate some line drawings to compare different parameterizations of our rendering. Figure 18.5 shows on the left a minimal line drawing illustrating the manual letter "A". Only the contour of each freeform patch is drawn. The same rendition but with a greater level of detail is given in Fig. 18.5 on the right.

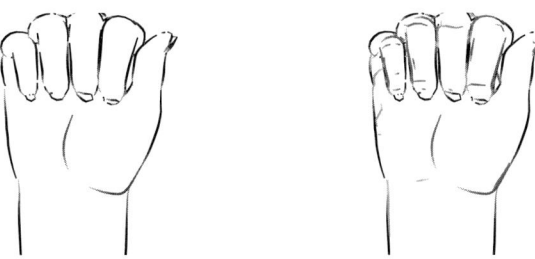

Figure 18.5: Presentation of the letter "A" in different drawing styles: (left) just outlines, (right) outlines and some simulated wrinkles, which are achieved by changing the level of detail

Figure 18.6 gives a comparison between a line drawing and a photorealistic presentation with shading performed in today's standard quality. The depicted hand posture can be recognized more easily in the line drawing, while the photorealistic presentation can convey more spatial details. The speed advantage is such that even if the photorealistic image is desired, the line drawing can be drawn first, followed by an interlaced transmission of the photorealistic image. The right image in Fig. 18.6 shows the overlay of the photorealistic image and the line drawing.

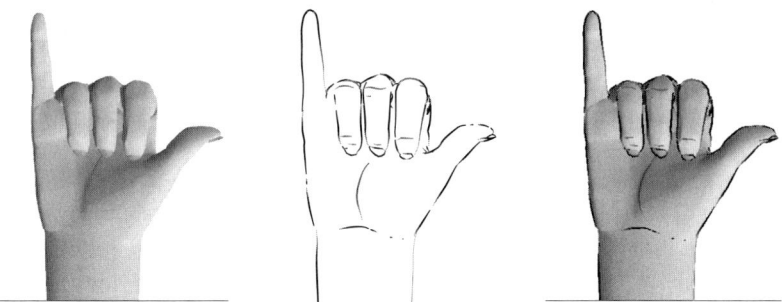

Figure 18.6: Presentation of the letter "Y" in different styles: (left) photorealistic, (middle) line drawing, (right) a line drawing laid over a photorealistic rendition can enhance the recognition of gestures

For users who prefer a more spatial presentation, we provide shaded line drawings where the shading is realized either by cross-hatching or stippling. Figure 18.7 contrasts line drawings with and without shading, and stippling is used as shading method in the left image. In the right image of Fig. 18.7, the index finger and the thumb are drawn with a thicker line width in order to direct the viewer's attention to this part of the picture.

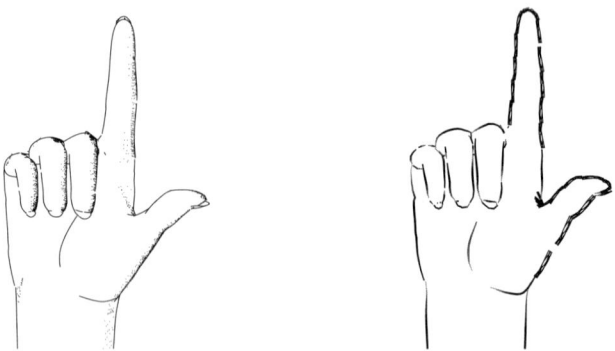

Figure 18.7: Presentation of the letter "L" in a shaded drawing style (left), and in a style where outlines of index finger and thumb are emphasized (right)

18.5 Conclusions and Future Work

We have introduced in this chapter an application for illustrating gestures either as images or as animation sequences. The most prominent characteristic of our system is the presentation of gestures as line drawings. Line drawings convey the important information when illustrating gestures (e.g., the hand posture or finger tension) better than photorealistic presentations. In a discussion, a specialized teacher of German sign language pointed out that line drawings are very convenient for gesture demonstration. A computer aided application with interactive, easy manageable tools for creating and presentating gestures would be useful for teaching sign language.

Furthermore, most illustrations in books intended to illustrate gesture language consist of hand-drawn line graphics. This is because line drawings have the advantage of effortless integration into black-and-white publications since no special print media are required. Another important characteristic of our application is its extensibility. Integrating new gestures does not require 3D modeling, because specification of view rotations suffices, for example, to define a static gesture.

In the future we intend to extend our system in several aspects. In its current state, only gestures performed with one hand are handled. We plan to gradually incorporate the presentation of both hands, arms, and even facial expressions. These extensions yield much more complex models whose handling requires improved support. In defining new gestures for complex models, automatic collision or touch detection would be very helpful. Sophisticated support in designing new dynamic gestures would also be desirable. Some guiding tools for the average user should be developed, especially if the underlying model becomes more complex.

Contributors of Chap. 18: Frank GODENSCHWEGER and Hubert WAGENER

Chapter 19

Animation Design for Simulation

While the previous chapter concentrated on how to *render* animations, this chapter deals with how to *create* them. It introduces a new method of generating the *animation content* mentioned in Chap. 15. That content can be presented using the techniques described in that chapter.

Since both chapters share the words *Animation Design* in their titles, it might be worthwhile to point at the distinctions. This chapter is concerned with the content (e.g., timing and positional parameters), not with the details of its presentation. Chapter 15, on the other hand, assumes the existence of a scene or an animation and derives presentation and emphasis techniques to aid the viewers' perception and understanding. Creation (modeling) and presentation represent different *levels* of animation design.

In contrast to the origin of the word animate (to bring to life, see previous chapter), for the computer, an animation can be described in more technical terms as a visible process that transforms an initial state (a *scene*) into a final state using a set of transformations (*animation actions*). However, this definition does not yet define the state or the transformations.

In computer graphics, we describe the scene as a set of graphics objects, each having a shape, appearance (color, texture, ...), and other attributes. Previous chapters discussed some of these attributes at the scene or object level (line styles, etc.) and how they affect the rendering process.

This chapter is focused on another aspect of animations: the actions. An animation action is a change in the graphics scene like an object movement, a turn or a change in color. In long and detailed animations, there are usually many animation actions involved. In traditional studio animation systems (softimage, Alias|*wavefront*, 3D Studio), the user has to specify these manually, albeit with sophisticated support from the system. But still, the manual design step makes the creation of computer animations very expensive. For another more automated approach – using a plugin based application framework – we turn to the domain of computer simulation where animated visualizations are also very desirable.

The next two sections will discuss the benefits and the problems of technical animations in the area of computer simulation. After that, we outline how plugins can improve the design process for these animations, and finally give an overview of VISMOD [HRI97], the visualization modeling system that implements these ideas.

19.1 Using Simulation to Create Animation Models

Despite what many people think, a computer simulation is not something one can see (this would be a *visualization*). Instead, the simulation is an abstract computational task that can, among other things, be used to generate data for the visualization.

Simulation models are usually created with the goal of analyzing and optimizing the real-world behavior of the modeled entities. They record data for statistic analysis that aims at providing answers to questions like "How many checkout counters should the supermarket have?" or "What is the optimum shape of the ship's hull to minimize overall fuel consumption?" Such questions must be answered through simulation, since there are usually no closed analytic solutions for the problem. Today, powerful simulation systems allow the creation of sophisticated models that can remove the need to actually build the modeled systems until they are thoroughly understood and optimized.

In many cases it is necessary to document this simulation process for people not directly involved in it. A good candidate for this is computer graphics, and since we are talking about dynamic processes, computer animation. There are several ways to create an animation from a simulation experiment:

- *Online animation*
  The simulation system shows an animation while the simulation is in progress. The user can monitor the running system and validate the model. This requires the simulation system/model to be efficient enough to run in real time (multiplied by the time factor used in the animation), but that's hardly a limiting factor these days. Since the animation system is part of the simulation environment, the animation design is always constrained by the feature set of the built-in animator.
- *Offline (post-run) animation*
  The simulation produces a trace file that records all relevant events that occur in the simulation experiment (see Fig. 19.1 (left)). An animation

19.1 Using Simulation to Create Animation Models

```
B+ 0.000000 173 143 0 158 0        hide 55.9103 0    4
BI 0.100000 173 143 0 158 0        key  55.9103 0.14 6        palette1       0.285
OW 0.200000  36 143 0  43 0        key  55.9103 0.14 8        palette1       0.285
B- 2.000000  36 143 0  43 0        show 54.7103 0    4
B+ 2.100000  43 143 36 44 0        move 54.7103 1.0  wagon    wagon-50-55    1
OW 0.200000  37 142 0  44 0        move 55.7103 1.0  wagon    wagon-55-60    1
B- 3.000000  37 142 0  44 0        move 57.7103 1.0  wagon    wagon-0-25     1
B+ 3.000000  44 142 37 45 0        key  60.7103 1.0  4        palette9       1
OW 0.200000  38 141 0  45 0        move 61.7103 1.0  wagon    wagon-35-40    1
B- 4.000000  38 141 0  45 0        move 61.7103 1.0  4        wagon-35-40    1
B+ 4.000000  45 141 38 46 0        show 61.9103 0    4
```

Figure 19.1: simulation trace (left) and animation trace (right)

system interprets these events directly or after a translation to animation actions (see Fig. 19.1 (right)). Since the animation is decoupled from the simulation system, the user can choose the animation system. Fig. 19.2 shows the information flow in such an environment. If the simulation system doesn't provide the trace file by itself, appropriate output statements must be added to the simulation model, which leads to significantly more complex models.

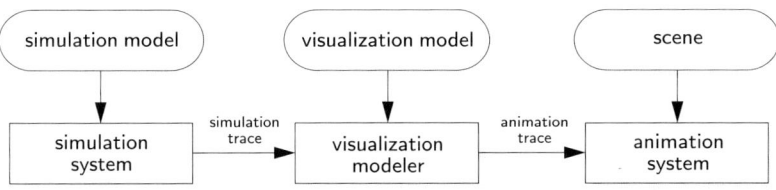

Figure 19.2: Relations between simulation and animation

The two tables in Fig. 19.1 show simulation and animation trace files. While the left listing contains information on what happens in some simulation elements, the right listing shows commands that alter graphics objects. Note that there are some similarities in the structure of the trace files. Both have analogous syntax elements like event types, time, IDs (name or number) of the entities involved, and auxiliary parameters. Translation mechanisms for the conversion of simulation traces for animation could exploit these analogies to yield simple and easy-to-implement solutions; one of them (and its related problems) will be discussed in Sect. 19.2.

The rest of this chapter is focused on offline animation. An online animation system is usually either very abstract and closely tied to its simulation system or requires a great deal of modeling to achieve a convincing and attractive animation. Simulation systems that provide both simulation and animation modeling capabilities tend to be very expensive and specialized. Offline animation, on the other hand, gives the user a choice as to which animation system to use and how to use its capabilities to achieve certain communicative goals pertaining to the simulation. However, this flexibility comes at the steep price of loosing the integration of both tools. The user must either generate an animation model during the simulation run or find a way to translate the simulation trace into an animation.

Considering all the new line-drawing algorithms and applications described in the other chapters, there is another point. Many of the drawing techniques mentioned before can be used once a proper interface is established that helps to harness and make use of the expressiveness of, say, the line styles and their potential to improve the viewer's perception. Some of these techniques are well suited for animation in the context of computer simulation, but none of their existing applications is part of an online animation system. So the coupling of previously unrelated simulation and animation tools via some interface is a very interesting field.

Readers familiar with computer simulation will notice some bias towards material-flow like simulations where transient objects move through the system. That is because this area of computer simulation is particularly amenable to animation not only as a visualization tool for the end-user, but also as a model validation and analysis tool. However, the methods presented should be applicable to other application domains as well.

19.2 Problems in Generating Animations

Even though animations help a simulation to gain acceptance, simulation experts try to avoid animation if it requires significant additional modeling effort. Some simulation systems aim to provide a combined modeling environment for simulation and animation aspects of the model, but there are many systems where this is not the case. These systems (GPSS/H, SIMPLE++, ...) are nevertheless capable of producing trace files that can be used to generate animations.

An additional modeling step, which we call *visualization modeling*, must bridge the gap that is caused by the diverging design goals of simulation and animation. The *visualization model* controls how the result (here: a trace file) of the simulation is converted into an animation. Therefore, together with the simulation trace and model, the visualization model defines the animation.

Creating this visualization model can be a very complex task depending on the desired amount of detail. This is because (despite some overlap) both simulation and animation present a very different view of the modeled system. Unlike a simulation that answers a given set of questions, an animation is expected to show a continuous, realistic, and convincing process. The realism often expected requires much detail to be added to the animation model. Since most of these details (e.g., colors, exact movements versus simple translations) are of no significance to the simulation, they will not be included in the simulation model, which means that they have to be added later when creating the animation. This is a problem when the simulation system is responsible for creating the animation trace file (as is the case with using GPSS/H to generate Proof animations), where it leads to increased modeling time and longer simulation runs. Ideally, the simulation expert should not be concerned with animation details and should create lean models that can be efficiently simulated.

Based on our experiences with the prototypical animation system ANIPLUS (see also Chap. 15) we found that the visualization model and the translation mechanism must be fairly expressive and flexible. Early versions of ANIPLUS employed a rule-based method of creating animations using a simple translation mechanism [LH95]. The rule interface was built for one simulation system (an element-oriented material-flow system DOSIMIS [DOS]) and allowed the specification of a parameterized animation action for each combination of simulation element and simulation event in the trace file. Since this rule mechanism was indeed very mechanical, it enforced a one-to-one relation of simulation event to animation action. Therefore, a simulation event could not be used to generate a series of animation actions. Since simulation events are somewhat high-level in terms of how much detail and how many animation actions a good-looking animation requires, convincing animations could not be achieved without animation-specific simulation modeling that provides this additional information. This extra modeling had to compensate for the limited versatility of the rule interface.

While it was in fact possible to build animations with this system, our experience with this approach led us to some important conclusions: The conversion interface must have considerably more built-in intelligence than the essentially table-driven rule-based conversion scheme. Also, the new conversion interface must consist of entities that have a state (internal variables), so that they can keep track of changes in the simulation model and emit animation actions according to their internal state. In other words, the animation elements monitor the simulation. Given the diversity of existing simulation systems, this requires a lot of flexibility. This flexibility is best achieved in a modular, user-extensible system.

The next section gives an example of how to implement such a system and proposes a possible application "infrastructure".

19.3 Plugins for Visualization Modeling

In some application areas, like image processing, WWW browsing, and animation, plugin concepts have gained wide acceptance. A plugin is a piece of software that communicates with a host application via a predefined interface that basically provides access to the current document (image, WWW page, animation model, ...). With plugins, a developer can avoid implementing a whole application with all the basic functions (file handling, editing, cut-and-paste, undo, displaying, ...) and instead focus on a few features only.

Users, on the other hand, can customize their application by selecting only the plugin that they really need.

But what can plugins do for visualization modeling?

The key idea is to move the simulation trace conversion to an application framework that implements the translation step in user-extensible plugins. By providing an open framework in which plugins can be integrated, a wide set of users has the opportunity to create or modify plugins to fit their specific requirements. When all relevant functionality is implemented using plugins, the host application itself remains highly flexible. System vendors can provide plugin libraries for specific target simulation and animation systems, but the user would still be able to implement his special requirements by further extending existing plugins.

Figure 19.3 shows the general system design. In the first stage, the input is scanned to create an intermediate model that hides the input file syntax from the following stages. The second phase converts the input trace events into generic animation actions (movements, rotations, ...) that are not yet tailored to a specific animation system. This is done in the last stage, where the backend writes animation actions to the output file.

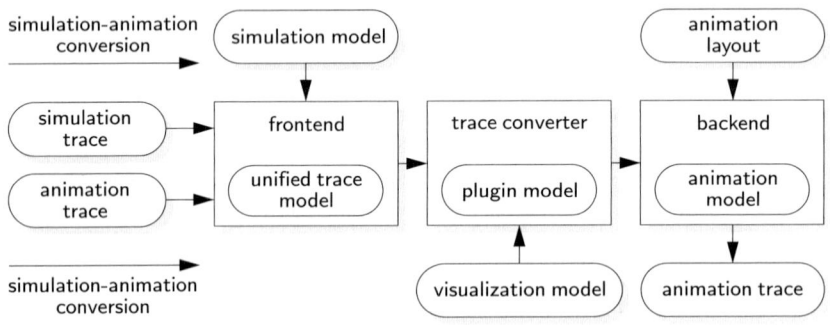

Figure 19.3: System architecture for a trace conversion framework

Using this approach one can derive any kind of information from a simulation trace, not only animation scripts; for example, it is even possible to generate explanatory annotations along with the animation actions that can be displayed when the user clicks on an animated object (see Chap. 15).

19.4 Trace Conversion in a Plugin Based Framework

This chapter gives a more detailed description of how animations are generated in this plugin environment. It also describes the requirements and responsibilities of the system components.

19.4 Trace Conversion in a Plugin Based Framework

For a trace conversion, three properties of the trace files must be taken into account:

- *simulation trace format syntax*
  Even if two simulation systems (or models) use the same simulation concepts and generate the same information, they can use different trace formats.
- *simulation trace semantics*
  Today's simulation systems allow many different problems to be modeled in many different ways. Capturing the simulation logic and translating into something else is the most interesting step and requires most of the intelligence.
- *animation trace syntax*
  By analogy to the simulation trace syntax, the output format depends on the target system.

Since the file format dependencies are only syntactical and do not vary between simulation models, they are not part of the visualization model which contains only the information needed for the semantic conversion.

Frontend. The primary purpose of the frontend is to collect all necessary information about the simulation model and the simulation run. Thus, the frontend extracts all "interesting" information from the incoming simulation trace file and builds an intermediate unified trace model that serves as an abstraction from the real simulation model (see Fig. 19.4). It contains all active entities from the simulation and their associated simulation events.

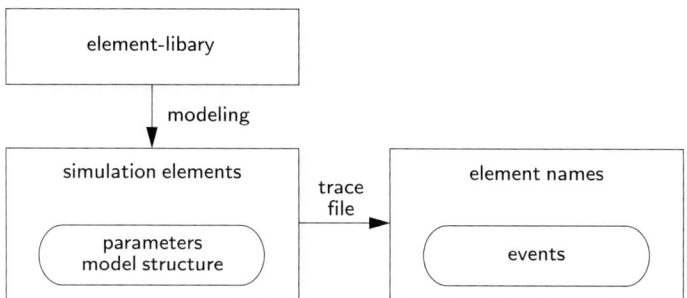

Figure 19.4: Information obtained from a simulation trace file

The goal in the design of this representation is to minimize the dependencies from the real simulation model so that simulation systems using similar concepts can be interfaced with different frontends, but (almost) the same conversion network.

To build this model, it might help to have access to the actual simulation model, but this would lead to much more complex frontend interfaces since the structure of models is very different in each simulation system. In most cases, the contents of the simulation model file(s) are not accessible to the trace conversion because of proprietary formats.

Many simulation systems provide a native trace capability. It was originally intended for debugging purposes and therefore reflects the simulation logic and the internal structure of the system. Other systems allow the user to include special output statements in the model (sometimes in addition to the built-in trace facility).

For those systems that give the user control over the contents of the trace file, it is important to understand the requirements for the trace file. Since they depend on how the conversion plugins work and how they access the trace events, this will be described in the next section.

Based on the unified trace model, the system decides which plugins are needed to convert the trace file. In preparation for the conversion pass, all conversion plugins are then instantiated and initialized.

Conversion Network. Once all plugins exist, the second pass through the trace file can begin. To generate animation actions, each plugin needs access to the trace events.

Consider a plugin that mimics a buffer in a simulation model. In a simulation, a buffer is something that can store an object until it can move on. They usually have a finite capacity as one of their parameters. Incoming objects can only enter if there is enough space left in the buffer and will be rejected otherwise. One can model a storage or a waiting room, etc., using this very generic buffer concept. In a simulation run, each buffer knows when an object enters, leaves, or is rejected. Each of these situations can result in a trace event generated by the buffer. Suppose the trace events look like this:

```
124.5    in       lid-storage-1    lid-press
134.8    out      lid-storage-1    lid-paint
144.0    reject   lid-storage-1    lid-press
```

The important information in a trace event is:

- the time when the event occurred
- the type of event
- the model element that generated (sent) the event
- auxiliary information that depends on the event type; in this case: where did the incoming/outgoing object come/go?

A plugin created because the trace analysis found the model element lid-storage-1 would listen to all trace events coming from this element.

To show objects going in and out of the buffer, the buffer must have a visual representation. Assume that the graphic scene contains a small rectangular area where the waiting objects are to be stored and that there are paths from/to the neighboring facilities lid-paint and lid-press. The plugin can maintain an internal list of used and unused spots within that area and assign unused spots to incoming objects. Likewise, when objects leave, it would free their spots for later reallocation.

Since the simulation guarantees that there will be no overflow, we can assume that there will always be a free spot for an incoming object. So when a new object wants to enter the buffer, it could simply be placed on a free spot. More detailed animations would have the object move from the entry point to the spot. Here, the buffer plugin would generate a request for the backend to place the object on the coordinate of the free spot. It does not issue any animation commands itself.

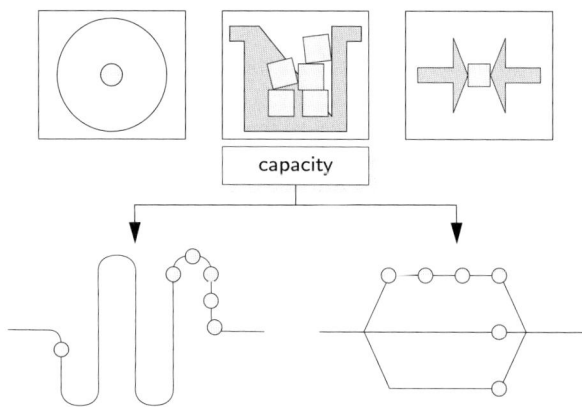

Figure 19.5: Above: a buffer in a simulation model (between a source and a server). Below: two possible visualizations in a 2D system. The path lengths reflect the buffer capacity

Note that in this example the simulation only provides very simple trace events. The important point here is that even in the simple case of a buffer, there is a lot of detail in the animation (where can objects enter/leave the buffer, spot allocation strategy, how exactly do objects move to their spot, ...) that is not part of the simulation model. Like many other simulation concepts, the concept of a buffer is applicable in so many different real-world situations (that require many different visualizations) that a one-size-fits-all solution for its graphical presentation is not possible.

The abstraction process that led to the use of the buffer as a simulation element is therefore reversed in the trace conversion by adding the required detail. Since this happens during the visualization modeling (i.e., after the simulation run), this allows the simulation expert to focus on the simulation modeling.

Backend. The backend accepts generic animation commands from the conversion plugins and forms the actual animation commands. This works like an "intelligent" dictionary. As in the frontend, decoupling the syntax from the semantics makes it possible to exploit more similarities in different animation systems. For instance, moving an object to another place is a common task in an animation, but each animation system has a different command syntax to specifiy a movement.

The other important function of the backend is the layout management. It maintains the graphics scene that contains all objects with their attributes. This has two main uses:

- The backend only issues animation actions when scene objects really change. This makes plugin design easier since it allows plugins to request animation actions that may or may not be carried out. Examples are the creation and destruction of graphics objects that could be handled with simple show/hide commands in the animation and movements to the same position.
- Given an appropriate data structure for the layout manager, it could store more object attributes than are really needed for the animation, thereby providing a simple communication channel for plugins. Plugins can query the layout objects for position and other properties. One plugin can use the "animation" objects to pass on information to the next plugin. The current implementation does not yet exploit this.

19.5 Future Work

It is still too early to realize and use the full potential of the plugin approach in this application, but there are some interesting uses.

In a computer aided documentation system, the animation can be commented with annotations that describe the ongoing action for the viewer (not only for the animation system). The annotations describe the same animation, only at a higher level. Therefore, they must be generated along with the animation actions when the knowledge about the simulated system is still available, i.e., in the conversion plugins.

This feature will be used in the VISDOK [HHRS98] system, an interactive documentation system that combines 3D animation and graphics with text generated in a knowledge based server. Not only can the user get technical data and descriptions by selecting 3D objects and their context menus, but also the generated text can contain references to the displayed objects as well as the discourse history. The response of the system to user interaction is not limited to displaying menus and text, but can also be an animation or camera movement. The plugin mechanism makes it possible to provide additional information that can be used to extend the text generation to reference actions taking place in an animation. Mere animation actions are too low-level to be referenced by the text-planning module. The additional high-level information can be fitted to the knowledge based concepts and thus be more easily integrated in the text-planning techniques employed by the system.

A similar use of this additional information is possible for some of the augmenting animation techniques described in Chap. 15. Here, the information about relevance or possible relationships between different actions in the animation can be exploited to apply the appropriate camera techniques and scene structuring methods to emphasize these non-obvious facts.

Contributor of Chap. 19: Ralf HELBING

Part VII

Abstraction for Specialized Output

Thus far in the book we have dealt exclusively with applications of abstraction to visualizations presented on a computer screen. However, the methods and tools we have developed go beyond the computer screen and extend to specialized output media, too. Indeed, certain output media have an even greater need for abstraction than images on a computer screen.

Perhaps the most widespread application area for methods of abstraction is cartography. While the methods of abstraction in cartography are often subtle, maps for blind people push the methods to the limit, as the tactile output medium has a very low resolution. Rainer MICHEL shows in Chap. 20 that the widespread use of inexpensive electronic maps makes it necessary to develop efficient algorithms which can be tuned by end-users.

The topic of synthetic holography, taken up by Alf RITTER and Hubert WAGENER in Chap. 21, is a pointer to the future. Synthetic holography is an attempt to go beyond today's display technology to achieve real 3D images. The challenges to be addressed on the way to commercial products are manifold; this chapter investigates efficient methods of rendering holograms of line drawings. The result is that textures, which can be implemented in hardware on graphics workstations, can be used as the basis for the rendering process. In addition, line-based synthetic holograms are of particular value when the display quality is not high enough to support holograms with complex details on the surfaces of objects. The method presented in this chapter represents a large improvement over the brute-force method of pixel-by-pixel rendering.

Chapter 20

Tactile Maps for Blind People

Like maps for sighted people, tactile maps are depictions of areas like countries or towns. However, they are not just embossed versions of the maps that sighted people are used to (see Fig. 20.1). A number of particularities have to be observed to ensure the tactual legibility of these maps, resulting in several restrictions to the map design (refer to [Edm91] and [Hud83] for more information). Since haptic perception has a lower discriminability, symbols have to be larger and simpler, e.g., point symbols should have a diameter of 3–5 mm. To avoid confusion, symbols must have a minimum distance between one another. While these distances are about 0.1 mm for visual features, tactile symbols must be at least 2–3 mm apart to ensure their separate perception. Braille texts have a fixed height of 6 mm and hence entail a street width of at least 8 mm to allow labeling of the streets. While color can be replaced by textures, the textured areas have to be very large to enable the differentiation of the different textures, and still there are only very few different textures easily recognizable even for larger areas.

The restrictions thus imposed by the properties of haptic perception require special attention to map design. Only few specialized institutions have the know-how and the experience for the design of suitable tactile maps as well as the necessary equipment. A common way to create a tactile map by hand is to glue pieces of fur, sandpaper, cloth, and wire to a cardboard or wooden base to represent the shapes of geographical features like lakes, forests, roads, etc. These hand-made maps are either usable as they are or serve as masters for a thermoforming process which allows production of several plastic copies from a master map.

Another common method is swell paper printing, where the map layout is printed on a plastic-coated paper that yields an embossed depiction of the black areas after being exposed to heat. While the latter technique imposes some restrictions on the durability and legibility of the maps, it allows their fast and inexpensive production, which makes it the preferred option for the quick creation of small lots of maps.[1]

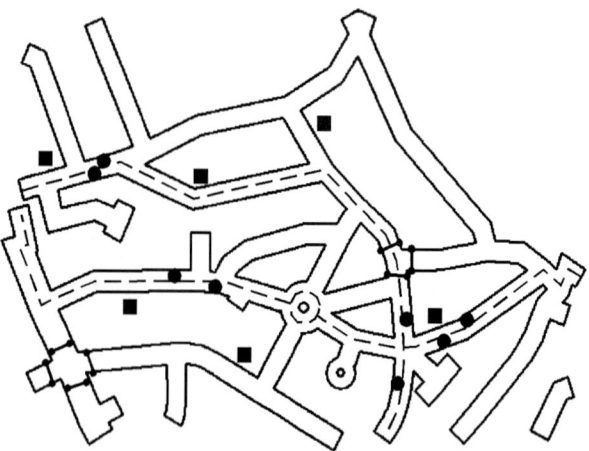

Figure 20.1: Sample tactile map of a part of Birmingham. Double-line symbols of 8 mm width represent the streets, dashed lines indicate public transport lines with stops shown as filled dots. Traffic lights are displayed as lines with dots at each end. The area of 1 100 m by 750 m is presented using a scale of 1:7 500

Although the techniques of thermoforming and swell paper printing are available for the creation of multiple embossed copies of a tactile map, the production of tactile maps currently needs tedious manual labor and is time-consuming and expensive. This prevents flexible and user-oriented creation and leads to insufficient availability. An improvement of this situation has become possible with the growing availability of digital geographical data in the last years. This lays the foundation for computer-based creation, which could lead to a dramatically reduced production time. In the long run, this would help to open up a similar variety of information to visually impaired people as there is for sighted. In addition, supporting the process of designing the map layout could enable persons without extensive cartographic knowledge, like friends or relatives of a visually impaired person, to create tactile maps. In consequence, the opportunity for a shift in the production process away from a few central institutions toward the map reader would become possible. It would even lay the foundation for creating customized maps.

---

[1] For a complete survey of the classical techniques see [Gil74].

20.1 Customized Maps

When exploring large information spaces, the screen real-estate problem arises as described in Chap. 2. A very similar problem is the design of suitable tactile maps supporting safe and independent mobility for blind people. Tactile symbols have to be very large compared to those in maps for sighted people, as described in the previous section. This makes cluttering a very evident problem. Preventing symbol confusion and observing the tactile minimum distances calls for large map scales. However, large map scales let the presentable area shrink, which in some cases may even lead to maps that can no longer cover a whole route.

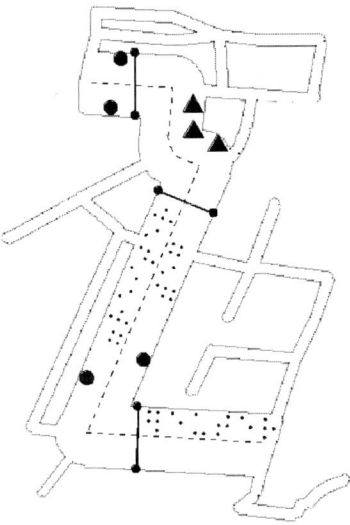

Figure 20.2: Example of a tactile route map. The street symbols forming the route have a width of 1–2 cm to allow labeling and the presentation of mobility information. The remaining streets are displayed in a simplified way. The size of the map on this page is reduced by four compared to the original

Another option is the reduction of the information contents. This is common practice, since apart from symbol size, the slowness of haptic perception makes this reasonable. Only a small fraction of the information that can be perceived visually can be perceived tactually by blind people in the same amount of time. In addition, the sensing finger (even if more than one is used) only allows a punctual sensation, preventing reception of the image as a whole at one time. Reducing the number of symbols in a map can, therefore, ease the effort of reading it.

However, this call for reduced information content collides with the need for information to enable blind people to walk safely and independently. Analyses of route descriptions by blind people have revealed that, in particular, they contain more details at decision points and mention more orientation cues along the way, resulting in route descriptions that are more than twice as detailed [Bra82].

With the automation of map creation on the basis of digital geographical data, the necessity to produce the same, general maps for a large readership diminishes. Thus, customized maps have become feasible which may serve just one person for one purpose ("one-time maps"). Such maps are comparable with the screen maps used as interfaces to geographical information systems. They can satisfy the reader's specific information need without presenting superfluous details which, in turn, would add further strain to the already strenuous haptic perception process.

The concept of customized maps allows the creation of maps supporting mobility for a certain route instead of a whole area. This opportunity is the basis for a new type of map – the *tactile route map* [HMS95]. Tactile route maps are an example of a customized map that can solve the conflict between information demand and symbol density for safe walking. While the route is presented with the necessary information for mobility, the surrounding streets are presented in a simplified way. The streets in the environment are preserved to aid the spatial integration of the route and to ensure that little detours can be planned if needed (see Fig. 20.1).

The concept of the tactile route map is comparable to fisheye techniques (see Chap. 2). The route as the main information carrier is presented in detail, while the context is simplified to give space for the route presentation. This allows optimal utilization of the available space on the map sheet, preventing the map from becoming too bulky to handle. But primarily it eases the time-consuming haptic perception process in restricting the amount of information to the necessary minimum.

Like the common fisheye techniques, it introduces a distortion to the whole map layout. Widening the street symbols along the route to gain enough presentation space for labeling and display of mobility information usually causes overlaps with symbols in the vicinity, e.g., parallel streets. This poses particularly strong demands for symbol displacement to unclutter the map. However, symbol displacement is already frequently necessary for the creation of tactile maps, as discussed in the next section.

20.2 Map Creation

20.2.1 Data Sources

The prerequisite for the computer-supported creation of the map layout for tactile maps is digital geographical data. In recent years, such data have become increasingly available due to the broader operation of Geographic Information Systems (GIS), e.g., in municipalities, environment protection institutions, and in fleet management and vehicle navigation systems. In these different application fields, there is a varying need for data content and accuracy. Large-scale, geometry-related data, which is suitable for land registries and urban data management, contain descriptions of buildings, land lot borders, sidewalks and curbs. These features are usually represented as polygons describing their contours.

In addition, data that is mainly used for vehicle navigation and fleet management systems describes the street network and part of the railway and water network. Unlike the above mentioned type of data, these data do not emphasize the actual 2D geometric extensions of the features but describe their connections within the transport network. Accordingly, the streets and rivers are represented by their central lines and centers of the junctions. This graph is usually supplemented by attributes defining relevant properties like street names, road classifications, and specifications of the traffic flow (e.g., one-way streets, forbidden turns). Among the more widely used formats for this type of data is the Geographic Data File Format (GDF). Figure 20.3 shows a simple visualization of a part of the data for Magdeburg.

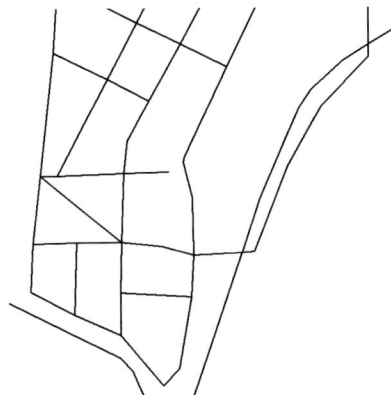

Figure 20.3: Part of vehicle navigation data for Magdeburg

Because of the data model as well as the contents, the GDF data forms a suitable basis for map creation. Central lines instead of polygons for the curbs facilitate symbol placement, and the utilization of a road classification allows a distinct presentation of the streets according to their importance.

The digitizing of analog maps is usually a manual process, which means the data may contain errors preventing the creation of a correct map:

- isolated vertices (e.g., junctions without streets),
- loops (edges having the same vertex as start and end vertex),
- multiple edges (two or more edges between the same vertices),
- non-planarity (edges intersect with no vertex at the intersection), and
- multiple subgraphs (two or more subgraphs run almost exactly on top of each other)

It is necessary to be aware of the existence of these errors since otherwise unpredictable effects may be noticed in a map which after expensive tracking down may reveal errors in the data source. Since these errors are independent of the map creation process, they can be removed during preparation of the data. All of them are automatically detectable, but some require human interaction for the correction to resolve ambiguities. Non-planarity, for example, leads to undefined data where it is not algorithmically decidable which road runs over the other; hence data models generally demand planarity.

Some of the errors can be removed without loss of information after their detection (e.g., isolated vertices and loops) but others need correction in accordance with their local surrounding (e.g., multiple subgraphs).

Another effect of human digitization is that due to psychomotor problems the digitized points do not always follow exactly the original line but have some offset to either side. This cannot be considered an error but it allows data reduction. Line simplification algorithms like the Douglas-Peucker algorithm [DP73] can be used to remove some of the superfluous points, speeding up the symbolization process.

20.2.2 Map Layout

The availability of geographical data lays the foundation for the computer-supported creation of tactile maps. However, the attempts so far have mainly been restricted to automation of the process of transferring the finished map layout to an embossed presentation. Thus, there are several approaches to processing graphical descriptions in order to control milling machines for the creation of a master for thermoforming [Dah97, SGD93, Lux88], whereas the labor-intensive process of generating a map layout on the basis of digital geographical data has been largely neglected so far.

One reason may be the need for cartographic generalization. As mentioned above, double-line symbols have to be 6–8 mm wide to allow the placement of symbols, e.g., for bus stops or crossings inside the street symbols, or to label streets with Braille, and symbols have to be 2–3 mm apart to ensure their separate haptic perception. Compared to maps for sighted people, these figures are about ten times larger. In consequence, the symbolization of the street network of a city at the scale 1:2 500 already requires symbol displacement. Given the restrictions imposed by the technology for embossing maps, generally only maps of size A4 (297 mm by 210 mm) or A3 (double that area) are feasible. The creation of tactile maps for a larger area, therefore, requires map scales of about 1:5 000 to 1:10 000. Because of the symbol size this would result in cluttered maps that show comparatively large overlaps. Hence, displacement becomes the central issue in the creation process.

20.3 Symbol Displacement

20.3.1 Overview

Symbol displacement is an important part of cartographic generalization – an abstraction process that adjusts the symbol presentation to the available presentation area and information needs. In the process of displacement, symbols are moved apart to gain space inbetween. It becomes necessary when symbols are no longer separately perceivable for a given map scale. Indeed, displacement becomes nearly unavoidable for the creation of maps for blind people due to the large symbol sizes compared to those in maps for sighted people.

Few attempts have been made so far to provide computer support for symbol displacement, though much work has been done for the automatic map generalization [MLW95]. Raster-based approaches have been investigated in which the raster format is used for the detection and analysis of symbol overlaps [Jäg90]. However, the matrices describing the amount of displacement necessary per pixel can become complicated and difficult to analyze.

A completely different approach has been devised by MONMONIER, who suggests the use of a few maps at different scales and describes an algorithm to interpolate maps at intermediate scales [Mon89]. Up to a certain extent, this algorithm can also be used to extrapolate to new scales.

POWITZ describes an approach to the displacement of streets and buildings [Pow93]. Resulting from the widening of street symbols, the algorithm uniformly moves all symbols inside the meshes of streets of a certain hierarchy level towards the mesh center. This mathematically demanding approach yields good results but does not allow to solve conflicts between streets of the same hierarchy level, which occurred frequently in our examples.

20.3.2 Requirements

The symbol displacement should preserve the topology and the shape of the traffic network. It should perform efficiently in a way that graphical conflicts are solved but the distortion introduced is kept to a minimum.

These objectives are difficult to meet with the increasing amount of necessary displacement. Considering the figures for the size of tactile symbols and the map scales required to present a larger area, it becomes apparent that a significant displacement is necessary to solve the graphical conflicts (in the example in this chapter of more than 8 mm). This large displacement has some implications for the design of a suitable displacement algorithm.

Often the effect of the displacement is faded out within a certain distance of the overlapping symbol to avoid a global distortion of the map. In effect, stopping a displacement after a short distance may, on the contrary, cause severe distortions; Figure 20.4(a) shows this effect. The solution is to use the whole map area to recover from the displacement, i.e., all displacements run

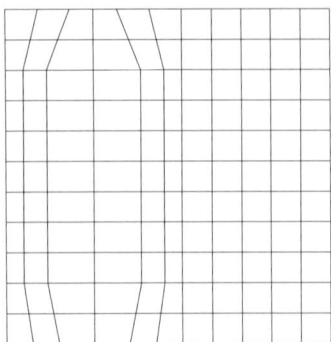 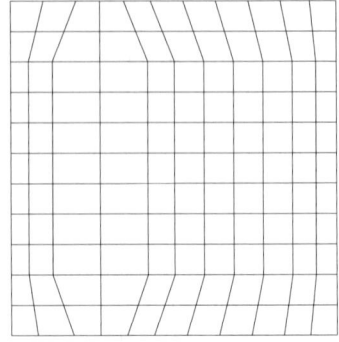

(a) Limited displacement zone: columns 5 and 6 are disproportionately squeezed.

(b) Unlimited displacement showing a less distorted grid

Figure 20.4: Different displacement methods applied to a regular grid

to the map edge (see Fig. 20.4(b)). This is also useful in another respect, since displacements in one area are likely to cause conflicts in another area and, hence, displacement propagation is needed.

It is common practice to carry out the displacement hierarchically to preserve the distinctive shape of some features and to ensure positional accuracy for important features [MLW95]. These hierarchies result in a sequence of actions. For example, first rivers may displace their surrounding symbols, then the main streets may displace the side-streets and buildings, and so on. However, it is doubtful that a hierarchical displacement is suitable for the creation of tactile maps for several reasons. First, it is not apparent how the hierarchy should be set up. Unlike road maps for drivers, it is not very likely that major streets are important for navigation by visually impaired pedestrians or that their shape should be maintained. Blind pedestrians frequently select streets on the basis of their safety; they sometimes prefer side-streets with less traffic or follow a route with safe crossings. The positional accuracy of highways or rivers becomes less important in this context.

Another aspect in favor of non-hierarchical displacement is the attempt to minimize the overall distortion caused by the displacement. Considering every conflict as equally important and displacing all surrounding symbols regardless of their classification leads to a mechanism where the whole traffic network is treated as if it were floating on a water surface. This paradigm minimizes the effects of local displacements in the immediate vicinity; the maximum changes to distances and angles are minimized. However, while this approach reduces the relative error, it increases the absolute error of the positional accuracy or, put in another way, it is best suited for preserving shape accuracy at the expense of positional accuracy. The actual results will be discussed in Sect. 20.4.

In addition, a non-hierarchical symbol displacement allows separation of symbols of the same feature class. This is no rare case, since for example junctions with streets of the same classification tend to overlap and need to be moved apart (see the conflict marked A in Fig. 20.5).

20.3.3 Detection and Analysis of Conflicts

A prerequisite for automatic displacement is the detection and analysis of graphical conflicts. As a result of this process, the center, the direction(s), and the magnitude of the displacement are determined. The algorithm presented here uses the vector format to analyze the areas of conflict and, hence, unlike the raster based approaches, yields an analytical description of the necessary displacement.

With respect to the detection, two classes of graphical conflicts between symbols can be distinguished: conflicts that are already detectable during the creation of a symbol and those that require a separate scan. The first class comprises those conflicts that are caused by overlaps with adjacent symbols (see Fig. 20.5). In these cases, the symbol polygon of the middle street segment cannot be correctly created because the symbols of the two adjacent street segments already overlap. To solve these conflicts, the adjacent street segments have to be moved apart and, thus, the middle segment is extended.

However, simply extending the middle segment may cause local distortions to the surrounding symbols. Figure 20.6(a) shows the result. In the

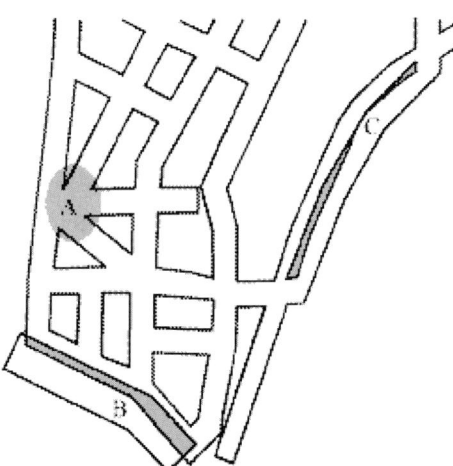

Figure 20.5: Graphical conflicts after symbolization of the area displayed in Fig. 20.3: segment A is hidden by its adjacent symbols; B and C mark overlaps between non-adjacent symbols

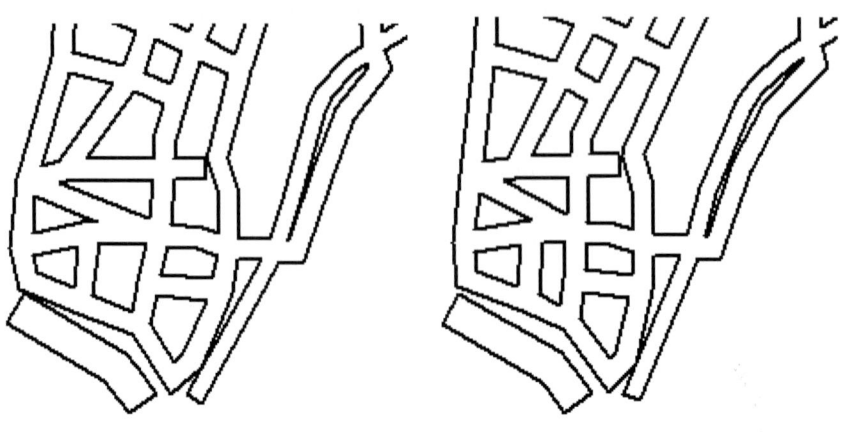

(a) Effect of locally resolving the conflict marked A in Fig. 20.5

(b) Context-dependent displacement; the left street running north-south was used as the anchor of displacement

Figure 20.6: Context-sensitivity of the displacement

example, segment A was extended by moving both end nodes apart. The resulting map shows bumps in the streets running in the north-south direction, the angles have been remarkably changed, and indeed the whole shape has been distorted. Avoiding these distortions requires a change from a local (blind) displacement to a global, context-dependent correction. For this purpose the graph structure has to be analyzed and subgraphs with suitable properties have to be identified.

Typical, easily recognizable shapes are long straight streets whose characteristics should be preserved during generalization. For this reason, major roads are sometimes placed at the top of the displacement hierarchy to prevent them from being subject to displacements. However, as already mentioned, these hierarchies have drawbacks when strong displacements become necessary. Thus, an alternative to a fixed hierarchy is required that is capable of preserving shapes. As a solution, part of the analysis of a local conflict has to be the detection of straight streets in the vicinity.

This can be accomplished algorithmically by examining the angles with adjacent street segments at both end points of a segment with overlaps. All segments with approximate right angles can be considered to be candidates. Each are then examined to determine whether it is an edge of a longer, nearly straight path that is perpendicular to the segment with overlaps. Selecting the longest of all potential straight subgraphs proved to yield the best results.

If such a path can be found, it is then used as the anchor for the displacement. The center of displacement can be described on the basis of this as an open polygon that runs through the middle of the segment with overlaps and parallel to the straight path. The direction of displacement should be perpendicular to this polygon. Using both sides of this line for displacement reduces the total displacement per point and, consequently, the absolute error. The third parameter of the displacement that needs to be determined is the amount of distortion. This can easily be deduced from the depth of the overlapping area.

Applying this algorithm for the analysis of graphical conflicts to the sample map results in a depiction without bumps (see Fig. 20.6(b)). Although segment A was prolonged by 8 mm, the context-dependency achieved a generalization that preserved the overall shape. The shape of the centers of displacement can be seen in Fig. 20.7.

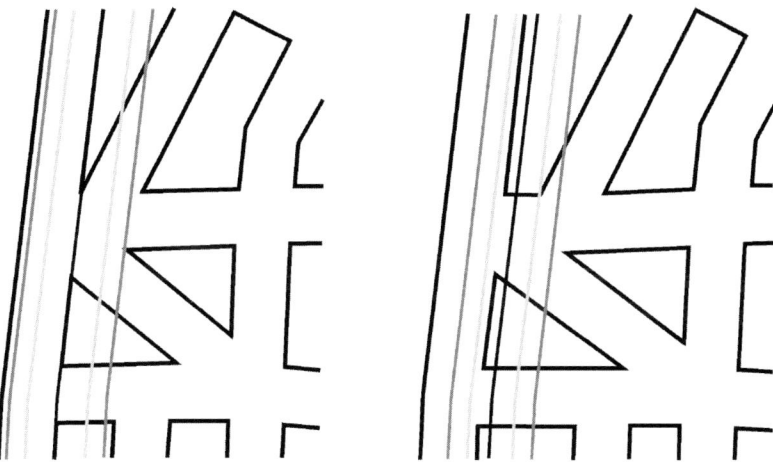

(a) Original image: the central line runs through the center of the middle segment, the inner pair of lines is set on its end points, and the outer pair marks the target position

(b) Corrected image: the middle segment has been prolonged to the distance between the outer pair of lines and has hence become visible

Figure 20.7: Using the *focus line* to correct overlaps between adjacent symbols

While the first category of conflicts is characterized by overlaps with adjacent[2] symbols, the second category comprises overlaps between non-adjacent symbols. These conflicts are not detectable during the symbolization phase but need a separate scan. Typical examples are parallel streets that come too close at some points (recall Fig. 20.5).

---

2 Note that here adjacent is used in the graph-theoretic sense where adjacent edges are those that share a common vertex.

Detection of these conflicts requires testing the symbol polygons for intersection. As a first step the resulting pairs of intersecting symbol polygons are checked to see if they are connected. If they are, they are merged to determine the whole area of intersection. Once the intersecting areas are detected, they need to be analyzed to determine the center of displacement as well as the directions and the amount of displacement. This can be accomplished by calculating the skeleton of the polygon enclosing the whole intersection area. As in the first case, the directions of displacement are reasonably set perpendicular to the edges of the skeleton to both sides. The amount of displacement can again be deduced from the area content of the intersection polygon, i.e., the height of the polygon at each point along the skeleton (see Fig. 20.8).

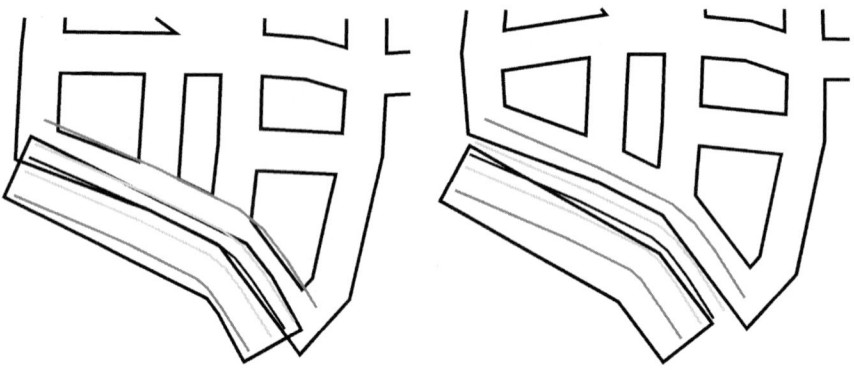

(a) Original image: the central line runs along the central axis of the overlap polygon, the inner pair of lines is set parallel on the minimum width while the outer pair marks the target position

(b) Corrected image: both symbols have been displaced perpendicular to the central axis, removing the overlap completely

Figure 20.8: Using the *focus line* to correct overlaps between non-adjacent symbols

20.3.4 Displacement

As a result of the analysis of the graphical conflicts, the center, the direction(s), and the amount of distortion are determined and the displacement can thus be performed automatically. The displacement should result in a smooth, continuous modification to the map. As discussed in Sect. 20.3.2, the modification should originate from the center of displacement and propagate the displacement toward the map edge, but should stop at the edge to avoid an enlargement over the given paper size. It should maintain relative positions and minimize the relative error.

This can be achieved using the *focus line* displacement algorithm that allows displacement perpendicular to a line (recall Chap. 8). The induced movement runs nonlinearly to zero with decreasing distance to the map edge. Hence, while symbols close to the line at both sides are moved away by the necessary amount, the displacement is quickly reduced for the symbols further away. But the displacement does not fade away before the border is reached, and hence preserves the relative positions.

The amount of distortion results from the necessity to move the symbols to the exact minimum distance apart. The *focus line* has to be placed and parameterized to achieve the necessary displacement. The need for space can be characterized by the depth of the overlapping zone and the minimum distance between symbols. Hence, when the central line is placed at the center of the displacement, a point with perpendicular distance s_0 to the central line needs to be moved until its distance becomes s_0' in order to fulfill the need for new space. The distance between points with a distance s smaller than s_0 must be increased, but decreased for those with a distance greater than s_0.

In order to remove the overlap of adjacent symbols, the middle segment has to be enlarged by the depth of the overlapping zone, i.e., both end points of the segment have to be moved by half of the depth. To achieve this, the *focus line* is placed perpendicular to the segment running through its middle. The parameter s_0 is set to the distance to each end point and s_0' is set to the new length (see Fig. 20.7(a)). The resulting displacement can be seen in Fig. 20.7(b). Note that all points that have been under the inner pair of lines are afterwards under the outer pair of lines, indicating that the displacement has enlarged the segment by exactly the difference between these two pairs of lines.

The overlap between non-adjacent symbols is characterized by a polygon enclosing the overlapping region. The amount of displacement can be deduced by the maximum width of this polygon. To resolve the overlap, the *focus line* is placed along the central axis of the polygon, s_0 is set to the minimum distance between the axis, and the polygon vertices and s_0' is increased by the maximum overlapping depth (see Fig. 20.8).

20.4 Communicating the Map Fidelity

Symbol displacement allows the creation of conflict-free tactile maps from digital geographical data (recall Fig. 20.3). Figure 20.11 shows the street layout for a tactile map at scale 1:7 500 where all overlaps have been removed. Street segments between junctions have been enlarged and parallel streets moved apart to separate symbols that came too close. While the resulting maps are free of graphical conflicts they are no longer accurate in every respect. The position as well as the shape of the street symbols was changed due to the displacement.

In the example (see Fig. 20.11) the maximum request for displacement was 8 mm. However, this resulted in a maximum positional error of only 4 mm due to the non-hierarchical displacement (remember the discussion in Sect. 20.3.2). Accordingly, the average positional error was 1.3 mm and thus significantly lower.

While the positional error is easy to determine, shape fidelity is not measurable [God97]. The preservation of the main directions is an important aspect of the quality of the method (recall Sect. 20.3.3) and may be used as an indicator for shape distortion. In this example the angles between all triples of points changed on average by $1.5°$, which is hardly noticeable. The maximum value $56.8°$ occurred in an area where two non-adjacent streets had to be moved apart to resolve their overlapping. As with the positional accuracy, no big changes occurred as unintentional side effects of the displacement method.

Although the overall shape was preserved to a great extent and the positional errors are minimal, it may be important to reveal these changes to the map reader. This is particularly important as MONMONIER points out that maps are usually accepted without question as being accurate [Mon96]. JOÃO argues that information about map fidelity is essential to the map reader since it affects map applicability [Joã95].

We investigated two ways to communicate the modifications applied to the map: visualization of generalization error and figure captions.

Visualization of Generalization Error. Figure 20.12 visualizes the distribution of the positional error over the whole map. In this presentation, gray shades correspond to the absolute error for each position; dark gray is used for strong displacements and light gray for light displacements, respectively.

This allows us to estimate the overall impact of the single displacements. Thus, it can be seen that the strongest displacement is achieved in the close vicinity of each focus line. The magnitude is reduced if an area is in the influence of two focus lines with opposite directions of displacement. Eventually, this leads to an area where the two focus lines compensate the effect of each other. This effect can easily be seen in the top right part of Fig. 20.12 where a white semicircle has developed.

In consequence, most of the extra presentation spaces that were necessary to ensure symbol discriminability have been taken from the sparse area close to the map area while the inner area of the map remains largely unmoved.

Figure Captions. As discussed in Chap. 12, figure captions are a common means to give additional information assisting in the interpretation of figures. This applies also for maps where their use has largely remained underestimated so far [Sch97]. Accordingly, JOÃO suggests textual reports about the map fidelity accompanying a map [Joã95].

20.4 Communicating the Map Fidelity

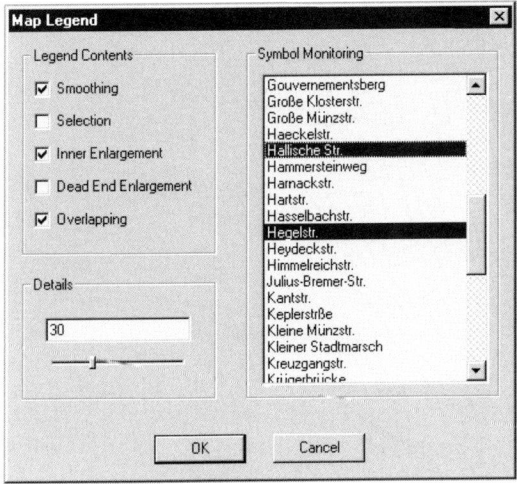

Figure 20.9: Dialog to adjust figure captions for maps

The generation of dynamic figure captions for maps follows the general scheme described in Chap. 12. Figure 20.9 shows the dialog to adjust figure captions for maps. The left part provides options for the customization of the content. This option allows a user to request a notification when a certain operation has been performed on the data, i.e., when streets have been smoothed or enlarged or when overlaps between non-adjacent symbols have been removed. The slider on the bottom left controls the amount of detail. In the example, only the most important third of all notifications are presented.

Often it is necessary to know all modifications that happened to a street. Hence, the right part of the dialog allows streets to be selected for monitoring. All operations that affect those streets are then recorded. However, since a street may be subject to several displacements and may be affected by displacements in the proximity, this requires some analysis. This is facilitated by generating events for each operation and collecting them centrally. The Context Expert (recall Chap. 12) manages these events. It sorts them by priority and analyzes them to detect logical relations.

Traced streets are set into a state where they detect any modification they are undergoing and generate a message accordingly. This message is then sent to the Context Expert for analysis. Thus, a street, for example, may register a repositioning and signal this. But the Context Expert receives in addition to this message information from another street stating that in order to solve a local graphical conflict with a river nearby the street has initiated a displacement. The Context Expert is now able to relate both events to one another and to inform the map reader that the street he or she showed particular interest in has been moved due to a displacement that was propagated throughout the map.

Figure 20.10 shows a sample caption summarizing the major generalization effects. In this example the user has expressed particular interest in

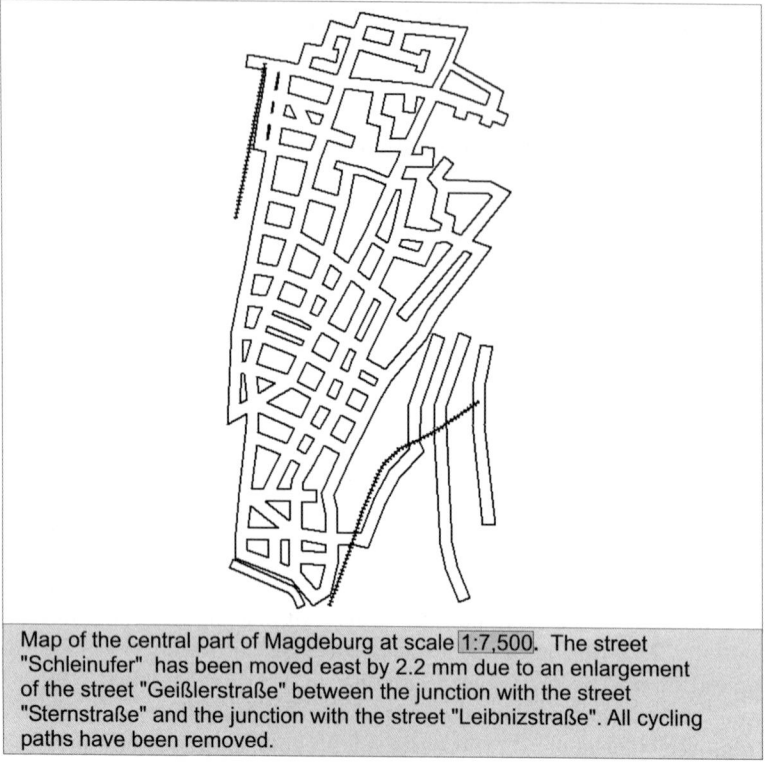

Map of the central part of Magdeburg at scale 1:7,500. The street "Schleinufer" has been moved east by 2.2 mm due to an enlargement of the street "Geißlerstraße" between the junction with the street "Sternstraße" and the junction with the street "Leibnizstraße". All cycling paths have been removed.

Figure 20.10: Tactile map of Magdeburg with an interactive figure caption describing the major generalization effects

the street "Schleinufer". The street may have been affected by several displacements, which in total moved the street east by 2.2 mm. The system has analyzed all operations and detected one that had the most impact.

Note that it is not always straightforward to describe a position in the map, which is internally represented as a node (latitude and longitude) or a street segment (edge between two nodes). So far, we have chosen to mention the linear feature to which it belongs, e.g., the junction if applicable or the part of a street between two junctions.

20.5 Concluding Remarks

The presented techniques have been implemented and integrated in the system called MAP WIZARD [MS97]. This system facilitates the creation of tactile maps. Figure 20.11 shows the street layout that was created automatically on the basis of the geographical data (recall Fig. 20.3) at scale 1:7 500. The conflicts partly shown in Fig. 20.5 were solved automatically. Overlaps have been successfully moved apart to the extent that they do not overlap any longer. They are still closer together than haptic discriminability requires, but the algorithm can be adjusted to heed these distances.

The displacement method based on the *focus line* technique as presented in this chapter proves to be a very flexible method that keeps the noticeable overall distortion to a minimum. The method rearranges the whole network as if it were floating on a water surface until all conflicts are removed.

However, if two or more almost parallel *focus lines* intersect substantially, they no longer function as they should. This is the case when the local symbol density is too high to be resolved by simply displacing the individual symbols. For the correction of these conflicts other generalization processes like selection, simplification, or classification become inevitable.

While the development of appropriate algorithms has already made dramatic progress in the last years, there are still many problems left for future research. Apart from improvements to the individual algorithms for generalization operations, their "orchestration", i.e., their coordination to solve the generalization problem is still an open problem. For more information on the current state of the art in automatic map generalization, see [MWLS95] and [MWB97].

Contributor of Chap. 20: Rainer MICHEL

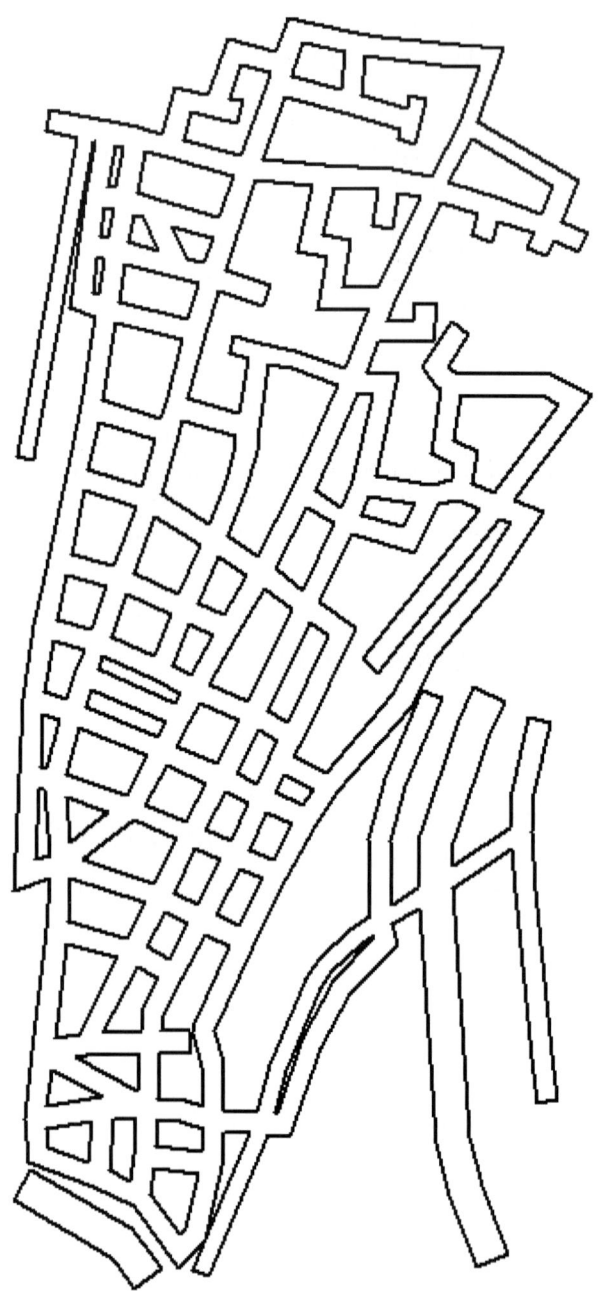

Figure 20.11: Final street layout. All overlaps have been removed

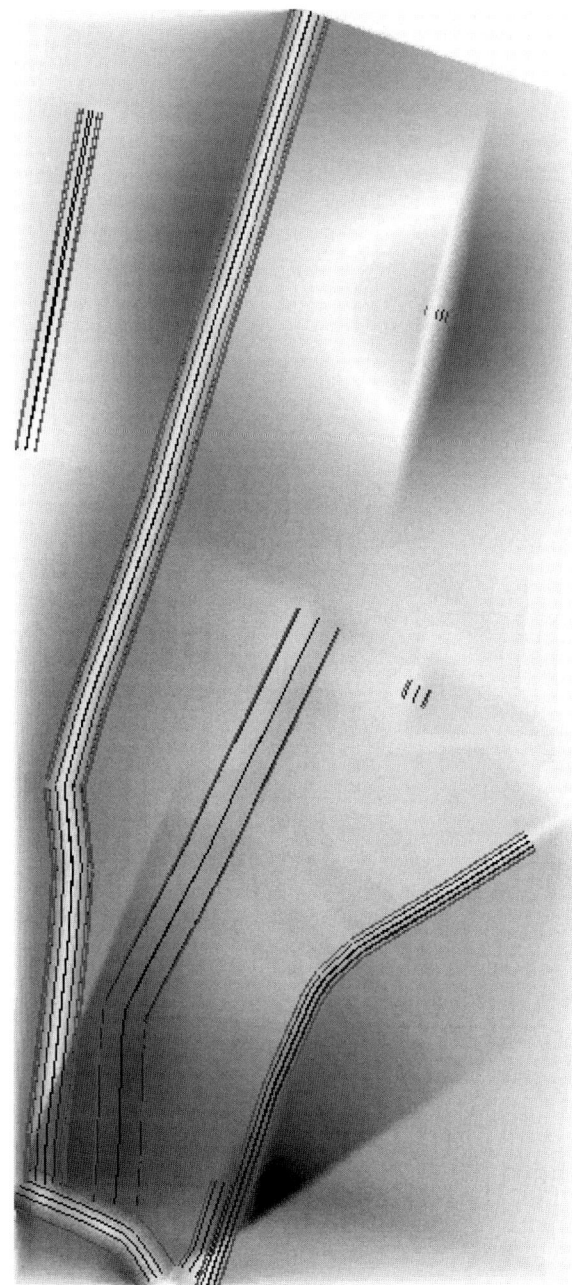

Figure 20.12: Effect of the displacements: Lines indicate centers of displacement, gray shades represent absolute positional error (increasing from light to dark gray)

Chapter 21

Synthetic Holography

Holography is a method for three-dimensional imaging of objects. It was first presented by DENNIS GABOR [Gab48] in 1948 and has expanded into various fields since then. In holographic interferometry, arbitrarily shaped diffusely scattering objects are examined. A description of this process can be found in LAUTERBORN, KURZ, and WIESENFELDT [LKW95] and EICHLER and ACKERMANN [EA93]. The same object can be compared with itself at a later time, allowing for the analysis of stress or deformations. Other applications of holography are in the design of diffractive optical elements, as described by AAGEDAL et al. [ABST94] or holographic storages [EA93].

21.1 Holography as a 3D Visualization Technique

In this chapter, we concentrate on synthetic holography as a 3D display method. It is used as a visualization technique for computer graphics to display objects in 3D. We focus on the holographic imaging of objects composed of line segments, since it allows for a decrease in computational effort. A new method is derived using standard computer graphics rendering.

21.1.1 Optical Holography

Holography, as described in physics text books, for example by BERGMANN and SCHAEFER [BS93] and FOWLES [Fow89], is a two-step process for the *recording* and *reconstruction* of three-dimensional objects. After DENNIS GABOR proposed his idea, holography attracted little attention until the laser became available as a source of highly coherent light.

The hologram is a special diffraction screen used to reconstruct in detail the wave field emitted by the object to be imaged. To make the hologram, the output from a laser is separated into two beams, one of which illuminates the object. The other beam (reference beam) is directed onto a fine-grained photographic film. The film is exposed simultaneously to the reference beam and the reflected laser light from the object (see left of Fig. 21.1).

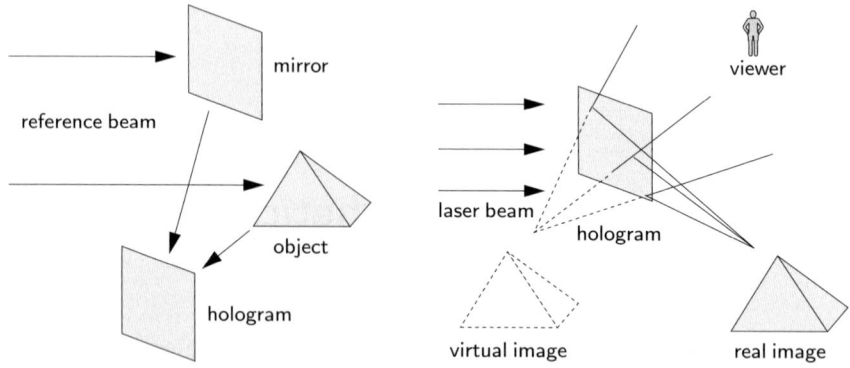

Figure 21.1: Hologram recording (left) and reconstruction (right)

A complicated interference pattern results. It is recorded on the film and constitutes the hologram. The hologram stores all the information needed to reproduce the wave field of the object as the magnitude and phase of the wave field. However, coherent light as provided by a laser is required for establishing a fixed phase relation between the reference wave and the wave reflected by the object. For reconstruction, the developed hologram is illuminated again with the reference beam (Fig. 21.1, right image). Part of the resulting diffracted wave field is a precise, three-dimensional copy of the original wave reflected by the object. The viewer looking at the hologram sees the image of the object in depth. The viewer can change the perspective of the view just by moving his or her head.

Holography is possible because, by Huygens principle, the known distribution of the field strength of a wave field *in a plane* determines the complete wave field. For recording a spatially distributed wave field, it is sufficient to store the wave field in a plane. If the wave field is reconstructed in this plane (wave front), Huygens elementary waves are propagating from this wave front, resulting in the reconstruction of the complete wave field. Therefore, holography is also known as *wave front reconstruction*.

There are several methods of hologram recording and reconstruction (see, for example, [LKW95]). They determine the hologram type: in-line holograms, reflection holograms, transmission holograms, and white light and rainbow holograms. The latter can be viewed just by illuminating the hologram with white light.

21.1.2 Synthetic Holography

Synthetic holography embodies the computer simulation of the overall holographic process or of parts of it. Synthetic holography differs from optical/experimental holography in two aspects: the transmission of a hologram is calculated by a computer, and its fabrication is done by special devices controlled by a computer (ZHANG in [Zha95]). The problems of simulating wave propagation on a computer and of synthetic hologram generation are discussed by SCHREIER [Sch84] and LAUTERBORN et al. [LKW95]. The major application of synthetic holography is the simulation of the hologram generation step. The computer calculates the transmittance of the holographic plate. This method has the advantage that holograms can be generated from objects for which only a mathematical description exists, such as CAD models, but also optical elements like lenses with multiple foci. The resulting hologram is in most cases transferred to photographic film and optically reconstructed.

The reconstruction step can also be simulated with systems like DIGIOPT, which is described in [ABST94]. The immediate display of images from synthetic holograms without using photographic film involves the transfer of a great deal of data from computer memory to a real-time display. It was implemented with the *MIT holovideo system*, which is described by LUCENTE and GALYEAN in [LG95].

21.1.3 3D Display Techniques to Provide Depth Cues

This section describes holography and other 3D display techniques in terms of how the perception of depth is provided. The description is based on the survey of imaging systems by MCKENNA and ZELTZER [MZ92].

Depth Perception. The perception of distance or depth is a complex phenomenon. Mechanisms of the eye as well as the brain are involved. A couple of cues, or patterns of stimuli, provide us with information about the depth and shape of objects in the real world, as well as objects presented to us in an image. Depth cues are categorized into *monocular* and *binocular* ones.

The eyes are displaced from each other. Thus, each eye sees a slightly different image of a scene. The difference in the resulting retinal images is known as *binocular disparity*. The depth perception due to binocular disparity is called *stereopsis*. In *convergence* the eyes rotate to center their viewing axes on a particular point in space to be able to fixate an object. In order to focus on objects at varying distances from the viewer, the shape of the lens is changed by means of contractions of the annular muscles in the eye. This monocular depth cue is called *accommodation*. Another monocular depth cue is *motion parallax*. It is generated as the viewpoint changes and objects at different distances move with respect to each other.

Pictorial depth cues belong to the monocular category. *Overlap, image size, linear perspective, texture gradient, shading* and *shadows* of objects, and *aerial perspective* are representatives of this category of depth cues.

Besides the depth cues mentioned above, a couple of technical attributes exist which determine the suitability of display devices for certain visualization tasks. These attributes encompass: *field of view, spatial resolution, refresh and update rates, levels of brightness, color, viewing zone/volume extent,* and *number of views.*

3D Display Types. Three-dimensional displays are classified into two major groups: *stereoscopic* and *autostereoscopic*. Both present different views to the eyes, but the latter do not require special viewing aids such as stereo spectacles.

In *stereoscopic displays* one 2D image for each eye is generated, providing a sensation of depth. If, in addition, head-tracking is available (interactive stereoscopic displays), views depending on the actual position and viewing direction of the user can be presented. Stereoscopic displays encompass monitor-glass combinations or boom-mounted displays. A well-known representative of stereoscopic displays is the CAVE, as described by CRUZ-NEIRA, DEFANTI, and SANDIN in [CNDJ93].

A *lenticular screen* consists of an array of cylindrical lenses. They generate an autostereoscopic 3D image by directing different 2D images into viewing subzones, which appear at different angles in front of the lenticular screen. The observer places each eye in a different viewing zone. Each eye sees a different image, and thus binocular disparity is achieved. Horizontally, a very high resolution is required to be able to image a large number of views at a high resolution.

A *parallax barrier* is a vertical slit plate placed in front of a display to block parts of the screen from each eye. As with a lenticular screen different 2D views are presented to the user.

Slice stacking or *multiplanar displays* build up a 3D volume by layering 2D images. A planar image can be created by a spinning line of LEDs, while a rotating plane of LEDs creates a volumetric image. A similar volume can be scanned using CRT displays and moving mirrors.

The principles of *holography* have been described above. Holography is capable of generating full-color, high-resolution images with wide field of view. However, the synthetic generation of holograms is expensive in terms of time and computational power, so only small volumes are imaged.

All of the 3D display systems mentioned above provide at least two different views, so they all support retinal disparity and convergence. The eyes pivot and change their convergence angles to fixate on objects at different depths in the 3D image, which is due to different retinal disparities. All the display systems generally support pictorial depth cues. However, slice-stacking displays do not support overlap, because a luminous volume is imaged creating transparent surfaces. To implement overlap, head tracking has to be added.

Aerial perspective is supported to some degree on all of the display systems. However, it cannot be accurately displayed on holographic and slice-stacking systems, since the image volume is relatively small. Motion parallax due to observer motion is supported by all of the display types, except for the non-interactive stereoscopic display. However, motion parallax is supported in the horizontal direction only by parallax barrier, lenticular, and some holographic displays, such as the MIT holovideo system. Parallax barrier and lenticular displays exhibit a "coarse" horizontal parallax, since only a limited number of views are imaged.

Holographic displays in general provide *all* the depth cues. They are autostereoscopic. For perceiving depth or motion parallax no further viewing aids are needed by the user. Thus, synthetic holography is a very attractive display method to study from the standpoint of computer graphics.

21.2 Methods of Synthetic Holography

This section gives a brief overview of hologram computation approaches. However, this is not a detailed review, and just a few characteristic methods from the computer graphics point of view are considered. The techniques are more thoroughly discussed by SCHREIER in [Sch84] and ZHANG in [Zha95].

Synthetic holography imposes high requirements on computational power and storage capacity. The reduction of effort is a common goal. In this section, several methods are described: the common point oriented approach and two other computation procedures which target on a reduction of effort. The outline of these techniques leads on to our line oriented approach, which is described in the next section.

Direct Simulation. The object to be imaged is represented by a number of radiating points. Each of these points is the source of a spherical wave. The complex amplitude of this wave is determined for all locations at the hologram plate, as illustrated in Fig. 21.2 (left).

To get the total amplitude of the object wave at the hologram point, all partial waves from the individual objects are summed. The intensity at each hologram point is computed, including the reference wave. Each object point emits a spherical wave generating a Fresnel zone plate (see Fig. 21.2 (right)). Thus, the hologram is an accumulation of all the Fresnel zone plates generated from each object point.

For the generation of synthetic holograms using this method, one computation step per hologram point (pixel) and luminous object point has to be performed. Each computation step includes complex additions and multiplications. Considering a hologram size of $5\,000 \times 5\,000$ pixels and an object consisting of 1 000 points, 25 billion steps have to be performed. According to

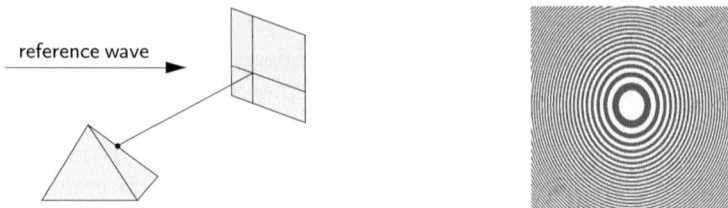

Figure 21.2: Calculation of the synthetic hologram (left) using the point oriented direct simulation, (right) the resulting Fresnel zone plate per point

LAUTERBORN et al. [LKW95], the approach allows for certain simplifications, e.g., setting an equal amplitude at each object point or assuming that the reference wave strikes the holographic plate at normal incidence. The computation is still very time-consuming. One possible solution to this problem is the determination of point contributions in a separate step.

Precomputing Point Contributions. In direct simulation discussed above, the object consists of luminous points, the contributions of which are summed up in the hologram. LUCENTE describes in [Luc93] a method approaching real-time computation and display of holograms.

The object space is organized in a 3D grid. The distance between the grid points is chosen such that the image points appear to be continuous, given a certain viewing distance. The human visual system generally regards as continuous two points that are separated by 3 milliradians of arc [Luc93]. The contribution of each 3D grid point is precomputed and stored in a lookup table. The table is indexed by the grid point's x and z position. In the actual computation, the analysis is performed to determine which luminous points comprise the object. Then the contributions of these points are taken from their corresponding look-up table cells and summed to generate the hologram. For further simplification, vertical parallax is neglected. Thus, the 3D grid is reduced to a layer of 3D points. For each hologram line the same grid can be applied. Computation is very fast compared to the approach introduced above. A massively parallel system consisting of 16K processors was able to generate a hologram in less than one second.

Stereograms. Stereograms consist of a set of 2D views. As in lenticular screens or parallax barrier displays introduced in Sect. 21.1.3, the 3D sensation is achieved by presenting a different 2D view to each eye.

Again, LUCENTE et al. present in [LG95] a method for the rapid generation of holograms. The look-up table approach described in the paragraph above can be extended to stereograms. Then, the table is indexed by the image's x position and viewing angle rather than by x and z. Furthermore, since the stereogram is based on 2D images, conventional computer graphics hardware and software can be exploited.

In the first step, different 2D view images are rendered. The views are combined with a set of precomputed basis fringes. These basis fringes are designed to diffract light in specific directions. One basis fringe is the holographic pattern that causes light to diffract from a particular view-image pixel location to a particular viewing subzone. The view images act as weights for the basis fringes. Thus, the final hologram pattern is composed.

The Line Approach. The methods described so far generate images of objects consisting of luminous points. The high computation effort is decreased by sophisticated methods for precomputing certain information, thus speeding up the actual computation process.

In cases where the 3D object consists of line segments, it is useful to decompose the object information into lines instead of points. A line can represent a large number of points. Composing the objects as lines leads to a considerable reduction in computational effort.

Since line drawings are a powerful method in computer graphics and since they can be effectively transferred into a holographic image, we focus on the computation of holograms taken from objects composed of line segments.

21.3 Where Holography and Common Computer Graphics Meet

In this section a new approach to the generation of holograms of line objects is presented. First, the physical background and the conventional approach are discussed. The setup for hologram generation (software architecture) and reconstruction is outlined. By analyzing the results of the conventional hologram computation a new method is derived which exploits computer graphics hardware and software and allows for rapid generation of holograms. The idea and implementation details, together with a critical evaluation of the results, are described in the second part of the section.

21.3.1 Holograms of Objects Composed of Line Segments

Objects to be imaged in a hologram consist of luminous geometric primitives such as points, lines, or surfaces. These primitives emit waves which during the hologram recording stage result in a certain pattern on the hologram. During hologram reconstruction, the waves are again generated and focus in the original primitives, thus reconstructing these primitives.

As stated for instance by Frère in [Frè88], a mapping of primitive and wave type exists:

- a point source emits spherical waves,
- infinite lines emit cylindrical waves, and
- plane waves are emitted by infinite planes.

This mapping is used in the conventional approach for generating holograms of line objects, which is introduced by FRÈRE et al. [FLB86]. Instead of representing a line by a set of points, which are sources for spherical waves (see Fig. 21.2 (right) for a spherical wave resulting in a Fresnel zone plate at the hologram), a line is treated as a source of a cylindrical wave. Thus, it can be processed in one step during hologram computation.

For the description of the holographic patterns generated by cylindrical waves originating from lines, we introduce a Cartesian coordinate system. The hologram is in the xy plane of the coordinate system. The z axis is the optical axis. If the line is parallel to the x axis and located at a distance $z = R$ from the hologram plane, the complex amplitude $u(x, y, 0)$ in the hologram plane is described by the Fresnel approximation

$$u(x, y, 0) = \exp\left(i\frac{\pi}{\lambda R}y^2\right), \tag{21.1}$$

where λ is the wavelength. This equation is sufficient for an infinite line but not for a line segment of finite length. For representing line segments, the line must not influence more than a rectangular area on the hologram. A clipping function $rect\left(\frac{x}{2a}\right)$ is introduced, extending equation (21.1) to

$$u(x, y, 0) = \exp\left(i\frac{\pi}{\lambda R}y^2\right) rect\left(\frac{x}{2a}\right). \tag{21.2}$$

This representation is restricted to line segments parallel to the x axis. An arbitrary line segment L is described as follows:

1. the angle α of L relative to the x axis,
2. the angle γ of L relative to the hologram plane, and
3. the coordinates (x_0, y_0, z_0) of the center point of L.

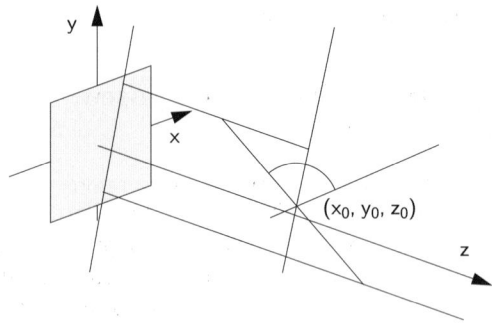

Figure 21.3: Line and its parameters determining position and orientation

21.3 Where Holography and Common Computer Graphics Meet

The point (x, y) on the hologram plane is transformed by a 2D rotation to a point (X, Y) with $X = x\cos\alpha - y\sin\alpha$ and $Y = x\sin\alpha + y\cos\alpha$. The angle γ is incorporated by

$$R(X, \gamma) = z_0 - X \tan\gamma. \tag{21.3}$$

The function $R(X, \gamma)$ describes the distance between the line and the hologram points (pixels). The reconstruction of lines outside the optical axis (z axis in Fig. 21.3) is achieved by introducing a linear phase factor

$$\exp\left[i\frac{2\pi}{\lambda z_0}(x_0 X + y_0 Y)\right] \tag{21.4}$$

The resulting complex amplitude is

$$u(x, y, 0) = \exp\left[i\frac{2\pi}{\lambda z_0}(x_0 X + y_0 Y)\right] \exp\left[i\frac{\pi}{\lambda}\frac{Y^2}{R(X, \gamma)}\right] rect\left(\frac{X}{2a}\right). \tag{21.5}$$

Combining the complex amplitude with a reference gives the hologram transmission [Sch84]

$$t(x, y) = \left\{1 + \cos\left[2\pi\nu_0 X + \frac{2\pi}{\lambda z_0}(x_0 X + y_0 Y) + \frac{\pi}{\lambda}\frac{Y^2}{R(X, \gamma)}\right]\right\} rect\left(\frac{X}{2a}\right), \tag{21.6}$$

where ν_0 is the spatial frequency of the carrier [FLB86].

Figure 21.4 shows an example of a holographic image obtained with the method described above. Three lines perpendicular to each other constitute a coordinate system (Fig. 21.4(a)). In the hologram (Fig. 21.4(b)) the rectangular areas representing the wave patterns are to be seen. Clipping is performed in the x and y direction to prevent spatial frequencies which cannot be transferred to the hologram anyway. The reconstruction (Fig. 21.4(c)) shows the image generated by the hologram. In this case the reconstruction is obtained by simulation and not by optical means. We use the DIGIOPT system which will be briefly described in Sect. 21.3.2.

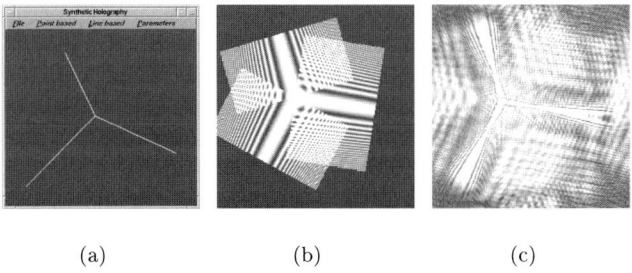

(a)   (b)   (c)

Figure 21.4: Image of a coordinate system: (a) original object, (b) hologram, and (c) simulated reconstruction at a certain depth

21.3.2 Implementation

This section describes our setup for the generation and reconstruction of holographic images. First, the architecture of our system for hologram computation is outlined. Second, the verification of holograms by means of optical reconstruction and simulation is discussed.

Software Architecture. Our system for the generation of synthetic holograms (see Fig. 21.5) has a modular structure. The modules form a holographic pipeline which is fed with the geometric data for the object and produces the holographic image at the end. The *viewing module* loads the geometric description (given in OpenInventor *.iv or Drawing Exchange Format *.dxf) of the object to be imaged. The object is rendered conventionally and can be arranged arbitrarily with respect to the camera (rotation, translation). However, the main task of the *viewing module* is to extract the information needed for the actual hologram computation, which is performed in the *generator module*. The *generator* implements several computation methods including point-based (direct simulation and using a look-up table, see Sect. 21.2) and line-based ones. It reads either line-based or point-based information given by the *viewing module*, depending on the computation method. The *output module* collects the computation results generated by the *generator* and stores the hologram in a file (pixel-based formats TIFF, BMP, Postscript, IRIS RGB).

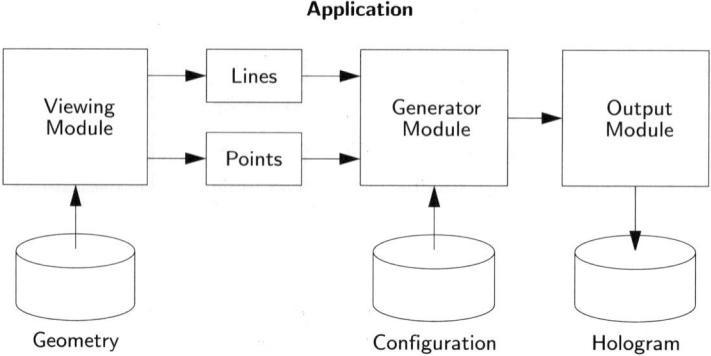

Figure 21.5: Software design: the modular architecture of our system

Hologram Reconstruction. To visualize the holographic image, the hologram generated with the system described above has to be reconstructed. The reconstruction can be accomplished in two ways:
- simulation with the DIGIOPT system, or
- optical reconstruction.

The results of a simulation are shown in Fig. 21.4. The advantage of a simulated reconstruction is that the results can be obtained quickly. On the other hand, only holograms of reduced resolution can be simulated because of memory limits.

Experimental Setup. The results of hologram computation have to be verified by optical reconstruction. In order to prepare the holograms for optical reconstruction, they are transferred to photographic material using a film recorder. The photographic material is processed conventionally. In our setup (illustrated in Fig. 21.6) for the optical reconstruction of synthetic holograms, we use an argon crypton laser which emits visible light at a wavelength of $\lambda = 514.5$ nm. The wavelength is selected by a prism. Since the space on the optical table is limited, the laser beam is redirected twice. It is widened by a telescope consisting of two lenses. The laser beam penetrates the hologram, and the real image of the object is reconstructed in the space beyond the hologram.

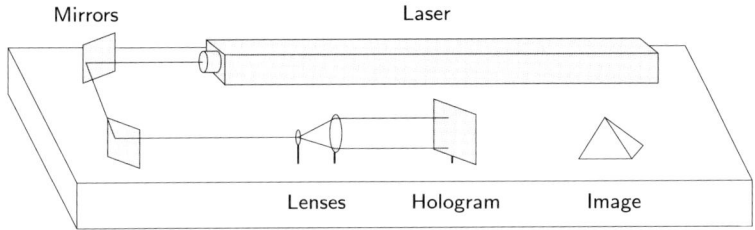

Figure 21.6: Setup for the optical reconstruction of holograms

The experimental setup for optical reconstruction was established by Dr. Thomas BENZIGER. His contribution to our research in synthetic holography is gratefully acknowledged.

21.3.3 A New Approach to Holographic Imaging of Lines

A straight line emits a cylindrical wave (see [LF87],[FLB86]) providing a constant phase distribution along the line. The phase of individual points on a line is a free parameter. Its modification does not alter the perception of the geometry in the optical reconstruction. The relationship between the line segment to be reconstructed and the conical wave is not uniquely determined. In the reconstruction step each line focus can be obtained by an infinite number of different conical waves. The cone angle β is the free parameter [Les87]. A boundary condition is that β has to be chosen such that in the recording step the light emitted by the luminous line segment reaches the hologram.

In particular we can assume a linear phase distribution along a line segment such that the hologram plane is parallel to a tangential plane of the emitted conical wave. Such a pattern is illustrated in Fig. 21.7.

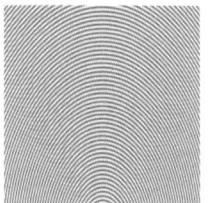 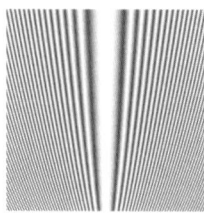

Figure 21.7: Hologram of an inclined line (left), the same line with a linear phase distribution applied (right)

The pattern in Fig. 21.7 (right) represents conic sections (the cone is cut). The pattern can be generated with the method described in Sect. 21.3.1. It represents conic sections the aspects of which are described by AUMANN and SPITZMÜLLER in [AS93].

How can these patterns be obtained using computer graphics methods? In a first approach, we explore the approximation of these holograms by "linear" patterns. A line parallel to the hologram emits a cylindrical wave (Fig. 21.8(a)). As soon as the line is inclined to the hologram, the pattern is more or less distorted (Fig. 21.7(right)). At first sight, the distortion seems to be similar to a *perspective projection*; this is the simulation which leads to our new method to render holograms of wire frame images. In order to simulate this behavior, the object to be imaged in a hologram is transformed into its *holographic geometric equivalent*. This equivalent consists of a set of textured rectangles which are constrained in their orientation. The texture represents the "reference pattern" (Figure 21.8(a)) generated by a cylindrical wave.

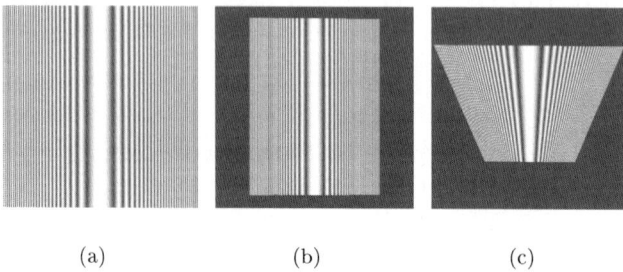

(a) (b) (c)

Figure 21.8: (a) Cylindrical wave, (b) rendering of a rectangle with the cylindrical pattern as a texture map, (c) the same rectangle inclined to the viewing plane, pattern (linearly) distorted

One textured rectangle (Fig. 21.8(b)) per original line represents the wave emission of the line. The rectangles are oriented and positioned in the same way as their line counterparts which build up the original object (Fig. 21.9, in which the rectangles are centered around the original lines). The rectangle orientation according to the original line leads to a distortion of the rectangle together with its texture (Fig. 21.8(c)) in the perspective projection. Thus, a line inclined to the hologram plane is simulated. The rectangles mimic the clipping of the wave pattern accomplished by the rectangle function shown first in equation (21.2).

Examples. We shall now show some holographic geometric equivalents. A first example showing the equivalent of a single line was already shown in Fig. 21.8(c). Figure 21.9 illustrates the transformation of three lines perpendicular to each other into their holographic geometric equivalent.

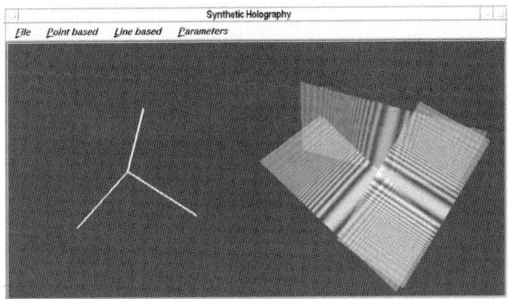

Figure 21.9: Three perpendicular lines forming a coordinate system (left) and the holographic geometric equivalent (right)

It consists of three rectangles which are rendered translucent. Thus, overlap of the three patterns is accomplished without introducing further disturbances in the reconstruction step.

A more complex example is shown in Fig. 21.10. The original object consists of about 100 lines. The hologram is generated just by rendering the equivalent. No further computation steps are required.

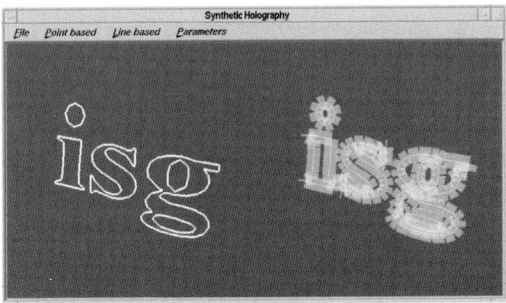

Figure 21.10: Lines which build up a logo (left) and their equivalent (right)

Implementation Details. Because geometric processing and texture mapping are implemented in hardware on computer graphics workstations, hologram computation is fast. It can be performed in nearly real time for reasonable resolutions. The "reference texture" showing the cylindrical pattern is computed using equation (21.1). The texture is generated in a separate pass and stored persistently in a file. It is loaded again as soon as the holographic geometric equivalent is displayed.

The geometry of the original object composed of line segments is stored in an IRIS Performer tree-like data structure, the *scene graph*. In the process of generating the holographic geometric equivalent, the scene graph is traversed to detect all line primitives. An additional scene graph is built up, which consists of rectangles possessing the same length as their line counterparts. The *equivalent scene graph* consists of similar branches to the original one. The precomputed textures are applied to the rectangles. Additional attributes which are assigned to the rectangle encompass the alpha value to control the translucent appearance and the rectangle width to control overlap and spatial frequencies in the hologram.

The length, position, and orientation of the rectangles is chosen in accordance with the lines from which they originate. However, the rectangles are constrained in their azimuthal orientation. First, the rectangle is centered around the line, and, second, the plane normal of the rectangle is mapped under parallel projection to a vertical line segment, i.e., it has an x-component of zero. Otherwise, distortions due to the perspective projection in the azimuthal direction introduce corruptions of the depth reconstruction of the line segments. Thus, as can be seen in Fig. 21.9, the rectangles are longitudinally inclined according to line orientation but normal to the viewing plane in the azimuthal direction. The object to be imaged can be interactively transformed, translated, and positioned relative to the camera. The equivalent is transformed in the same way. During rotation, the rectangles of the equivalent are tilted. The tilt with respect to the axis specified by the original line has to be compensated in order to obey the azimuthal orientation constraint. This is accomplished by using a special node provided by IRIS Performer. *Performer Billboards* are utilized to guarantee the desired orientation of the affected geometry (the rectangles).

As stated above, the hologram is generated just by straight rendering of the equivalent. However, viewport dimensions are constrained to fit typical computer graphics applications. Since holography requires much higher resolutions, the viewport constraint prohibits results in a reasonable hologram resolution. To remedy the situation, the image is tiled. Each tile is rendered in one step within the given constrained viewport dimension. Figure 21.11 illustrates the approach.

The camera is centered for each tile. The rendering setup (camera and viewport) has to be chosen carefully to prevent aliasing effects. Aliasing at the tile borders of the final image would destroy the hologram, making a suc-

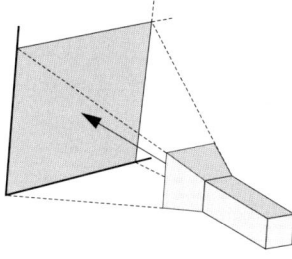

Figure 21.11: Rendering of tiles that build up the hologram

cessful reconstruction impossible. The problem is the same as when setting up a picking region in OpenGL (see [NDW93]). This solution was successfully adapted to our problem. It requires an additional matrix multiplication per tile rendering. After all the tiles are rendered, they are collected and combined into the final hologram which, thus, can be of very high resolution.

21.3.4 Results

The verification of the holograms generated was performed by means of simulation and optical reconstruction. The first example is shown in Fig. 21.12. In the simulated reconstruction (Fig. 21.12(b), 21.12(c)) the line focus "travels" over the extent of the line. In this case the simulation was performed for two distinct depths. If the whole series of simulations of the line hologram were shown, the line focus would travel almost continuously over the reconstruction. The different line foci appear as "sharp" regions in the reconstruction. In regions out of focus the line appears not as a narrow slit but rather widened and blurred.

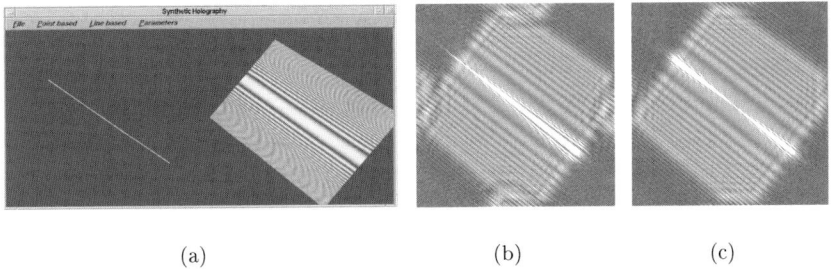

(a)   (b)   (c)

Figure 21.12: Hologram "rendering" of a line and its reconstruction results: (a) the original line and the holographic geometric equivalent of the line, (b) and (c) two reconstructions at different distances from the hologram

Another example is shown in Fig. 21.13. Again, it is the coordinate system. For comparison, the same object with a conventionally generated hologram and its reconstruction was shown earlier in Fig. 21.4. In the equiv-

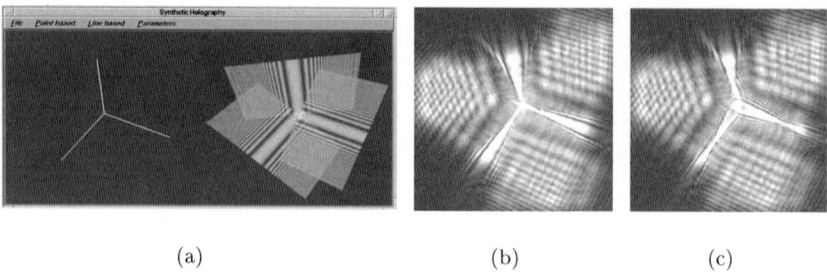

(a)   (b)   (c)

Figure 21.13: Three lines forming a simple representation of a coordinate system: (a) original object and the equivalent, (b) and (c) reconstructions

alent shown in Fig. 21.13(a), each line of the original object is represented as a textured rectangle.

In this example, these rectangles have the same "starting point", the origin of the coordinate system to be imaged. The major requirement in this example is that the reconstructed foci of each line converge at this starting point. This requirement is fulfilled in the holographic geometric equivalent: the rectangles have one common point at the origin of the visualized coordinate system. Furthermore, the rectangles are of the same size. The textures projected on the rectangles are identical. Thus, by means of perspective projection, the textured rectangles are distorted consistently. That is, the distances between pattern maxima (black stripes in the texture) are equal for equal depths in the equivalent. The reconstruction proves that this assumption is viable. Also, in the reconstruction of the "coordinate system example" the three reconstructed lines converge at one common point, the "origin". Figure 21.13(b) illustrates this feature of the holographic geometric equivalent by choosing the foci close to the origin in this example.

The holographic equivalent of a house composed of lines together with its reconstruction is shown in Fig. 21.14. The reconstruction illustrates how the front lines appear in different foci due to different reconstruction depths.

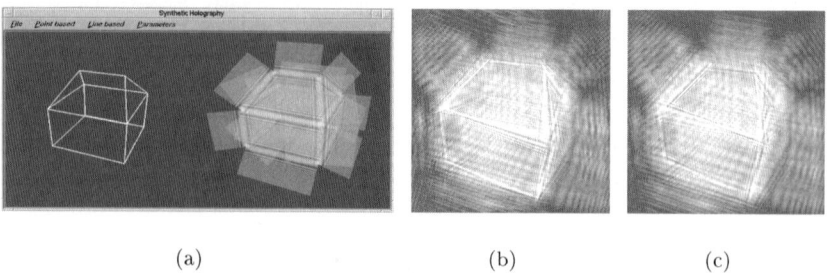

(a)   (b)   (c)

Figure 21.14: Example of a house composed of line segments: the reconstructions show different foci of the front lines

However, not all lines are reconstructed with the same quality, i.e., the same contrast and brightness. Though the front lines in Figs. 21.14(b), 21.14(c) are of good quality, the lines on the left hand side are barely visible in the reconstruction. This is because not all line equivalents contribute in the same magnitude to the hologram. The intensity of their holographic representation depends on the drawing order. Since they are translucent, the appearance of the line equivalents, and thus their reconstruction quality, can be improved by alpha blending techniques as described by NEIDER et al. in [NDW93], which are currently under investigation.

The examples shown in this chapter are all reconstructed by means of simulation using the DIGIOPT system. An optical reconstruction using the experimental setup described in Sect. 21.3.2 was performed as well. It verified that, basically, the input line objects are reconstructed properly. The reconstructions are of considerable depth, which is typical for conical waves as stated by LESEBERG in [Les87].

Conclusions. The holograms obtained with the method of rendering of holographic geometric equivalents reconstruct basically the original objects. The reconstructions are of relatively good contrast compared to the results obtained with the conventional approach. However, a thorough examination of the underlying principles of the holographic geometric equivalent and its projection to the hologram reveal a weak point of the approach. As stated in Sects. 21.3.1 and 21.3.3, cylindrical and conical waves focus on the lines to be reconstructed. The mathematical description of these waves is based on equation (21.1), which is a quadratic function. The patterns generated on the hologram are similar to conic sections. However, since the textures used in the hologram represent a cylindrical wave and are projected onto the hologram plane, a linear distribution results. The patterns converge linearly (Figs. 21.12–21.14).

Clipping (equation (21.2)) is implemented by using rectangles as basic primitives for the holographic geometric equivalent. It turned out to be a reasonable approach to clipping. Since the textures and the rectangles are of finite extent, high spatial frequencies which occur at distances from the texture center are eliminated. The varying point distance to the hologram (equation (21.3)) along the line is accomplished by the longitudinal tilt of the rectangles in the holographic geometric equivalent. The reconstruction of lines outside the optical axis (equation (21.4)) is accomplished by positioning the rectangles in the holographic geometric equivalent at the same location as their line counterparts in the original object. All these "computer graphics" procedures turned out to be valid approximations of the physical background described by equations (21.2–21.4) in Sect. 21.3.1.

However, as mentioned above, the approximation of conical waves (patterns similar to conic sections at the hologram plane) by linear distributions is not proven to reconstruct *straight* lines. In optical and simulated reconstruction, no image artifacts occurred (see Sect. 21.3.4), but a precise theoretical analysis still needs to be carried out.

21.4 Future Work

Further developments include primarily refinement of the existing approach to eliminate the weak points described above. The conversion of an object composed of line segments into its holographic geometric equivalent is kept in principle. However, a simple rendering of the equivalent in a perspective view is an illicit simplification of the hologram generation process. The shape of conic sections is approximated by a linear distortion of a cylindrical wave pattern. In a refinement step, the shape of conic sections (see Fig. 21.7 (right)) has to be simulated, resulting in a more exact contribution of the particular equivalent to the hologram. Two steps need to be performed:

- rendering the equivalent in a *parallel projection*, and
- applying the distortion according to the line inclination angle by altering texture mapping coordinates.

This achieves exact control of the rendering result. When exactly simulating conical waves, the reconstruction of straight lines is guaranteed.

The feasibility of the new approach has to be demonstrated on more complex input objects. Such objects can be found in the chapters on line graphics in this book. However, the objects have to be given as sets of 3D lines. Regarding more complex objects, the holographic display of models given in a spline representation is desirable. A spline can be approximated by short segments of straight lines. Straight line segments can be directly processed by the system introduced in this chapter. However, the reconstruction of short line segments is likely to be degraded due to clipping. The shorter the line segments, the more artifacts are introduced due to clipping. Another possible solution would be a distortion of the wave pattern according to the shape of the spline as shown in principle by FRÈRE et al. in [FB86].

The holographic imaging of splines and, in addition, line styles (Chap. 4) enables us to give a 3D insight into techniques applied to computer generated line drawings. An interesting question is how holographic images including line hatchings are perceived by the observer of a hologram. Thus, line drawings and holographic images "live" in a symbiosis.

Contributors of Chap. 21: Alf RITTER and Hubert WAGENER

Part VIII

Epilog

The final part of this book serves to take a step back from the nitty-gritty details of the algorithms in order to think about what has actually been accomplished.

In Chap. 22, Jörg SCHIRRA and Martin SCHOLZ study issues related to the question whether abstraction and (photo-)realism in fact exclude one another or not. Drawing on principles of design, communication theory and philosophy, they argue that indeed an abstract image may in fact be realistic at the same time.

In the final Chap. 23, Thomas STROTHOTTE takes a look at some of the fundamental issues addressed when mixing spatial and non-spatial data in rendered images. In particular, he considers the design of a specific visualization for a model as akin to producing an instance of an abstract data type. Just as certain operations are not possible on abstract data types, certain renditions of a model do not enable the viewer to answer all questions which he or she may have about the objects being portrayed. The author takes this analogy one step further and argues that a good image conveys to its viewer which questions can be answered (correctly), and which ones cannot be answered. He shows ways in which this information can be conveyed to users and discusses the implications of this point of view.

Chapter 22

Abstraction Versus Realism: Not the Real Question

When browsing through a book on computer graphics, one usually finds a lot of more or less interesting pictures that are produced by means of computers. These pictures are embedded in pages of technical texts describing how this image generation was performed and why it provides a better way to do so than other methods. Less space is usually given to the methodological background and the motivation underlying the preoccupation with computer visualization. In this chapter, we want to complement the more technically oriented part of this book with some reflections as to why such techniques can be interesting not only for computer graphics researchers, and where, from a communication-theoretic point of view, they might be of use in our society.

22.1 The Naïve Opposition of Abstraction and Realism

As already mentioned in Chap. 1, most approaches in model-based computer visualization carry a more or less implicit dedication to naturalism, often named the ideal of "photorealism". Realism is seen as the ultimate goal of any effort to create pictorial representations of reality as it is or could be, and naturalism as the single stylistic method to achieve realism. In photography, for example, realism is seemingly guaranteed by a particular kind of causal relation holding between the scene represented and the image produced. By means of this causal relation, any aspect relevant for realistic representation seems to be automatically covered.

Abstraction appears, in contrast, as the intentional omission of aspects that would have to be present for a realistic representation; or, in an extended sense, also as the pictorial representation of aspects that are actually not visible at all. Some applications, however, call for images that include some abstraction, images that are usually seen as less realistic, in consequence. For example, in a textbook on anatomy, what is mostly used is not a photo, which could be taken quite easily, but a sketch that has been produced with much effort (see also Sect. 1.1.1): The effort is not only a manual one, but essentially one of deciding whether the aspects to be communicated can be "read" from the sketch in an unambiguous, clear manner that simultaneously matches the variation in appearance the anatomist might see in reality. The sketch is intended to refer to all instances of what it shows by means of a typical instance that is stripped to the essentials: this "stripping" is far from trivial.

In the following, we refer essentially to functional pictures. Interrogating the fine arts in this respect is less fertile since, first, such an investigation would have to refer to the same basic distinctions as discussed here. But, second, those distinctions are played with in the fine arts in a complicated manner and on much more reflected levels that are seldom involved in computer visualization. The central theme of the American "photorealism" of the 1960s and 70s, for example, is an indirect critique of the visual access to reality in the modern industrial societies: an access that is almost totally mediated by technical reproductions, and thus open to all kinds of hidden manipulations (see [Hel75]). The images of artists like CLOSE, BELL, and MORLEY do not try to show reality in a photo-like realism; their subject is the mediated access to what is believed to be reality by media that are assumed to present subjects realistically. The classical "abstract art" – of KANDINSKY, DUCHAMPS, ARP, GROSZ, to name just a few – can be understood as a reflection about the reference relation of pictures, too: a reaction against the earlier, academized forms of naturalism. People interested in computer visualizations usually have less ambitious goals: their aim is basically to make "useful graphics" with more or less straightforward purposes.

In the context of the traditional view of a strict opposition, we have to ask whether or in what degree abstraction and realism exclude each other mutually; or alternatively, whether they mark two different dimensions of pictorial information presentation, and hence may co-occur. A clear analysis of the relation between abstract and realistic depiction is to provide essential hints and restrictions for the construction and application of useful computational visualization methods.

22.2 Three Examples of Functional Pictures

Let us have a look at some typical contexts of using functional images in our culture: architecture, engineering, and advertising.

Example 1: Architecture

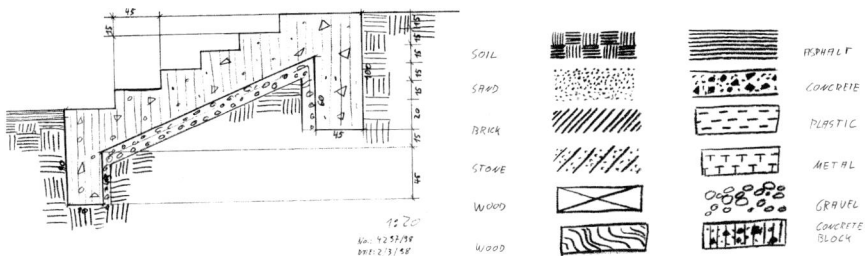

(a) Construction plan for a stairway   (b) Conventions used in (a)

Figure 22.1: Images in architecture: examples of construction plans

As a rule, the images drawn by architects have two different purposes, at least: either to give the client an impression of the object under consideration by means of an *architectural sketch* (look again at Fig. 1.2 on p. 6); or as a draft used for the realization, i.e., to impart the correct data to the constructional engineers by means of an *architect's plan*, a *construction drawing*, etc. (Fig. 22.1). While architectural sketches are used as a relatively unrestricted medium of communication between the architect and his client (drawn ideas, so to speak), building plans are legally binding for everybody involved. The purposes clearly affect the kind of rendering:

- Architectural sketches are notoriously changed and redrawn, starting from the first rough lines up to the final refined version. Apart from the fact that a refinement takes place, no generally applicable rules can be ascertained for the kind of representation to be used. The final version is the basis for the rendering of a building plan.
- In the building plan, strict representational conventions between the users have to be applied.[1] The single tasks of representation are again divided into clearly defined drawing types, such as overview, sectional view, site plan, ground plan, etc.

Thus, although strong conventions of representation may be useful, they do not yet exist in an explicit form for architectural sketches. On the other hand, the building plan is a legally binding basis for the realization exactly because those conventions of representation are codified as a result of the necessity for clear preconditions for realizing a building, the educational standard in our society, and the tradition of this trade.

---

[1] For example, the kind of lines is regulated by German Industrial Norm DIN 15, the way to specify the measurements on a blueprint in DIN 1356, and the legibility of the numbers, the uniformity of the scale, and the arrangement of the views in DIN 6.

Example 2: Maintenance Instructions in Engineering

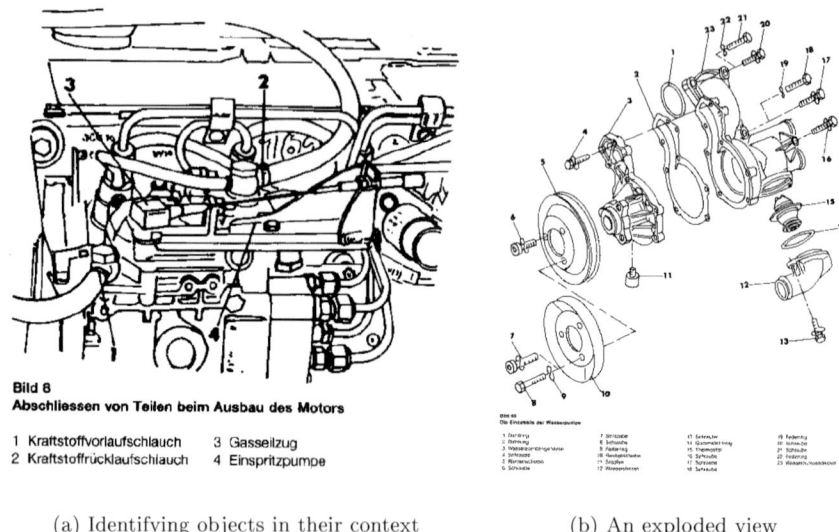

(a) Identifying objects in their context   (b) An exploded view

Figure 22.2: Pictures in maintenance instructions

In engineering, two major tasks for pictures used in maintenance instructions can be observed: one is to help identify objects in complex environments that are difficult to comprehend or see clearly. Or the function of an object or part is to be clarified in relation to the spatial configuration of the whole system. Designers of maintenance instructions follow certain heuristics:

- A naturalistic representation like a photo of an engine with lots of parts does not usually enhance the clear and easy identification of objects in a complex environment. A schematic representation of the objects' places and their rough forms is often enough: all irrelevant aspects that may distract the viewer are eliminated (Fig. 22.2). The point of view is determined by the perceptual situation of the person performing the maintenance: he or she must be able to map the sketch onto what is perceived.
- For proper identification, the parts or objects are labeled with numbers or letters that are explained by noun phrases in a legend (see Fig. 22.2(a)). The text of a repair instruction refers to the arrangement of the parts in the representations by using those noun phrases directly.
- To clarify the function of parts of an engine, documents for repair and operation include isometric sketches and illustrations of objects simultaneously in two ways: on the one hand, the objects are shown in isolation; on the other hand, the spatial relations between the parts are illustrated with the help of *exploded views* where the single parts are connected by dashed lines (see Fig. 22.2(b)). Understanding these pictures presupposes

a lot of knowledge about those parts and their typical shapes. The point of view must be carefully determined in order to present typical outlines, and avoid irritating the observer with an unusual view of an object.

Engineering has to use some conventions of representation when functional connections are to be shown. If the pictorial representation is employed to make clear the function of the objects within the whole system, it is not important exactly how the objects look, i.e., what color or texture their surfaces have, or which light produces what reflections. Those aspects can be abstracted – even to such a degree that mere icons (pictograms) are used (as in electrical engineering, e.g., the symbols for a capacitor or a transistor).

Example 3: Product Advertising

As a third example, we examine functional *photos*, i.e., a kind of picture usually rated naturalistic in contrast to the former examples. Typical situations for using such photos are the realistic representations of products in advertising or on the outside of a sales package, e.g., a photo of a coffee maker.[2] The task of the photo of a product in this context is (a) to promote sales of the object depicted, and (b) to cultivate the image of the trade name. Both purposes are usually intertwined and shown in the presentation:

- The photos printed on the packages of consumer goods are standardized by the specification of the particular line of products given by the manufacturer. All products of one such product line are exemplified by one common "image" regardless of actual differences in form, size, color, or function of the concrete object. Thus, a type is constituted that allows the customer to distinguish the products of that producer from comparable appliances of competitors.
- A photographic image is conceived as the only presentation achieving sufficient quality (with relatively low costs) to show clearly the colors, forms, and features that distinguish this product from its rivals.
- Over and above showing the pure appearance, photographic naturalism gives the observer two important pieces of information. The photographic image is read as a proof of the existence of the object shown. And the image is seen as a first visual indication of the functional potential of the product. The latter point is visualized by emphasizing the differences in form between this product and other products.
- The photographer can choose among several types of parameters to enhance the customers' ability to "read" the picture: for example, he or she may set a clearly directed light and use the resulting shades to demonstrate the spatial extension of the object in question – a wrong or illogical shadow destroys the intention of the image. Reflections can be employed for visualizing the condition of the surfaces; the addition of well-known objects into the set – e.g., a cup or a book – helps to clarify the proportions of the product, as well as its purpose.

---

2 Similar considerations hold, by the way, for portraits as used by casting agencies.

The communication of the correct spatial extension of an object is only one special case of pictorial information: in such functional photos, the mental representations of object types and of the producer's company image or product line are evoked by means of the typical appearance of an individual object. Moreover, to a significant degree the idea of that object is originally defined using such photos.

In general, the producers of pictures have tried for a long time to create "realistic" and "naturalistic" images, for example in photography. But from the artists' point of view, the intention guiding this kind of "realism" was rather to elaborate a "construction of (our perception of) reality" than to "represent reality *per se*", as can be clearly observed in the development of perspective in the Renaissance (see, e.g., [KL89]). As images were used in mass media more and more extravagantly, the creators, who were no longer artists but designers, technicians, and marketing specialists, ignored the restrictions inherent to images. But in the end, we have to realize that the original communicative intention, namely to present "the reality" and the essence of the objects as given by means of a naturalistic representation, has failed – indeed had to fail due to the very character of pictures and their role in communication.

22.3 Several Kinds of Realism

Speaking of realism in the singular seems to imply that there is exactly one kind of realism, the climax of which is reached in photography and similar representations (Fig. 22.3).[3] But why should we rate examples like Figs. 22.4 and 22.5 as being less realistic? Certainly, visual aspects have been omitted, like color, or added, like lines as the edges of objects. But those pictures can very well serve a lot of purposes related to corresponding real scenes: for instance, recognizing the objects represented (Otto von GUERICKE's vacuum experiment of 1659) or classifying something as of the same type (a bison).[4] The preceding section gave some further examples.

Putting it simply, "realism", as we understand the expression here, is the property of a representation that it gives an impression of a configuration of spatial objects that is or could be in the world. "Naturalism" in our sense refers to the quality of a pictorial representation that it evokes a visual impression as close as possible to that of the scene depicted. The naïve opinion is that realistic images have to be naturalistic. In a reverse deduction, it was often assumed that non-naturalistic pictures are therefore not realistic,

---

[3] Actually, a color photo was meant to be used here; we abandoned that plan for technical reasons and now show a digitized black-and-white version of a photo as a mere hint at full photographic naturalism.
[4] We do not state that the function of the paleolithic painting given was to classify; but it could at least be used for that purpose, as well.

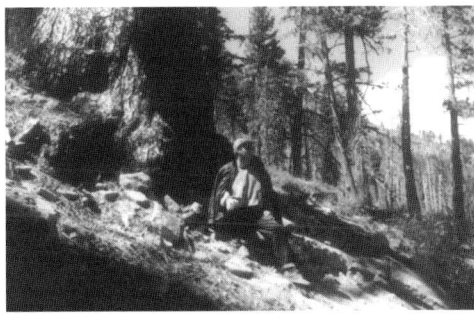

Figure 22.3: Example of a photograph

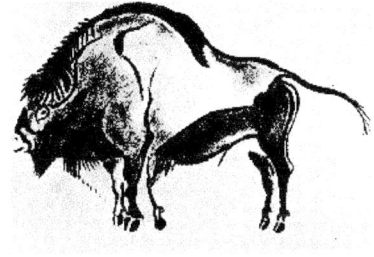

Figure 22.4: Paleolithic drawing of a bison [Altamira, Spain]

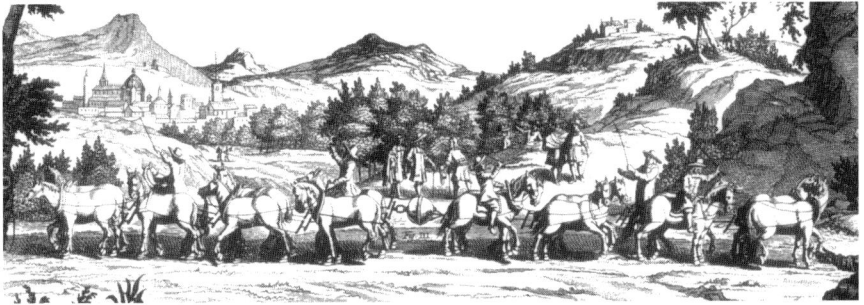

Figure 22.5: Engraving illustrating one of von GUERICKE's vacuum experiments

nurturing the traditional opposition of the latter to abstraction.[5]

Figures 22.4 and 22.5 indicate, however, that there is a (potentially unlimited) number of distinct kinds of realism; only some of them are naturalistic presentations, as well. The clue to the choice must basically lie in the particular communicative intention and the restrictions of the situation at hand. Where do computational visualizations fit in here?

The construction process for traditional "photorealistic" model-based computer visualization consists essentially of two phases:

1. providing a three-dimensional geometric model (modeling),
2. projection of the model onto a two-dimensional image plane (rendering).

In the ordinary understanding, the projection phase imitates photography. The geometric model stands for the photographic motif "in reality". Pictures produced in that manner can be easily changed and redone. In contrast to manipulations of the real world, changes in the geometric model or projection parameters are essentially reversible without problems, an advantage over and above photography that seems to make computational visualistics attractive

---

5 There are, of course, a number of different determinations of the meaning of "realism" and "naturalism" depending on the context of discussion (e.g., in literature or epistemology). Those used here are particularly fertile for considering functional pictures.

for the production of naturalistic quasi-photos (or even of artificial cinema). Nevertheless, we have no hint so far that naturalism is the only possible goal, or that it can be achieved particularly well in contrast to other styles by model-based computational visualization.

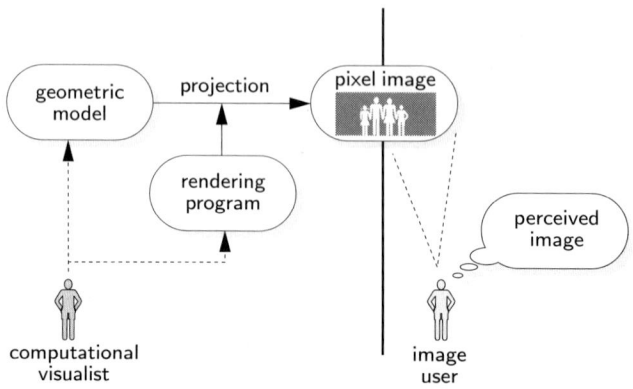

Figure 22.6: Phases and interfaces of standard model-based computer graphics

In fact, the geometric model is a (formalized) description based on a data structure that allows the computer scientist to describe three-dimensional geometric objects. In contrast to a real object, the object model, i.e., the description of the object's geometric and optical properties, already includes an abstraction; it concentrates on certain aspects of the object described. Its descriptive character is also the reason for the model to be changeable so easily and reversibly. From that description, the projection creates another description on the basis of a data structure that allows us to represent two-dimensional matrices of points with color attributes. It is a certain presentation of that second description that, finally, can be perceived as an image (Fig. 22.6). The projection algorithm, too, is primarily given as a description of what is to do in which cases, thus focusing on merely those aspects of the pseudo-optical projection that were rated as relevant. Again, it can be changed so easily because it is originally just a description.

The abstractions underlying the model and the projection method suggest once more that the relation between realism and abstraction cannot be a pure opposition. Abstracting as we understand it in this book is the process by which an extract of all the information available for some theme or scenario is refined so as to reflect the importance of certain aspects for the communicative situation at hand (see again Sect. 1.3.2). Descriptions of the geometric and optical aspects of a scene are just one kind of information that can be considered by computational visualists, and this type of information is as abstract as any other description. Moreover, constructing the model could focus on different aspects as well, and variants of the rendering program could "translate" those aspects into visible features of pixel images.

When dealing with computational visualisations in interactive systems, the schema of Fig. 22.6 has to be changed in a particular manner without altering the characterizations of the data structures given above: the picture is in fact produced by means of the rendering algorithm at some point in time and place apart from the original image creator (Fig. 22.7). Again, it is the descriptive nature of geometric model and rendering program that makes possible this *tele-rendering*, as we may call the situational separation of the computational visualist's design activities and the actual image production finally induced by the image user. However, we have to expect consequences for the communicative function of the picture created by tele-rendering.

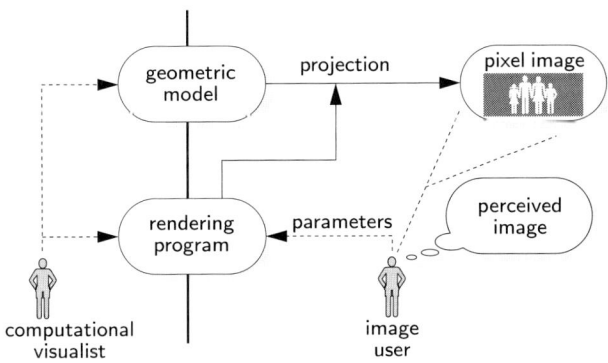

Figure 22.7: Phases and interfaces of tele-rendering

In the light of these considerations, we investigate the following theses:

Thesis 1
Realism and abstraction are not incompatible; they are relatively independent dimensions of the characterization of a picture; in particular, realistic images include abstractions, and vice versa.

Thesis 2
Naturalism provides merely one form of realistic presentation; it is an abstract one, as well: the abstraction in it focuses on the aspect of visual appearance of a scene. Other aspects necessary for the interpretation of such an image as realistic are not represented and appear only indirectly as inferred.

Thesis 3
Using naturalistic representation for the communication of other aspects (in particular, non-visual aspects like function) is dysfunctional: the focus of attention is directed to the visual appearance instead of the aspects to be actually communicated. The bodily basis of those non-visual aspects must not form the foreground of the presentation; it merely serves as an anchor point for the communicative intention.

In the following three sections, we examine the communicative conditions of images with respect to the three theses, and add particular conclusions as for the case of tele-rendering.

22.4 Images as Signs: Considerations from Communication Theory

Any serious effort to discuss our theses has to consider that images are signs, i.e., are used in communication. Determinations of abstraction or realism depend essentially on that characterization (cf. [vS74]):

> A sign is a material object that is used in a communicative act by somebody in order to direct the awareness of somebody to something – the signified subject.

An important consequence of this determination is that signs do not refer to anything by themselves. It is always the sign user who refers *with* them. This holds for images as a particular kind of signs as well; that is, we must not consider a picture alone, but have to include those who use the picture in our considerations.[6] To ask why a picture "works" is to ask why the communicative act works, i.e., why somebody can use the picture to communicate with somebody else. Obviously, this question is of particular interest in the case of tele-rendering, i.e., if the actual rendering process is performed autonomously by the computer, and the original image creator is not present any more, as in the ZOOMILLUSTRATOR, for example (Chap. 13). The computational visualist can be conceived in this case as providing indeed a large set of pictures together with options for the image user to choose one or the other. That the user in fact changes parameters of the image production within certain limits is not so important.

The link between abstracting and communicating already appeared at the very beginning of picture production, as the paleologist A. LEROI-GOURHAN, for example, observed:

> *Apparently, paleolithic art branches off from a real written language, so to speak, and follows a path on which, starting from the abstract, the ways of representing shape and motion are elaborated step by step; and at the end of that path, art finds realism* [in the sense of "naturalism"], *and finally dies away.* [LG83, p. 243, translated by the first author]

Visual art and written language have – as far as we understand today – a common communicative beginning, and due to the intimate relation to (oral) language, that starting point is closer to abstraction than to naturalism. The relation between pictures and language is interesting for us also for another reason: How could we rate the quality of functional pictures, like those shown

---

[6] In particular, this has effects on the discussion of "resemblance" as the primary mechanism of reference for images, which we do not want to discuss further here.

in Sect. 22.2? An obvious way is to use the verbal description of what purpose the image has, what is to be communicated by its use; that description would have to be compared with another verbal description of what an observer (image user) – possibly some kind of "standardized user" – can recognize as the picture's communicative function (i.e., what it "says" to him or her).

In the following, we summarize some basics of verbal communication, and try to transfer them to pictorial communication. The fundamental element of descriptions is the utterance of a singular declarative sentence about concrete things, sentences like (S 1) and (S 2):

S 1

The on/off switch is situated at the back of the device, on the lower left, close to the power line.

S 2

In Fig. 22.3 on page 385, the person I mean is sitting below a large tree.

Logically, singular assertive utterances are divided into several functional components (see [KL73] and [TW83]): one is called the involved set of singular terms, or *nominators*, which refer to some given (i.e., already mutually known) individual objects. Nominators, like "the on/off switch", "the device", "the power line", and "the person I mean" in the examples above, are used to identify something already known to the other interlocutors that is to serve as an anchor point for further information. The second component is called the general term, or *predicator*. The function of predicators is to introduce a standard gauge with respect to which the objects considered are rated: a dimension of distinction to be communicated (i.e., not known before to the other interlocutors). In the examples above, we employ the predicators "to be sitting below a large tree", and "to be situated at the back, on the lower left of something and close to something". Nominators and predicators cannot stand alone – they only make sense when combined in an assertion.[7] A *logical copula* is the third component of any assertion with the function of binding the nominators as arguments of the predicator, and, even more important, of performing the act of assertion.[8]

---

[7] More precisely speaking: predicators and nominators are only defined in that context. One-word utterances of infants ("holophrases") belong to a different, more elementary category of communication; see [Dor75]. In comparing the logical and the linguistic terms, the nominators correspond mainly to the definite noun phrases of the sentence; predicators are given mostly by means of the predicates (verbs, adjectives, adverbs, indefinite noun phrases, and prepositional phrases); however, logical and grammatical functions do not necessarily map one-to-one.

[8] See [KL73, I.4 and p. 90]. The logical copulas have to be distinguished from the linguistic copula, which essentially has the function of a non-specific verb binding adjectives as predicates to a subject; the logical copulas correspond to FREGE's "⊢", but carry in addition a polarity correlated to truth values; see [Sch94a, Chap. 6]. Traditionally, two copulas are studied in logic, corresponding to the two sides of a (binary) distinction: one for ascribing the predicator to that set of nominators, and the other for denying it ("internal negation"); see also [SW75, p. 239].

How can we associate the function of pictures with this short detour through the fundamental logic of assertions? Are pictures equivalent to nominators, i.e., used as acts of reference in order to identify things? Are they equivalent to predicators, i.e., used to communicate dimensions of distinctions? Or are they equivalent to assertions, i.e., whole propositions, especially compound propositions (conjunctions), like those used in verbal descriptions of an image?

All three possibilities mentioned above are apparently realized. We can use a picture of the Golden Gate Bridge to identify that object to somebody and then utter "Built in four years and finished in 1937". We also can use a picture in a book for mushroom determination to tell the doctor what kind of toadstool was in the lethal ragout: "This one". And finally, a picture can be employed to tell a whole story, as in a comic, thus being equivalent to a proposition. Note that in the first two cases, it is not merely the image use that mediates the communicative act: a predicative act, or a nominative act respectively, must be added to complete the pictorial proposition.

Here we run into a particular characteristic of images: they are open to interpretations and do not contain an unambiguous clue as to how to understand them; for example, captions have to be employed to clarify the interpretation (see also Chap. 11). A picture showing a large red suspension bridge could be used to identify a certain single object, or the place, or even the place at a particular time; or it may serve as a communicative tool for classifying suspension bridges in general, or red large suspension bridges in particular, or being red, etc. And in the right context, the very same image may even tell a story, like "It was a beautiful evening without fog, when they reached the Golden Gate, and on their bike, they crossed the bridge and finally entered the city of their dreams". Thus at first sight, a picture is in general used as a proposition – where sometimes additional nominators or predicators are applied, and apparently overwrite the corresponding component of the image.

The question is whether the three cases of use mentioned above are possibly derived, secondary applications of pictures. The "true nature" of pictorial representation, it seems, is not really grasped yet on that level. Indeed, that compound propositions can be used to describe what a picture shows does not already mean that this picture is logically equivalent to the proposition, although in some applications the relation to the proposition may dominate its use. When a verbal image description is produced, the image, more precisely speaking, takes the part of the referential context, it provides the situation to which the verbal description refers.

In fact, the analysis of the logical form of assertive utterances given above is not complete: assertions are necessarily uttered in a certain *situational context* that determines their meaning, and hence has to be conceived as a fourth functional component (see [Sch94a, Sect. 3.4]). The nominators in particular cannot be understood without the context: following STRAWSON's explications of the reference relation, a nominator does not simply represent an object by means of a one-to-one relation, like a name tag, but *picks out* an object from a certain given finite contextual domain of discourse objects, therefore conceptually requiring a one-to-many relation ([Str71, p. 17ff] and [Tug82, Sec. 21ff]). In an utterance, the context usually remains implicit, but as in example sentence (S 2) above, it can be explicitly mentioned: the expression "in Fig. 22.3 on page 385" refers to the (nested) context in which the rest of the proposition has to be interpreted.[9]

Two types of contexts have to be distinguished: the *lexical* context and the *referential* context. The lexical context is used in explanations of the connection between several assertions uttered in sequence: it is mainly viewed as the comprehension of the text communicated up to that moment. Understanding an assertion is conceived as transforming its context to the context that has to be used for any subsequent utterance [Kam90]. A novel is a perfect example for a fictional lexical context: the assertions of the text refer essentially to objects introduced earlier in the context of the novel.[10] The transformation of contexts by understanding an assertion is not simply the addition of the proposition uttered literally. The logical interaction of the new information with the contextual information changes the latter and leads to information not explicitly mentioned. There is a transputed message beside the one transmitted, as STROTHOTTE and STROTHOTTE have put it in [SS97, p. 98ff]. Any speaker has to be aware of these implications of what she utters (see [Gri75]): although she did not explicitly say that p her interlocutor has understood that she told him that p by what she said, and in the following will act and interpret accordingly.

In contrast to lexical contexts, the referential context of an assertion appears in explanations that anchor propositions in "what they actually mean", i.e., reality (or perception of reality). With respect to its referential context, an assertion can be true or false: for example, one has to look at the world in order to determine whether an assertion that ascribes some color to some object is true or not. Therefore, questions of realism involve referential contexts. A sketchy analysis of referential contexts is given in the next section. At this point, it may suffice that the referential context most important for us is the visual context, i.e., what is visually perceived by the interlocutors.

---

9 More precisely speaking: it establishes a connection between the current context of the discourse and the context to be used to understand the proposition; see [Fau85]. Already the distinction between nominators and predicators indicates the existence of contexts, since the nominators' function, namely to identify objects already known as anchor points for a new dimension of distinction communicated by the predicators, is particularly needed in cases where the logical context differs from the actual situation of the interlocutors, i.e., when they speak of something not present, past, hypothetical, or fictional (see [Tug82, Sec. 26.I]).

10 A special kind of assertion can be used to introduce an object for the first time (e.g., existential assertions); we do not deal any further with them here, although they may play an important role for image interpretation, as well, since this function can be integrated in the general function of nominators as outlined here (see [Tug82, Sec. 22]).

With respect to the immediate visual context, pictures, in particular naturalistic pictures, are similar to novels and their relation to the immediate dialog history: they are *fictional visual contexts*. However, in contrast to novels they are referential, not lexical.

This is not the place to elaborate further the relation between referential and lexical contexts (see [Sch93] and [Sch94a, Sec. 5.4]). But it should be clear that the relation between an image and a verbal description of that image provides the essential information if our goal is to improve the communicative quality of a functional picture: the description of what is to be communicated, and what is actually communicated. Unfortunately, this relation is not unique: only if conventions of pictorial representation are used that are sufficiently agreed upon and well known can the contents of an image be deciphered correctly by the viewer, that is, in the way intended by the producer. Therefore, the producers must be as clear as possible about what they want to communicate, and how their interlocutors in the pictorial communication act might interpret – and possibly misunderstand – the picture.

This is also true in the case of tele-rendering, where techniques anticipating or tracing the end-user's actual interpetation of the image can be employed to adapt the tele-rendering's parameters. Mechanisms for controlling generalized fisheye presentations are prominent examples given in this book; information used primarily for the rendering, like that encoded by G-buffers, may also be useful for the image producer when he or she wants to take into consideration what a distant observer might see in a picture ("viewpoint descriptions" as in [SS97, Chap. 9]). In any case, it is the original image producer who has to decide what picture the end-user gets in which situation.

22.5 Abstraction in Realism

With this theoretical background, let us now investigate the aspects of abstractness that appear in realistic pictures.

The essential aspect of abstraction in a realistic depiction – a successful photo like Fig. 22.3, for example – becomes clear as soon as we ask what is actually seen there: spots of color? Or geometric entities? Or spatio-temporally extended material objects ("spatial objects" for short)? Or persons? And so on. Although we usually do not deny the first two answers, the latter two are primarily expected. But how can that be? Spatial objects have more sides than are *de facto* depicted – therefore the technique of perspective is important for realistic depiction. And "person" is a concept with a structure that is even much richer and more complicated: a lot of aspects of a person have to be omitted in the pictorial representation. Most features necessary to identify something as a spatial object (and even more so for a person) are actually not transmitted by the pictorial communication, but transputed in the sense of STROTHOTTE mentioned above: they are added by the observer when looking at and interpreting the picture. Since the step to spatial objects is the crucial one, we ignore in the following the case of persons and deal with pictures of humans only as instances of images of a particular kind of spatial objects.

What we usually see on/in [*sic!*] a realistic image – the image content – are spatial objects, i.e., entities that are quite clearly separated spatially and temporally from their surrounding; entities that have parts[11] and distinguishable visual aspects: one can view them from several perspectives, and thus one can recognize the very same object even if it looks different at different times (from several viewpoints). However, there cannot be any doubt that the image shows basically a colored surface only. The expression covering the important dependencies between the image surface and the image content is *object constitution*: usually it refers to the "invention" of spatial, persistent, identifiable, and countable objects in the mental development of infants (see [Pia37] and [Tug82, Sect. 25]) – the growth of the ability to recognize individuated objects in the colloquial meaning, that is; but it is also used in a more general sense for naming the relation between geometric Gestalts (behaving like shadows) and spatial objects in the proper sense.

The relation of object constitution may best be explained by means of the current understanding of vision in AI: we here present as an example the perception of spatial objects by motion as demonstrated by the systems ACTIONS and XTRACK.[12]

In most computational approaches to visual object recognition, the signal from a video camera, i.e., essentially a temporal sequence of matrices of intensity values similar to the pixel images mentioned in Sect. 22.3 (see also Fig. 22.6 on p. 386), stands at the beginning. On a general level, two structurally different phases of subsequent processing can be distinguished: in the lower phase, the primary data is processed "bottom up" (data-driven): the results depend essentially on the original data and Gestalt factors alone (see also [Kof35]).

In the higher phase, intermediate data is related to other sources of information; this integration is usually performed "top down" (goal or expectation driven). On the lower level of our particular system (see Figs. 22.8–22.10), candidate spatio-temporally extended objects are calculated by means of several layers of grouping criteria depending on similarity of the entities grouped (including spatial and temporal closeness).

However, these candidates are not yet spatial objects in the usual sense. This can be clearly seen in situations like that shown in Fig. 22.11: do object candidates A and D belong to the same spatial object, or is it A and E that

---

11 At least, they have geometric parts, like the left part, the middle part, etc., and material parts, i.e., they are distinguished from their material.

12 See [Kol92]; an elaborated description and further references are to be found in [Sch94a, Chap. 9]. Considering motion in this context emphasizes particularly the crucial aspect of object constitution: such an object is identified in several situational contexts where it may appear quite differently.

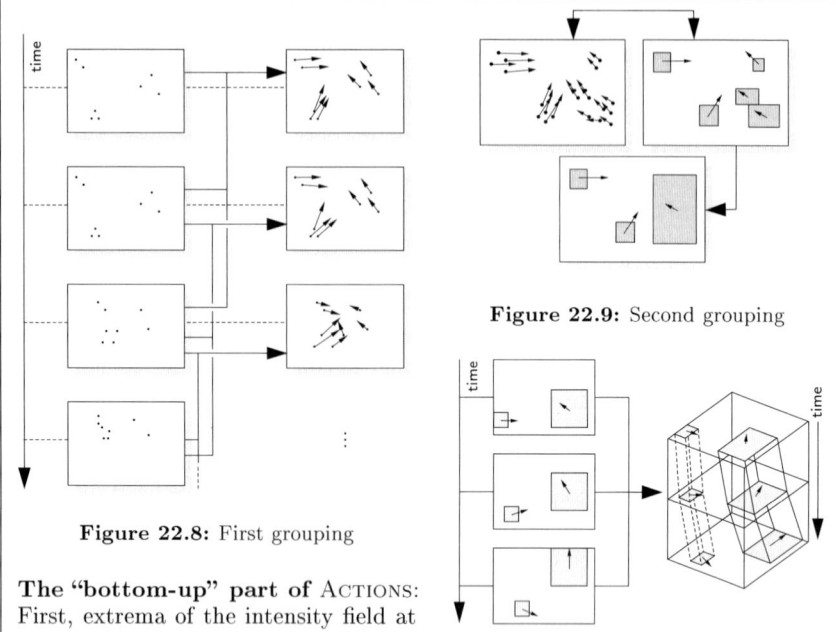

Figure 22.8: First grouping

Figure 22.9: Second grouping

Figure 22.10: Third grouping

The "bottom-up" part of ACTIONS: First, extrema of the intensity field at consecutive instants are grouped into instantaneous (velocity) vectors, if they are of the same kind and at almost the same position (Fig. 22.8); then, closely positioned similar vectors at one instant are grouped into spatially extended entities; if several of these still instantaneous entities happen to be close to each other and have similar velocity vectors, they are merged (Fig. 22.9); finally, another temporal grouping of the development of those entities is applied, resulting in entities that are also extended in time (Fig. 22.10).

have to be associated? It is impossible by means of Gestalt factors alone to identify the corresponding object candidates before and after the "melting" – and thus, to find the correct two spatial objects. The pure "bottom up" grouping has to be complemented by additional "teleological" knowledge providing the conditions under which deformations, loss or exchange of parts and substance, etc., do or do not alter the identity of an instance over time.

The established way to do this is using "object models": they essentially describe which geometric configurations of parts form an instance of a particular type of object.[13] The projection of the object models to the object

---

[13] See, e.g., [Mar82]. The geometric models used in model-based computer visualization are usually more closely related to the geometric descriptions resulting from the bottom-up phase than to the object models in the sense of MARR: information about part-whole structures are only seldom integrated, the models are "flat" (see Chap. 3). It should be obvious that meronomical information, i.e., the hierarchies of model components in the geometric models of computer graphics, play an essential role in computer animation; see Chap. 15.

22.5 Abstraction in Realism   395

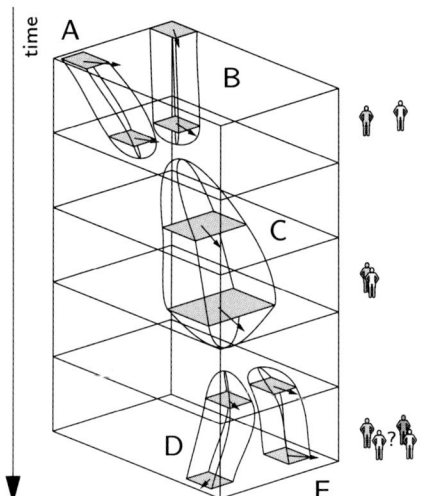
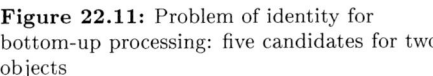
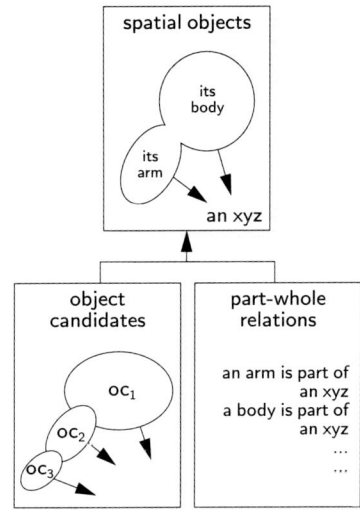

Figure 22.11: Problem of identity for bottom-up processing: five candidates for two objects

Figure 22.12: Sketch of object constitution: relating perceptual geometric and functional part-whole relations

candidates perceived finally establishes the perception of spatiotemporally extended, persistent, and localizable entities – exactly the type of objects involved in spatial descriptions and realistic pictures.[14] The largely geometric information about the *actual* configurations from the bottom-up phase is combined with information about part-whole relations governing the *possible* range of configurations (Fig. 22.12). In general, the constructed descriptions of what is seen form distinct contexts on different levels; perception can be conceived as the systematic relation between these contexts: the description of one level is used as the referential context for the description of the next higher level in the sense mentioned in the preceding section (Fig. 22.13).

It is an important logical characteristic of those calculi that geometric Gestalt principles allow us to formulate descriptions that organize individual geometric shapes ("object candidates") within a coordinate system of locations of *one* perceptual situation. But it is not possible in general to associate those shapes as the same individual in different contexts: if an object candidate goes out of sight, it "dies away" and can never come back. If the corresponding spatial object again enters the field of sight, a completely new object candidate is born (see also [Vie91]). Among other effects, the trans-

---

[14] This projection is, in a way, analogous to the projection described by the rendering program in model-based computer visualizations; see again Fig. 22.6 on p. 386: but here, the projection is used to decide whether a given picture could or could not be the picture of a certain object model.

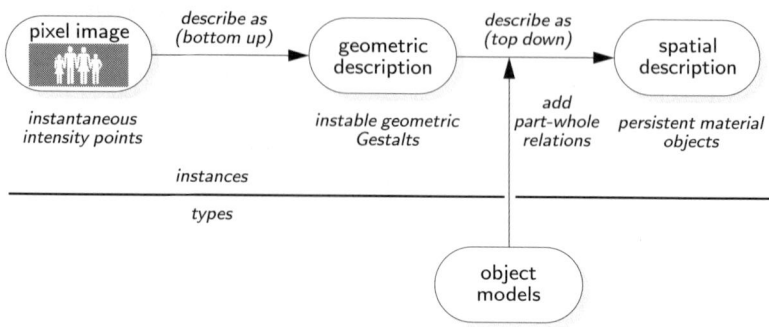

Figure 22.13: Conceiving perception as a cascade of descriptions

formation to a description based on spatial objects enables us to originally integrate several perceptual situations and their corresponding coordinate systems of places and times, and thus to speak at all of persistent objects, that is of objects that do not disappear when we do not look at them (see [Tug82, Sect. 26]).

After all, what an image contains primarily is, at best (when reached merely from data), a configuration of visual Gestalts that may serve as the referential context for a description involving spatial objects: that is, the spatial objects are never contained explicitly. Any picture user has to infer (more or less implicitly) that spatial objects are meant at all with the configuration of light intensities presented. This is true for naturalistic images, as well. In contrast to other (i.e., non-naturalistic) realistic pictures, a naturalistic depiction concentrates particularly on the accuracy of the geometric/optical aspects of spatial objects, thus directing the focus of attention of any image user primarily to those aspects. Furthermore, an image user usually assumes in that case that this emphasis is intentional: therefore he or she assumes, too, that it is exactly this aspect – the visual appearance of a configuration of objects – that the image producer wants to convey.

Since we have determined realistic representations as representations that deal essentially with a configuration of spatial objects as it is or could be in the world, we now have to concede that realistic pictures indeed are never immediately realistic in that sense. They are linked to a (verbal) realistic representation by means of an abstraction: some crucial aspects of spatial objects that are not geometric are in fact omitted in any "realistic" image (and hidden surface removal is merely the tip of that iceberg; see also [Sch94a, Note 64]). Only the automatism of our perceptual capacities enables us to "undo" that abstraction and see there spatial objects, like trees or houses.

22.6 Realism in Abstraction

At this place, an interesting question arises: how much "geometric naturalism" (just to coin an expression) is involved in the first four example pictures of Sect. 22.2, pictures that are clearly rated to be abstract, i.e., architectural sketches, construction plans, or drawings in maintenance instructions? How much of the visual appearance can (and should) be omitted? And what exactly is the communicative function of the remaining naturalistic parts, a function that makes it necessary to keep those visual aspects in the depiction? This section presents only some first considerations on those questions.[15] In order to have a handy term in the following, let us call that remainder of the visual appearance of the scene depicted "the picture's *naturalistic residue*."

Of course, the function of the naturalistic residue depends on the general communicative intention guiding the picture's use. In particular, it depends on what is to be actually communicated, and also on what the "sender" can do to ascertain that the "receiver" gets that message correctly. As a first observation in the light of the distinction between nominators and predicators in verbal communication as mentioned in Sect. 22.4 we find that the naturalistic residue is essentially associated with something analogous to a nominative function: it anchors some new aspects to be shared in those aspects that are already known, for example, by means of immediate visual perception, as in the example of a maintenance instruction (see again Fig. 22.2a on p. 382): such a picture is used within the corresponding real situation. The objects' identity with respect to the instruction is to be communicated. That information is given by means of the legend and labels anchored in a rather simplified sketch that shows essentially the very scene the reader sees. Without the reader's ability to match the sketch with the objects, the picture would be not really helpful. However, it is not necessary that the corresponding predicative part of the picture is as abstract as in that example: the focus may be on merely one particular part of the visual impression. In most cases, the picture is not immediately confronted with what it is assumed to depict. The following list is a first collection of such cases without any pretence of completeness:

- If the *shape of one object* (already known otherwise) is to be communicated, the visual context of the object may be completely reduced. In some cases, however, some clues for the situational setting must be included, e.g., a horizontal line for the vertical orientation of the object, or some familiar objects as an implicit scaling. As for the representation of the object, the main outline from a certain (typical) perspective is often sufficient for communicating the shape.
- If the *spatial configuration* (of objects already introduced as theme of the conversation in some way) is the aspect in focus, representations of the

---

15 We leave it to the reader to consider these questions for the other abstract pictures in this book.

objects forming that configuration are secondary and may be suppressed just sufficiently for identifying the objects' identity, and thus serve as an anchor for the information to be actually transmitted. Often, as in a subway connection map, the objects forming the configuration (the subway stations in the example) are pictorially reduced to a mimimum, e.g., an icon, that is actually explained by some piece of text.

In addition, a non-visual aspect may be closely tied by convention to the spatial configuration in certain communicative settings: a mechanical engineer may indeed "see" more or less effortlessly the function of some part of an engine just by its spatial position with respect to the whole configuration.

- If the *spatial distribution of one particular visual aspect* in some context is what the image producer wants to convey by means of the image, e.g., the places of red things in a certain scene, it is usually not sufficient just to put some red pigment at about the places of the objects in the image plane: the contours should be given as well, as an anchor for the interpretation of the color spots.

  Due to the very nature of our conception of spatial objects (which also forms the basis for colored objects in this context), the colors have to be spatially bound to an object carrying them. Again, the geometric aspects of spatial objects serve not as the main content of the message, but as a necessary condition for the communication of that content.

- Similarly, the *numerical distribution of visual aspects* in some context could be concerned, e.g., the number of red things compared to that of blue things in a certain scene; again, the naturalistic residue serves as an anchor, which is an idea related to the nominators of assertions.

- If the *spatial distribution of a non-visual attribute* in a scene is to be communicated, rudiments of the shapes of objects can carry the function of anchoring the distribution, again similar to the nominators' function in an assertion. A minimal requirement is that the image observer must be able to identify the objects in question: a precise reproduction of the appearance of those objects is not necessary, and may even interfer with the visual encoding (e.g., by color) of the non-visual attributes concerned. A typical example is provided by communicating air temperature in a weather map, where some geographic shapes are visible in order to identify the locations. The sketches in maintenance instructions for identifying the relevant objects as mentioned above also belong partially to that class.

Note that in the latter cases, it is possible to first show the reduced shapes, and then add the (possibly visually encoded) attributes in question: but it would usually not work the other way round, first presenting the mere attributes and then merging in the geometric base. In these cases, only the first type of presentation supports the interpretation as intended: an assertion with nominators that refer to objects already known in order to anchor new information communicated by predicators.

Obviously, spatial objects are a central category for a lot of non-visual aspects. By means of representations of the geometric component of spatial objects it is possible to communicate those other aspects with pictures using the particular scheme of organization inherent to geometric Gestalts – namely that they are integrated in the coordinate system of perception. There is still, quite obviously, a lot of room for future research.

22.7 Abstraction *and* Realism: Conclusions for Computational Visualization

Where do we stand at the end of our examination?

First: literally each of the pictures presented in this book is in fact an example of a realistic depiction as we understand this term: it gives an impression of the configuration of spatial objects. Most of the pictures in this book are also the result of abstraction: namely the process of generating an extract of information according to the communicative situation.[16] They are, thus, illustrations of our *first thesis*: realism and abstraction in the senses considered here are not incompatible concepts (see p. 387).

Second: in most cases, the representation of the spatial configuration is used as the basic scheme of organization in which the most relevant information to be communicated is placed. Sometimes, the spatial configuration *per se* is the content to be transferred to the image user; the spatial objects in that configuration are, then, depicted so that they could be identified – but usually not naturalistically. Only if knowledge of the precise appearance of the objects is the central goal of the communication is the naturalistic style appropriate. In this case, too, merely one aspect of spatial objects is the focus of an abstraction, others are omitted: this is our *thesis 2*.

Third: in the framework of intentional communication, *thesis 3* is in fact an immediate consequence of thesis 2: if a naturalistic presentation directs the focus of attention of an image user particularly to the appearance of spatial objects as stated by thesis 2, it should rather be avoided if other aspects are to be communicated, especially if the aspects intended are not related to the visual appearance of the objects presented. Stylistic elements of naturalism should be used only to the extent that aspects of the visual impression are necessary for identifying those objects and their spatial configuration of which some other aspects are to be communicated.

Abstraction and realism, thus, are definitely not just opposite concepts, and do not form the end points of a more or less continuous linear scale: the naturalistic and non-naturalistic representations we have observed are simultaneously abstract and realistic. They form a loose structure of clusters

---

[16] In some cases (e.g., the photo in Fig. 22.3 on p. 385), it is not clear whether the extract of information was intentionally produced for a particular communicative situation; therefore, we hesitate to ascribe our concept of abstraction to all the pictures given in this book.

that are more or less closely related to each other. Only if we understand "abstract" in a *secondary* sense as "non-naturalistic" may we project those clusters onto a linear scale, with the naturalistic pictures at the zero point, and the other forms more or less distant from that point. This is, of course, the more colloquial meaning of "abstraction" with respect to pictures, but it is less productive in discussions on computer visualization, as we have seen.

For somebody applying computational visualizations, basically two questions have to be answered in advance:

1. What aspects of the scene or configuration of objects have to be communicated, i.e., should be easily and clearly "readable" by the interlocutor / end-user?
2. How much of the naturalistic residue, i.e., the set of geometric and visual properties of the objects, has to be present in order to anchor sufficiently the (potentially non-visual) aspects to be originally communicated, without putting too much stress on the mere anchor?

The computer cannot and should not take over the task of determining what is important, what has to be communicated in a particular situation. Even in the case of tele-rendering, the computational visualist who has designed the program has to determine under what circumstances the computer is to show which aspects as the important ones.[17] Of course, the machine also cannot add the creative potential of an artist, who succeeds in directing the attention of her public to some hitherto ignored aspects (be they visual or not) of something by means of an innovative form.

What computers can provide, and this is essentially what computational visualists should concentrate on with their work, is the following:

1. A broad set of methods for rendering pictures that are not naturalistic;
2. Rules for assisting the decision as to how much of the geometry and the pure appearance is enough for the purposes at hand and the rendering methods applicable;
3. Strategies for testing whether the communicative intention could be fulfilled by means of an image in the actual situation.

The latter point directs us toward an analogy to listener models or, more generally, partner models as they are commonly used in systems for generating natural language utterances: an "observer model". As it is so easy to misinterpret pictorial communication, it is even more necessary to keep control of what potential observers in the context of the image observation will presumably understand immediately or only after several false tries. For the image producer, it is crucial to adopt the perspective of the potential image observer, which is usually not that easy since the background and the

---

17 Techniques like the application of a *degree of interest* (*DOI*), *focus points* (*FP*), or *aspect of interest* (*AOI*) as defined in Chap. 2 allow the computer visualist to have some influence of what a user of his system is going to see. Saying that the system chooses by means of *DOI*, etc., is only a shortened way of speaking.

present context of action may be pretty different for those two people. Algorithmic strategies will accordingly be hard to develop and implement.[18] FURNAS' technique of generalized fisheye presentations and their extensions and applications in this book (see [Fur86] and the subject index) can be conceived of as a simplified, but computationally more tractable approach. Of course, the most interesting results are to be expected from techniques for the enhancement of tele-rendering.

As for the second point mentioned, few solutions have been brought forward yet: at least, some effort has been made to find rules that suggest whether some part of a compound structure to be communicated is to be transferred as text, and which other part should be given as a picture (see Sect. 13.1). Rules governing the decision between several graphic styles were not considered. However, designers have proposed heuristics for their work that could be adapted to computer visualizations, as well.

Ultimately, inventing rendering algorithms for automatically producing corresponding images is certainly the task currently most directly associated with the work of computational visualists. Of course, enriching or differentiating the geometric models underlying the computer rendering is one aspect of that task (as already mentioned in Chap. 1 and exemplified in Chap. 3). As for the rendering part in the light of the above considerations, the trend might be to divide that part of computer visualization into two phases: one for generating the geometric basis of the objects' configuration as far as necessary to serve as an anchor for the information to be mainly communicated (the nominatoric component of that picture, so to speak); and another one for adding that latter information in an appropriate manner (in a way, the predicative component of the pictorial assertive act intended). Whereas the first phase is to find a minimum of representation for the aspects concerned, the second is to give a corresponding maximum.

What we might expect from computer visualists, after all, is essentially a skillful toolbox, an *organon* of visualization, containing as its core a set of methods to be combined for the actual production of an image or sequence of images. It would also provide assistance for the correct and even advantageous use of those methods. And finally, some instruments ought to be available for rating and even controlling the success of the methods. There is a vast field waiting.

Contributors of Chap. 22: Jörg R. J. SCHIRRA and Martin SCHOLZ

---

[18] As a matter of fact, one of us has earlier dealt with a listener model for generating spatial descriptions in German that involves the production of sketch-like graphics as an intermediate representation, see [Sch94a, Part II] or [Sch95a]; the "observer model" projected here could, in a way, be seen as the inversion of that project.

Chapter 23

Integrating Spatial and Nonspatial Data: A Challenge in Computational Visualistics

Our book has dealt with selected aspects of what we call computer visualization. Indeed, we use the term Computational Visualistics[1] for the scientific study of how visualizations are captured, stored, processed, produced, and conveyed to users, as well as how computer users interact with, perceive, understand, and store pictures. The characteristic aspect of computational visualistics is that we always consider algorithms running within the computer in unison with what the user will do with the resultant graphical output. We have dealt with only one specific aspect of the topic of computational visualistics, that of producing and interacting with images of a particular kind. In this chapter, we shall now take a fresh look at the technical results presented, strive for an insight into what is actually happening when producing such images, and work toward placing the results into a wider context. In doing so, we shall also suggest some new concepts and terminology which will guide future work in the area.

23.1 Pictures, Lies, and Abstract Data Types

A frequently asked question is whether it is possible to still "believe" what one sees in a picture [GCEG93, DG97]. Such questions pertain in particular to methods of image processing applied to pictures. Commercially available tools based on such methods enable laypersons to modify photos and other pictures so as to change their message. This issue is of particular relevance for practically all methods introduced in this book, as the processes

---
[1] Computational Visualistics is also the name of a new undergraduate degree program introduced at the University of Magdeburg in 1996, and a graduate program introduced in 1997.

of abstraction which we treated from a technical point of view can lead to misunderstandings on the part of users. For example, enlarging a part of a geometric model using the 3D zoom (recall Chap. 9, in particular Fig. 9.4) may suggest to a viewer that the part is larger than it actually is. This is particularly the case when a printout of a modified image is made and examined later by someone who was not involved in the process of its production.

Sometimes the style in which the image is conveyed to the viewer can encode information about what can be taken literally ("at face value") and what not. For example, a pencil sketch probably suggests that the sizes and other details of the image do not correspond exactly to the attributes of the objects being displayed (SCHUMANN et al. [SSRL96]), while a photograph is generally accepted as an exact, objective image of a real-life situation. Of course, such hints as to the validity of a picture may be incorrect, and it is indeed only a myth that a picture can be taken as a reflection of reality. The sketch alluded to above could have been produced by the software introduced in Part II of this book, and the photo could be a photorealistic rendition of a non-existent scene. The point is that a viewer may in fact use pictures to seek answers to questions which cannot be ascertained using these pictures.

A similar situation arises within another branch of computer science. Recall the notion of an abstract data type (ADT) (see for example AHO, HOPCROFT, and ULLMAN [AHU83]). An ADT can be thought of as a mathematical model with a collection of operations defined on that model. For instance, sets of integers, together with the operations *union, intersection,* and *set difference* is a simple example of an ADT. A user wishing to apply the operation "sum" on the integers of an instance of this ADT will not receive an answer, but an error message at best.

By analogy, we propose that pictures be thought of as instances of ADTs on which certain operations are defined, while other operations are not defined. For example, for many maps the operation *measure distance* is not defined because these maps are not drawn to a uniform scale (recall Chap. 20). If a viewer measures a distance on the map and computes the distance between the points in reality on the basis of the scale, a wrong answer will undoubtedly result. However, there are a number of significant differences between the ADTs generally used on computers and pictures as ADTs:

1. *Need for ADT not conveyed*
   The general myth pertaining to the objectivity of pictures leads some viewers to the conclusion that information which can be "read" from an image is, in fact, correct. If this is not the case, viewers are quick to use terms like "falsification" or "manipulation" for the effect of the pictures.
2. *Available ADTs not known to the viewer*
   The contours of the various possible ADTs have not been formalized. Nonetheless, rules of interpretation do exist explicitly for some areas of endeavor. For example, a radiologist painstakingly learns what artifacts in an x-ray must receive attention, and which kinds of information cannot

be extracted from such an image. The reader of a textbook on mechanical engineering will also develop a feeling for the kind of information which can be extracted from the images accompanying the text.

3. *Choice of ADT not clear*
   Users sometimes do not know to which ADT a particular picture belongs, and hence which operations are defined and which ones are not. This may be because viewers do not know the conventions of the context for which the picture is intended, or because the style of the picture suggests to the viewer the wrong set of conventions (recall the sketch and photo example above).

4. *Missing feedback*
   ADTs implemented on computers generally punish users who apply undefined operations by returning an appropriate error message. However, viewers applying undefined operations to pictures tend to receive either a wrong answer or, in the extreme case, no answer at all. In the case of maps of cities mentioned above, a viewer measuring a distance is quite likely to calculate an incorrect distance. Alternatively, the viewer may be frustrated by not being able to find a small part of a town on a map with too coarse a scale, despite knowing that it must be represented in the underlying data.

It is instructive to look at important properties of ADTs to see the extent to which these are true of pictures, too. One such property is that of *encapsulation* (AHO, HOPCROFT, ULLMAN [AHU83]) in the sense that an ADT can be localized to one part of a program. Analogously, the operations "allowed" on a kind of picture may be known only to a small population of viewers who are familiar with the context in which this kind of picture is used. For example, drawings in some medical books simply assume that the viewer is highly specialized and take certain background information for granted. The difference to the encapsulation from ADTs in programs is that laypersons may happen to look at pictures intended for the specialist, while an ADT may be kept strictly local and invisible to other programs.

Another property of ADTs is that the operations defined in them generally operate on *instances* of the ADT. Indeed, it is assumed that for every operation, at least one instance of the ADT must be either an argument of an operation or the result of that operation. This is analogous to the way viewers deal with pictures: operations dealing with pictures may produce pictures (such as rendering, or painting by a human), or they may analyze pictures (such as image processing software, or a radiologist producing a diagnosis). In most cases of these examples, certain conventions are followed in the tasks. Picasso painted human faces in such a way that they are recognizable even though some of the features are juxtaposed.

In summary, we conclude that it is generally not the right terminology to say that a picture lies, gives false information, has been manipulated, or is falsified; a false interpretation of a picture may well be made on the basis of applying an operation to the picture which is not defined. Knowing this, the producer of an image has an obligation to convey correctly to the viewer which operations are in fact defined, and which ones are not. This is where manipulations and falsifications take place, when viewers are intentionally or accidentally not informed of the ADT to which they belong. The picture itself is not at fault.

23.2 Spatial and Nonspatial Data

We shall now analyze in more detail the process involved in abstraction, as we have introduced and studied it in this book. The fundamental task in generating computer visualizations is to write programs to map some arbitrary input data onto a two-dimensional space (the image represented as a pixel matrix). The dimensionality of the input data is important: If the data is already inherently spatial, there exists a straightforward mapping onto the two-dimensional space of the image. For example, recall that the process of *rendering* was defined by WATT [Wat93] as "...the overall process of going from a database representation of a three-dimensional object to a shaded two-dimensional projection on a view surface." There the perspective transformation together with a shading approach is used to go from a three-dimensional model to the two-dimensional image:

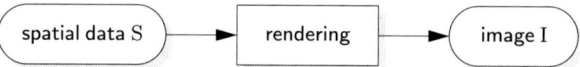

By contrast, recent research has focused on the area of information visualization, which has been defined as the task of "converting data which is not inherently spatial into spatial data" [CEG96]:

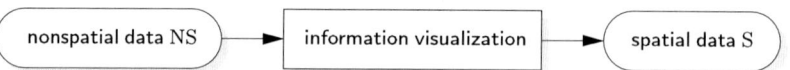

We are now in a position to interpret the process of abstraction which we have studied in this book as a function which converts an (enriched) geometric model into spatial data using a non trivial mapping:

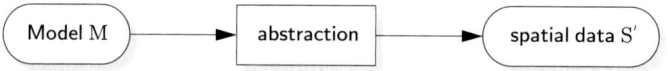

For example, the 3D zoom changes the sizes of parts of an object without changing the spatial nature of the data. After this process of abstraction, the usual rendering process is applied to carry out the actual visualization.

How can the computer decide which abstraction to carry out? The algorithms we have introduced in this book carry out such operations as modifying the sizes of parts, and adding or removing features. We contend that such information cannot be deduced from the geometry of the spatial input data alone. Indeed, in looking at the wide range of methods and applications described in this book, one can observe that it is always nonspatial data which is used by the algorithms for abstraction to compute how the spatial part is modified to produce other spatial data:

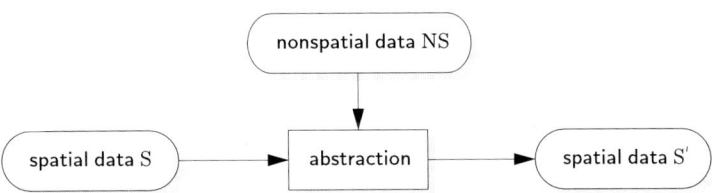

In the terminology of Chap. 3, S corresponds to the geometric information G and the graphical information R. We see basically two major sources of nonspatial data needed to carry out the process of abstraction:

1. *Enrichment to the spatial data*
   Recall the process of enrichment which we described in Sect. 3.1.1: three-dimensional geometric models are structured, and additional information can be associated with these structures. It is this information which is then used, for example, to define the units of the model which are treated uniformly by the algorithms for abstraction.

2. *Interaction*
   In the course of human–computer interaction, further information can be gathered by the system with respect to the model. User input defines such parameters as the degree of interest and the aspect of interest of parts of the model. The user indicates interest for certain objects by carrying out operations on the visualization; these operations can be noted by the system and used later on the interaction to select which abstraction to carry out.

We are now in a position to analyze the process of abstraction by studying properties of its input in terms of spatial and nonspatial data.

23.3 Continuity and Discontinuity in Abstraction

We can observe that the process of abstraction is, in some cases, a *continuous* process in the sense that small changes in the input yield small changes in the output. On the other hand, the process of abstraction is sometimes a *discontinuous* one in which the smallest possible changes to the input can lead to fundamental changes to the output. It is instructive to study these differences in detail.

23.3.1 Continuity

We contend that the basic prerequisite for continuity in the process of abstraction is that the nonspatial data serving as input to this process is itself continuous or at least has significant continuous components. For example, if the nonspatial data consists simply of an integer within a predefined range, the abstraction can, in principle, be defined such that a small change in the input produces only a small change in its output. This, in turn, can lead to a smooth animation when adjusting the input in a monotone manner.

Let us study some examples. RAAB devised an algorithm for incrementally adding lines in a drawing depending on a numeric value t ($0 \leq t \leq 1$). Starting from the contour lines of an object for a value $t = 0$, he shows how to move to a full wire-frame visualization for $t = 1$. For each edge in the polygonal 3D model, the parameter t is mapped linearly onto the angle α ($0 \leq \alpha \leq 90°$) between the adjacent faces. The edge is drawn if α lies beneath the corresponding value of t. Figure 23.1 shows a number of examples where t is input by the user with a slider. Note that for small values of t, the images still look esthetically pleasing, while there exists a value $t \geq t'$ for which the output gets cluttered with lines and no longer has a particular appeal. No algorithm has been found to determine t' except by user inspection and input.

In a similar manner, DEUSSEN has made use of G-buffers (recall Chap. 6) to include an edge in the interior of an object in a line drawing when the regions separated by the line belong to different objects, and the z-coordinates of these regions differ by more than a certain threshold, dictated by the input parameter t. This algorithm is not relevant for a 3D model like that of Fig. 23.1, but works well for other kinds of models like trees where there are many small distinct objects. His results are shown in Fig. 23.2.

It will be a challenge in the future to derive appropriate mappings from numerical input to (appropriate) attributes of the 3D model or the resultant image to carry out the process of abstraction. Each application will require its own mapping.

23.3.2 Discontinuity

If a more complex data structure like a semantic net is used as the nonspatial data, the algorithms for carrying out the abstraction are unlikely to be able to tune the spatial data in a continuous manner. Instead, they classify the symbols of the semantic net in a discrete manner, leading to discontinuities in the output. Some of the smallest possible changes in the input may lead to significant changes in the output, so that it may be difficult to produce smooth animations without additional in-betweening techniques.

We have seen of examples of this phenomenon in particular in Part IV of this book on textual methods of abstraction. Text as input to the abstraction algorithms is generally used to select certain graphical attributes to

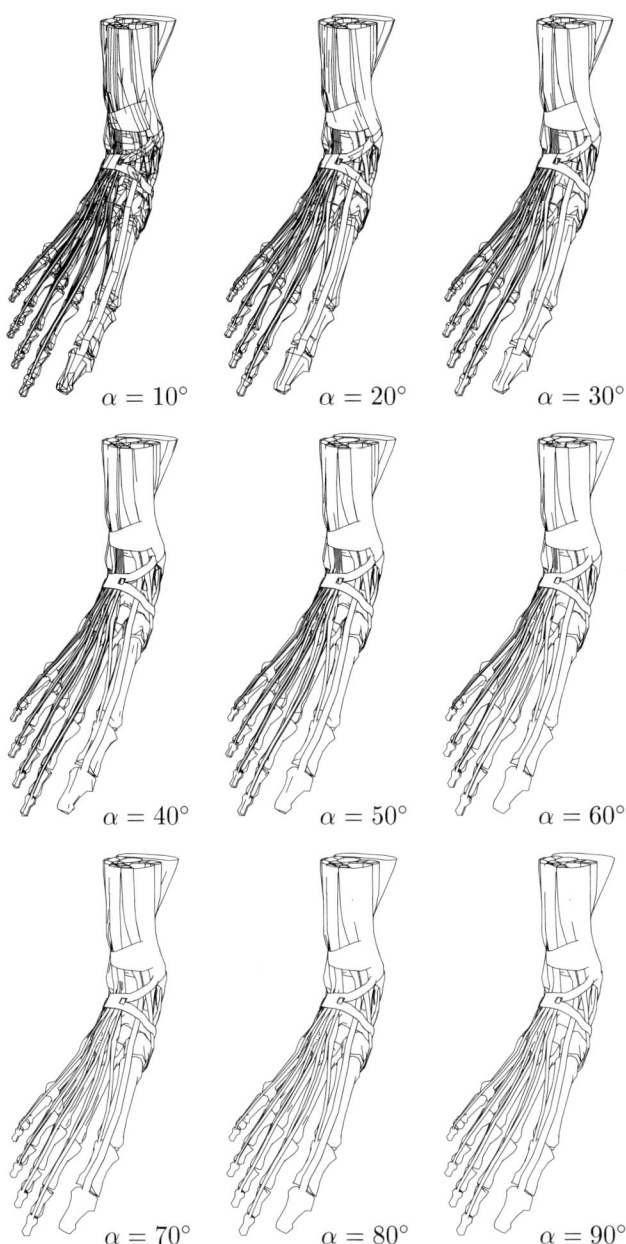

Figure 23.1: Several examples of line drawings visualizing a 3D model with more or less lines, depending on an angle α between adjacent surfaces (courtesy of Andreas RAAB)

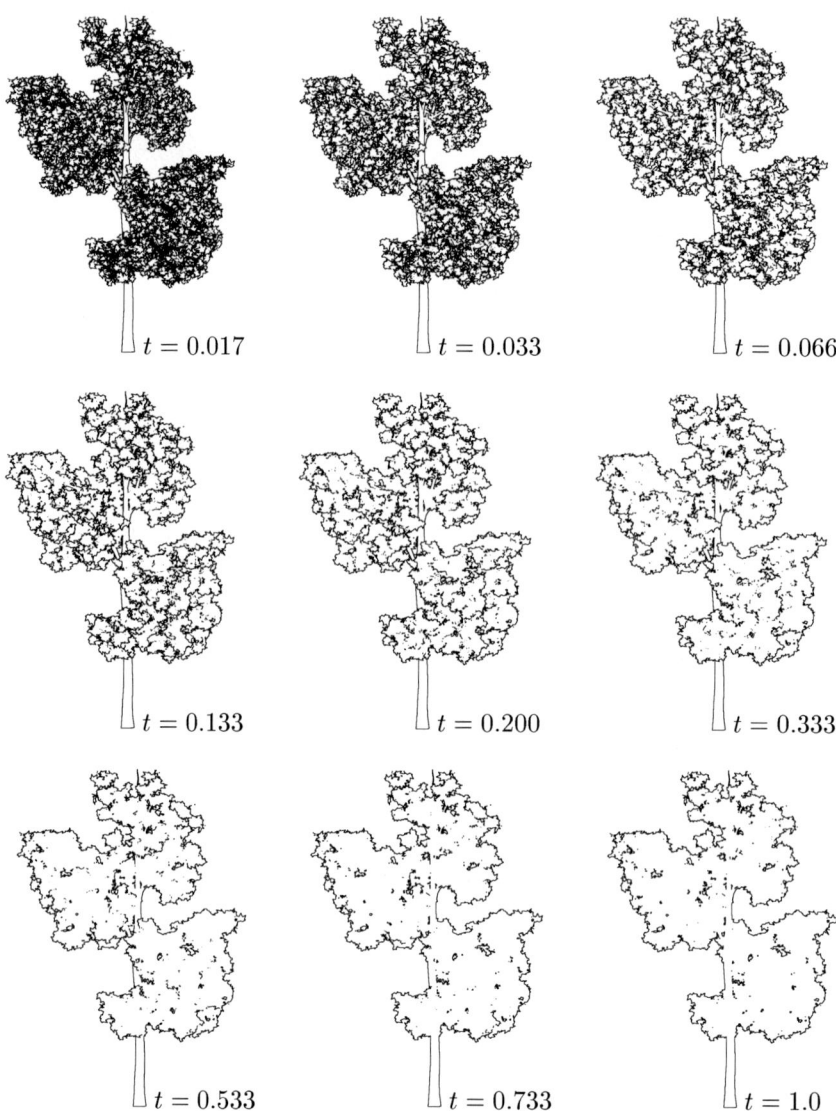

Figure 23.2: Several examples of line drawings visualizing a 3D model with more or less lines, depending on a parameter t mapped onto the difference in depth separated by internal contour lines (courtesy of Oliver DEUSSEN)

be included in the image. For example, if the objects in the 3D model are classified as to their type (e.g., bones, muscles, tissue, etc.), certain colors or a degree of transparency may be assigned to each of these types. However, it is a matter of either using these attributes or not using them, rather than adjusting their qualities continuously. Similarly, an object can either be labeled or not, while providing only part of a label generally does not make much sense. If more explanation is required for a particular object, the user can zoom up the label, but a discontinuity will result as soon as the label is large enough to accommodate the next longer explanation.

Smooth transitions can be devised, in principle, even for the cases described above. For example, labels can be faded out and replaced by others. However, the words of a label being faded out do not change their meaning during this process to the same extent as, for example, when morphing one object into another; changing from one text to another is a process which is inherently discontinuous, both graphically and semantically.

23.3.3 A Comparison Between Image and Language Generation

Language generators produce text based on symbolic input (see [DHRS92]). This process is often called *linearization* of the input structure, hence we can refer to the output as being *one-dimensional*. This input is discontinuous in the sense that the term is used above. The smallest possible changes in the input, i.e., manipulating a link in the representation (e.g., a semantic net) or making small changes to individual nodes, may have a significant effect on the output. Such small changes in the input may lead to whole words or word phrases being changed in the output.

Rendering, on the other hand, produces output which is inherently *two-dimensional*: The output, which can conveniently be represented by a matrix of pixels, only makes sense when its two-dimensional nature is preserved. To a human viewer, these pixels must be visualized on a surface with the pixels very close to one another, while for pattern recognition algorithms, the pixels must be stored such that there is fast access from any pixel to its four, eight, or 24 neighbors in the plane. As we saw above, it is the nonspatial data from which the choice of the algorithm and its parameters within the process of abstraction of the 3D model are derived. The output can vary continuously, in that small changes in the input may in fact result in small changes in the output (only a few pixels may be affected).

We have now arrived at the fundamental difference between the study of computational *linguistics* and computational *visualistics*. The former deals with inherently *one-dimensional* structures, while the latter deals with inherently *two-dimensional* structures. To avoid confusion, it must of course be noted that the objects of study of each of these areas can also have a higher dimensionality: In spoken language, for example, the intonation can be regarded as an additional dimension, while in images the color of the pixels can be regarded as playing a similar role. However, the point is that language can be reduced down to a linear sequence of tokens, while images cannot be reduced down further than a matrix of pixels.

It is interesting to note that the one-dimensional objects of study of computational linguistics tend to be discontinuous in the above sense, while the objects of study of computational visualistics can be continuous (although they may also be discontinuous). We hypothesize that there are properties inherent in the second dimension which enable the continuity, while one-dimensional structures lack the necessary degree of freedom to be continuous. These properties are what enable the concept of animation in two-dimensional structures, while there is no analog for one-dimensional structures. This is a fundamental observation which will require further study in the future.

23.4 Conveying Allowable Operations to Viewers of Images

Using the notion of nonspatial data alluded to above, we shall now go back to see how this relates to the idea of regarding images as ADTs. We contend that it is precisely this nonspatial input data to the process of abstraction which defines which operations can subsequently be carried out by users on the resultant images. It is this data from which the algorithms deduce what is to be changed in the spatial data S to produce the modified spatial data S'. Hence to avoid misinterpretations on the part of viewers of the images, attempts should be made to convey its effect. Two methods of conveying this information are envisioned at present: graphical comprehension cues encoded in the image, and linguistic comprehension cues accompanying the image. We will look at these in turn.

23.4.1 Graphical Comprehension Cues

The most direct way of conveying to a user information about the process of abstraction which has taken place to arrive at the output image I is through graphical comprehension cues. They are encoded within an image – either by producing an extra image I' or by modifying the primary image I.

1. *Accompanying graphical comprehension cues*
   The program carrying out the abstraction can produce an additional image encoding information as to what went on during abstraction. Figure 23.3 shows an example of such an image, illustrating one of the experiments of Otto von GUERICKE. Due to the rather low contrasts in the picture, the airpump is not recognizable well enough. An enhancement process has thus been carried out to emphasize the pump. To see what has actually been changed in the image, the third image of Fig. 23.3 has been created showing the difference in the color values of the two images.

23.4 Conveying Allowable Operations to Viewers of Images

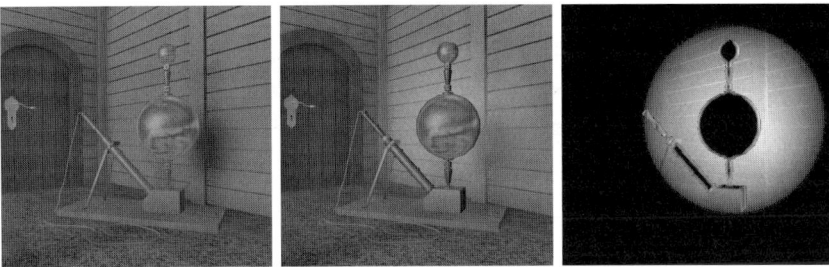

Figure 23.3: Example of accompanying graphical comprehension cues. The primary image produced by a rendering process is shown to the left. Certain parts of the airpump are hardly recognizable and have thus been emphasized in the middle image. The accompanying graphical comprehension cue is shown on the right and gives information on what has been changed in the middle image (courtesy of Axel HOPPE)

2. *Augmented graphical comprehension cues*
   In some situations, it can be helpful to produce additional information in the primary image to yield an augmented one with some additional information pertaining to the process of abstraction. This information does not interfere with the primary image, though there may be a certain lack of esthetic appeal in the resultant image. Figure 23.4 shows an example.

3. *Integrated graphical comprehension cues*
   The most interesting option for conveying information to users about the process of abstraction is to encode this directly in the image. The methods of non-photorealistic rendering can be used by employing parameters that do not obstruct the primary visualization. For example, when rendering the primary image as a line drawing with a uniform line thickness, the

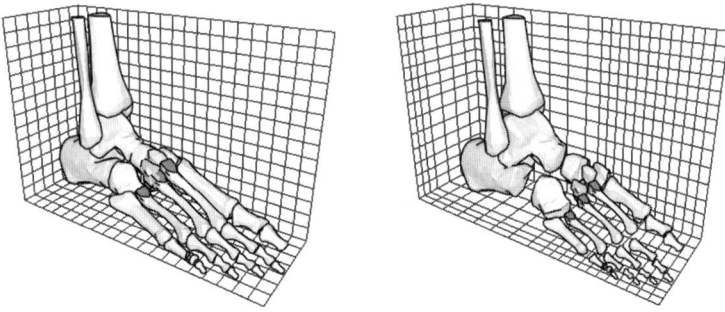

Figure 23.4: Example of an image (left) and an image of the same object with an augmented graphical comprehension cue (right). The 3D grid is included to indicate where parts have been enlarged (courtesy of Andreas RAAB)

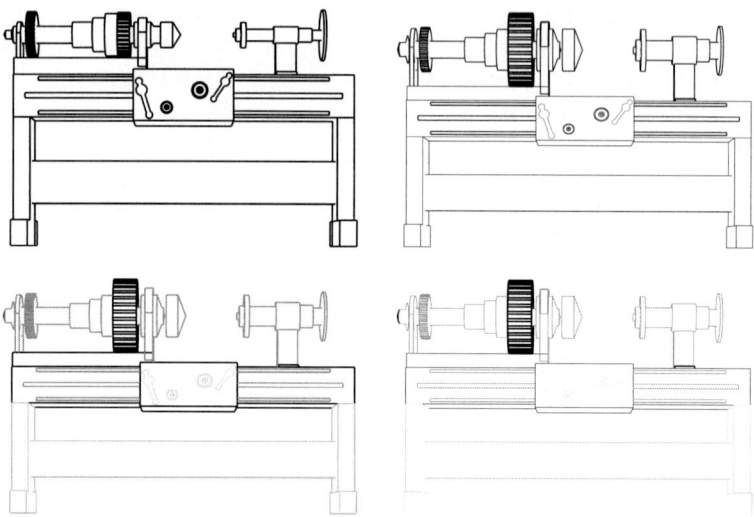

Figure 23.5: Example of integrated graphical comprehension cues. The primary image is shown in the upper left, while in the other images, a certain object has been zoomed up in size. The enlarged object is highlighted graphically, while the objects made smaller are drawn with less conspicuous lines using one of several line parameters (courtesy of Andreas RAAB)

scaling factor for individual objects (recall the 3D zoom) can be mapped onto the line thickness: the larger the scaling factor of an object, the thicker the lines defining its contour. The result (see Fig. 23.5) is a subtle way of communicating information to the user as to the process of abstraction.

Particularly the latter method can be used in many variations. Figure 9.4 already showed the use of transparency to indicate the scaling factor; other parameters which can be affected are the gray-scale of lines (Sect. 4.5.2), the density of cross-hatching (Sect. 5.2), or the font size used for labels (Chap. 13). If parameters which clearly do not belong to the primary visualization are used, the additional information can be encoded in the image without disrupting the viewer.

23.4.2 Linguistic Comprehension Cues

A less subtle, but in many situations very effective way of communicating information about an image was already presented earlier in this book: figure captions. These are what we refer to as linguistic comprehension cues about the image, its meaning, and its interpretation. Indeed, Chap. 13 emphasizes the difference between instructive and descriptive figure captions, where instructive captions tend to capture the intended effect or meaning of an image, while descriptive captions tend to convey information about the image. A careful analysis of this classification leads to the conclusion that descriptive figure captions contain precisely the information which is used to carry out the process of abstraction on the 3D model. Such captions aid the user in his or her interpretation by pointing out such information as which parts have been enlarged, rotated,[2] moved aside, or removed entirely.

The technique of giving linguistic comprehension cues can also be useful in connection with graphical comprehension cues. In the absence of a graphical comprehension cue, an appropriate linguistic cue might be to point out, for example, that the left ventricle in a drawing has been enlarged. If the line thickness is used as the graphical comprehension cue to indicate the scaling factor, an appropriate linguistic comprehension cue could be to point out that the line thickness indicates the relative sizes of objects being visualized. However, the use of graphical comprehension cues can be standardized for a particular context (such as blue and red for veins and arteries, respectively) and the necessary linguistic comprehension cues given in a legend pertaining to a whole collection of images.

An aspect of linguistic comprehension cues not explored systematically here is that of generating verbal explanations to accompany computer animation. Future multimedia systems will most certainly call for such facilities. Care will have to be taken to integrate linguistic and graphical comprehension cues; however, the simultaneity of these two kinds of cues opens up significant chances for improving the quality of presentations.

23.4.3 Comparison

It is interesting to analyze situations in which it is possible to generate effective linguistic comprehension cues and those in which graphical comprehension cues are the method of choice. Perhaps most fundamental is that linguistic comprehension cues are needed to name the object depicted in an image. This may be particularly useful in situations in which the object cannot be recognized readily out of its context by the user, or where an unusual viewing angle or perspective has been chosen. Graphical comprehension cues can sometimes be devised to convey the required information, but may be unnecessarily awkward. Linguistic comprehension cues are also particularly useful to explain to a user *why* a particular abstraction was chosen, whereas the result of the abstraction may be shown more aptly with a graphical comprehension cue.

We contend that there is a relationship between the appropriateness of the type of comprehension cue (linguistic or graphical) and the continuity of the nonspatial data determining the abstraction.

Our experience shows that linguistic comprehension cues are particularly useful for describing the nonspatial input to the process of abstraction when

---

[2] We have yet to solve the algorithmic problems associated with *selective* rotation of parts of an object. To date, we deal only with rotations of the entire object being displayed.

this is *dis*continuous. An example is when certain objects are cut away so as to be able to visualize objects of interest which are found at the rear; this information is conveyed more effectively with a linguistic comprehension cue (i.e., a figure caption) than with a graphical comprehension cue. Indeed, we discussed earlier in Sect. 23.3 the linearizability of nonspatial data lends itself well to generating linguistic comprehension cues, while the encoding of such data in a two-dimensional structure is difficult to compute.

By contrast, if the nonspatial data serving as the input to the abstraction process is continuous by nature, it can easily be mapped onto parameters of the rendering process, yielding effective graphical comprehension cues. For example, the focus line method of uncluttering maps discussed in Sect. 8.3 lends itself well to generating a graphical comprehension cue, whereas generating a linguistic comprehension cue is computationally difficult. It would be inappropriate to mention the focus line itself in a figure caption for end-users of a map but good to point out its effect. This, however, would have to be connected conceptually to the underlying geographic data, like street names. No such algorithms have been identified to date which would not be very vulnerable to misinterpretation.

A final point about the relationship between linguistic and graphical comprehension cues is interesting to note. Our emphasis in this book has been entirely on the process of abstraction, starting from a spatial model; we have searched for methods and tools to help in this process, and have identified that nonspatial data is the key to abstraction. However, it is a completely different topic to focus on the nonspatial data and to try to visualize this with the help of 3D models. While in this book the spatial data has been the "constant" and the nonspatial data the "variable", this observation instead suggests treating the nonspatial data as the "constant" and the spatial data (i.e., 3D models) as the "variable" used to achieve an appropriate visualization. This is a variation of some of the problems treated in the area of information visualization.

23.5 The Bottom Line

Our work in this book has focused on a particular aspect of the area to which we refer as *computational visualistics*. Indeed, in a sense our topic is analogous to some of the work in computational linguistics, except that we deal with images rather than language. More precisely, we have focused on the two-dimensional nature of pictures presented on computer screens, rather than the linear structures of language. Many of the results presented here can be seen as consequences of trying to endow such two-dimensional structures with some of the same flexibility linear structures have already attained. Future research will have to investigate in more detail the relationship between pictures and language by analyzing techniques and methods on the one hand and the dimensionality of the objects of study on the other hand.

The fundamental problem which we set out in Chap. 1 to study is that of extending the process of visualization of 3D geometric models over and above the standard rendering algorithms and software which we have been taught to master. The process of computer visualization was to make inroads in application areas in which generated computer graphics up to now have played practically no role. These areas have in common that the visualizations are typically carried out by hand and require considerable creativity, focus on the informative nature of the images, and can deal flexibly with incorrect and incomplete data. We thus construed the process of computer visualization as one of exploration of a complex information space, one which contains much more than only geometric data. The process to be carried out was defined as one of abstraction, encompassing adjusting, e.g., the size, shape, and orientation of detail, devising the rendering style to suit the situation, and to bringing images and text into unison with one another.

We have made modest progress on each of these topics. Highlights are the new interactive facility to zoom selectively on 3D objects, a flexible new repertoire of rendering techniques for medical illustration, new techniques for animation of 3D models, and new interactive tools for individualized maps. Furthermore, we have discovered the inherent need for text to accompany images, both within images as labels, and in addition to images as figure captions. Indeed, despite the very diverse requirements of the different application areas, we have been able to cast the methods developed into the framework of abstraction.

A significant result is that rendering and visualization must be treated as a highly interactive process, rather than the more batch-oriented process as which it has been viewed. The interaction provides an important source of information for algorithms which carry out abstraction. Indeed, we have met situations in which only through interaction can certain decisions be made by the abstraction software; we contend that no amount of data in the underlying information space would suffice to carry out the abstraction in the general case. Yet, abstraction in itself is only a tool for enhancing users' comprehension of images, and care must be taken that the interaction on which it is based does not become a burden for the users.

A decisive role in carrying out a process of abstraction is a flexible repertoire of visualization techniques. In particular, non-photorealistic rendering using lines is an effective way of expressing data which has been altered in some way over and above the physically correct geometric model so as to suit the dialog situation at hand. But note that the visualization in the form of non-photorealistic images does not itself constitute the process of abstraction: it is an expression of this process which has computed new geometric data to be conveyed to the user.

We have made progress in visualization techniques for non-photorealistic rendering, but more attention must be focused in future work on interactive techniques to enable users to select features from the repertoire available.

It will be interesting to design editors for material visualization and crosshatching styles, as well as for tuning and fine-tuning images. It will also be a challenge to develop style formats for images, similar to those for document and font format used in popular text processing systems.

The process of abstraction bears in it the danger that users will be misled by images which suit the dialog context at hand, but are, strictly speaking, neither complete nor correct in the sense that photographs or photorealistic images are perceived to be. We have used the concept of abstract data types to explain why users sometimes draw the wrong conclusion from images which have undergone a process of abstraction. To tackle the underlying problems, we have shown that the flexibility of non-photorealism comes to the rescue in many cases by enabling a rendering tool to encode information about the abstraction process within the image itself, without distracting from its overall message. These graphical comprehension cues provide viewers with help to decide how to interpret an image. Furthermore, we have identified a class of algorithms for abstraction for which linguistic comprehension cues must accompany an image if misinterpretations are to be avoided.

We contend that abstraction is one of the fundamental tasks which must be mastered in computational visualistics to extend the scope of rendering to areas of its application which have to date defied algorithmic treatment.

Copyrights

Fig. 1.1, p. 5	From [VKPW82]. Copyright Verlag Georg Thieme 1982
Fig. 1.2, p. 6	Courtesy of Martin SCHOLZ
Fig. 1.3, p. 7	Copyright Berliner Verkehrsbetriebe
Example I, p. 10	From [VKPW82]. Copyright Verlag Georg Thieme 1982
Example III, p. 10	Courtesy of Bert SCHÖNWÄLDER
Fig. 2.1, p. 23	From [Ris95]. Copyright Thomas RIST 1995
Fig. 2.2, p. 26	From [SB94, p. 75]. Copyright ACM 1994
Fig. 2.3, p. 27	From [SB94, p. 78]. Copyright ACM 1994
Fig. 2.4, p. 27	Courtesy of Rainer MICHEL
Fig. 2.5, p. 31	From [KS96, p. 31]. Copyright ACM 1996
Fig. 2.6, p. 32	From [CCF95, p. 224]. Copyright ACM 1995
Fig. 2.8, p. 34	From [RMC93, p. 67]. Copyright ACM 1993
Fig. 2.9, p. 35	From [RMC93, p. 67]. Copyright ACM 1993
Fig. 2.10, p. 35	From [RM93b, p. 105]. Copyright ACM 1993
Fig. 2.11, p. 38	From [KR97]. © 1997 IEEE
Fig. 2.12, p. 38	From [LRP95, p. 404]. Copyright ACM 1995
Fig. 2.13, p. 40	From [HV96, p. 391]. Copyright ACM 1996
Fig. 2.14, p. 41	From [BK96, p. 248]. Copyright John Wiley & Sons Limited. Reproduced with permission.
Fig. 3.5, p. 56	Courtesy of Steffen HEISE
Fig. 4.12, p. 83	Courtesy of Lars SCHUMANN
Fig. 4.13, p. 85	Courtesy of Bert SCHÖNWÄLDER
Fig. 4.14, p. 86	Courtesy of Bert SCHÖNWÄLDER
Fig. 4.15, p. 87	Courtesy of Bert SCHÖNWÄLDER
Fig. 4.16, p. 88	Courtesy of Bert SCHÖNWÄLDER
Fig. 6.10, p. 117	From [Gra90, pp. 44, 45]. Copyright Dover Publications, 1990
Fig. 11.1, p. 180	From [Ken80]. Copyright Academic Press 1980
Fig. 11.2, p. 182	Redrawn after [Mar78]
Fig. 14.4, p. 251	Redrawn after [Mei96]
Fig. 15.1, p. 262	Courtesy of Andreas BUTZ
Fig. 22.2, p. 382	Mit freundlicher Genehmigung aus: Reparaturanleitung Nr. 842/843, VW Golf Diesel erschienen im Bucheli Verlag, CH-6304 Zug

Fig. 23.1, p. 409   Courtesy of Andreas RAAB
Fig. 23.2, p. 410   Courtesy of Oliver DEUSSEN
Fig. 23.3, p. 413   Courtesy of Axel HOPPE
Fig. 23.4, p. 413   Courtesy of Andreas RAAB
Fig. 23.5, p. 414   Courtesy of Andreas RAAB

Bibliography

[Abm94] W. ABMAYR. *Einführung in die digitale Bildverarbeitung*. B. G. Teubner, Stuttgart, 1994.

[ABST94] H. AAGEDAL, T. BETH, H. SCHWARZER, and S. TEIWES. Design of paraxial diffractive elements with the CAD system DigiOpt. In I. CINDRICH and S. H. LEE, editors, *Diffractive and Holographic Optics Technology II*, pages 50–58, 1994.

[ADHC94] F. ARMAN, R. DEPOMMIER, A. HSU, and M.-Y. CHIU. Content-based browsing of video sequences. In *ACM Multimedia '94 Proceedings*, pages 97–103. ACM, 1994.

[AHU83] A. V. AHO, J. E. HOPCROFT, and J. D. ULLMAN. *Data Structures and Algorithms*. Addison-Wesley, Reading, MA, 1983.

[Ali94] ALIAS RESEARCH. *Alias 5.0 Essentials*. User Manuals. Alias Research Inc., 1994.

[AMR96] E. ANDRÉ, J. MÜLLER, and T. RIST. WIP/PPP: Automatic generation of personalized multimedia presentations. In *Proceedings of the 4th ACM Multimedia Conference*, pages 407–408. ACM Press, New York, 1996.

[AR94] E. ANDRÉ and T. RIST. Multimedia presentations: The support of passive and active viewing. Technical Report RR-94-01, DFKI, Deutsches Forschungszentrum für Künstliche Intelligenz, 1994.

[AS93] G. AUMANN and K. SPITZMÜLLER. *Computerorientierte Geometrie*. BI Wissenschaftsverlag, Mannheim, 1993.

[AT94] A. AKUTSU and Y. TONOMURA. Video tomography: An efficient method for camerawork extraction and motion analysis. In *ACM Multimedia '94 Proceedings*, pages 349–356. ACM, 1994.

[BBK82] T. BERK, L. BROWNSTONE, and A. KAUFMANN. A new color-naming system for graphics languages. *IEEE Computer Graphics and Applications*, 2(3):37–44, May 1982.

[BC94] L. BARTRAM and T. CALVERT. Evaluating the role of intelligent support in user interfaces to supervisory control systems. In *Proceedings of IEEE International Conference on Systems, Man and Cybernetics*, pages 717–722, 1994.

[BDD85]   K. F. BURY, S. E. DAVIS, and M. J. DARNELL. Window management: A review of issues and some results from user testing. IBM Human Factors Center Report HFC-53, IBM, San Jose, CA, 1985.

[Ber90]   R. M. BERNARD. Using extended captions to improve learning from instructional illustrations. *British Journal of Educational Technology*, 21(3):215–225, 1990.

[BFM+97] M. BORDEGONI, G. FACONTI, M. T. MAYBURY, T. RIST, S. RUGGIERI, P. TRAHANIAS, and M. WILSON. The reference model for intelligent multimedia presentation systems. *Computer Standarts & Interfaces: The International Journal on the Development and Application of Standards for Computers, Data Communications and Interface*, (18):477–496, 1997.

[BFP86]   K. S. BOOTH, D. R. FORSEY, and A. W. PAETH. Hardware assistance for Z-buffer visible surface algorithms. In *Proceedings of Graphics Interface '86*, pages 194–201. Canadian Information Processing Society, 1986.

[BH94]   B. B. BEDERSON and J. D. HOLLAN. Pad++: A zooming graphical interface for exploring alternate interface physics. In *UIST: Proceedings of the ACM Symposium on User Interface Software and Technology '94*. ACM, 1994.

[BK96]   A. BUTZ and A. KRÜGER. Lean modelling – The intelligent use of geometrical abstraction in 3D animation. In *Proceedings of ECAI '96*, pages 246–250. John Wiley & Sons, New York, 1996.

[BK97]   A. BUTZ and A. KRÜGER. Zur Auswahl von Abstraktionsgraden. In O. DEUSSEN and P. LORENZ, editors, *Proceedings Simulation und Animation '97*, pages 147–158. SCS Europe, Erlangen, 1997.

[BOD+94] L. BARTRAM, R. OVANS, J. DILL, M. DYCK, and W. S. HAVENS. Contextual assistance in user interfaces to complex, time-critical systems: The intelligent zoom. In *Proceedings of Graphics Interface '94*, pages 216–224. Canadian Information Processing Society, 1994.

[Bra82]   M. BRAMBRING. Language and geographic orientation for the blind. In *Speech, Place, and Action: Studies in Deixis and Related Topics*, pages 203–218. John Wiley & Sons, New York, 1982.

[Bri90]   M. H. BRISCOE. *A Researcher's Guide to Scientific and Medical Illustrations*. Springer-Verlag, Berlin, 1990.

[Bru95]   R. BRUGGER. *Professionelle Bildgestaltung in der 3D-Computergraphik: Grundlagen und Prinzipien für eine ausdrucksstarke Computervisualisierung*. Addison-Wesley, Bonn, 1995.

[BS93] L. BERGMANN and C. SCHAEFER. *Lehrbuch der Experimentalphysik*, volume III, Optik. Walter de Gruyter Verlag, Berlin, 1993.

[But94] A. BUTZ. Betty – planning and generating animations for the visualization of movements and spatial relations. In *Proceedings of the Workshop on Advanced Visual Interfaces, AVI '94*, pages 53–58. ACM Press, New York, 1994.

[But97] A. BUTZ. Anymation with CATHI. In *Proceedings of AAAI/IAAI '97*, pages 957–962. AAAI Press, Menlo Park, CA, 1997.

[BW95] A. BRUDERLIN and L. WILLIAMS. Motion signal processing. In *Proceedings of SIGGRAPH '95*, Computer Graphics Proceedings, Annual Conference Series, pages 97–104. ACM SIGGRAPH, 1995.

[Car96] S. K. CARD. Visualizing retrieved information. *IEEE Computer Graphics and Applications*, 16(2):63–67, 1996.

[Cat74] E. CATMULL. *A Subdivision Algorithm for Computer Display of Curved Surfaces*. PhD thesis, Computer Science Department, University of Utah, Salt Lake City, 1974.

[CCF95] M. S. T. CARPENDALE, D. J. COWPERTHWAITE, and F. D. FRACCHIA. 3-dimensional pliable surfaces: For the effective presentation of visual information. In *UIST: Proceedings of the ACM Symposium on User Interface Software and Technology '95*, pages 217–226. ACM, 1995.

[CCF96] M. S. T. CARPENDALE, D. J. COWPERTHWAITE, and F. D. FRACCHIA. Distortion viewing techniques for 3-dimensional data. In *Proceedings of the IEEE Symposium on Information Visualization '96*, pages 46–53. IEEE Computer Society Press, Los Alamitos, 1996.

[CEG96] S. CARD, S. G. EICK, and N. GERSHON, editors. *Proceedings of the IEEE Symposium on Information Visualization '96*, Los Alamitos, 1996. IEEE Computer Society Press.

[CNDJ93] C. CRUZ-NEIRA, T. A. DEFANTI, and D. J.SANDIN. Surround-screen projection-based virtual reality: The design and implementation of the CAVE. In *Proceedings of SIGGRAPH '93*, Computer Graphics Proceedings, Annual Conference Series, pages 135–142, 1993.

[Cul90] S. CULHANE. *From Script to Screen*. St. Martin's Press, New York, 1990.

[CVM+96] J. COHEN, A. VARSHNAY, D. MANOCHA, G. TURK, H. WEBER, P. AGARWAL, F. BROOKS, and W. WRIGHT. Simplification envelopes. In *Proceedings of SIGGRAPH '96*, Computer Graphics Proceedings, Annual Conference Series, pages 461–468. ACM SIGGRAPH, 1996.

[Dah97] M. DAHLBERG. Tactile mapping – an unusual GIS application. In *Proceedings of the 18th ICA/ACI International Cartographic Conference*, volume 3, pages 1417–1421. Gävle, Stockholm, 1997.

[Dat96] V. DATALABS. *Viewpoint Catalog*, 1996.

[DB88] T. DEAN and M. BODDY. An analysis of time-dependent planning. In *Proceedings of AAAI '88*, pages 49–54. AAAI Press, Menlo Park, CA, 1988.

[DBHH94] J. DILL, L. BARTRAM, A. HO, and F. HENIGMANN. A continuously variable zoom for navigating large hierarchical networks. In *Proceedings IEEE Conference on Systems, Man and Cybernetics*, pages 386–390, 1994.

[DG97] J. DILL and N. GERSHON, editors. *Proceedings of the IEEE Symposium on Information Visualization '97*, Los Alamitos, 1997. IEEE Computer Society Press.

[DHL+98] O. DEUSSEN, P. HANRAHAN, B. LINTERMANN, R. MECH, M. PHARR, and P. PRUSINKIEWICZ. Realistic modeling and rendering of plant ecosystems. In *Proceedings of SIGGRAPH '98*. ACM SIGGRAPH, 1998.

[DHRS92] R. DALE, E. H. HOVY, D. RÖSNER, and O. STOCK. *Aspects of Automated Natural Language Generation*. Springer-Verlag, Berlin, 1992.

[DL97] O. DEUSSEN and B. LINTERMANN. A modelling method and user interface for creating plants. In *Proceedings of Graphics Interface '97*, pages 189–197. Canadian Information Processing Society, 1997.

[Dor75] J. DORE. Holophrases, speech acts, and language universals. *Journal of Child Language*, 2:21–40, 1975.

[DOS] Fraunhofer Gesellschaft. *DOSIMIS-3*.

[DP73] D. H. DOUGLAS and T. K. PEUCKER. Algorithms for the reduction of the number of points required to represent a digitized line or its caricature. *The Canadian Cartographer*, 10(2):112–122, 1973.

[DZ94] S. M. DRUCKER and D. ZELTZER. Intelligent camera control in a virtual environment. In *Proceedings of Graphics Interface '94*, pages 190–199. Canadian Information Processing Society, May 1994.

[EA93] J. EICHLER and G. ACKERMANN. *Holographie*. Springer-Verlag, Berlin, 1993.

[Edm91] P. K. EDMAN. *Tactile Graphics*. American Foundation for the Blind, 1991.

[EE68]   D. ENGELBART and W. K. ENGLISH. A research center for augmenting human intellect. In *Proceedings of the Fall Joint Computing Conference '68*, pages 395–410. AFIPS Press, Montvale, NJ, 1968.

[ELMS91]   P. EADES, W. LAI, K. MISUE, and K. SUGIYAMA. Preserving the mental map of a diagram. Technical Report IIAS-RR__91-16E, Fujitsu Laboratories, 1991.

[Far91]   G. FARIN. *NURBS for Curve and Surface Design.* SIAM Activity Group on Geometric Design, 1991.

[Fau85]   G. FAUCONNIER. *Mental Spaces – Aspects of Meaning Construction in Natural Language.* MIT Press, Cambridge, MA, 1985.

[FB86]   C. FRÈRE and O. BRYNGDAHL. Computer-generated holograms: reconstruction of curves in 3-D. *Optics Communications*, (60):369–372, 1986.

[FBCT95]   J.-D. FEKETE, É. BIZOUARN, É. COURNARIE, and T. G. F. TAILLEFER. TicTacToon: A paperless system for professional 2D animation. In *Proceedings of SIGGRAPH '95*, Computer Graphics Proceedings, Annual Conference Series, pages 79–89. ACM SIGGRAPH, 1995.

[Fei85]   S. FEINER. Apex: An experiment in the automated creation of pictorial explanations. *IEEE Computer Graphics & Applications*, 5(11):117–123, 1985.

[FLB86]   C. FRÈRE, D. LESEBERG, and O. BRYNGDAHL. Computer-generated holograms of three-dimensional objects composed of line segments. *Journal of the Optical Society of America (JOSA)*, A3(5):726–730, 1986.

[FM93]   S. K. FEINER and K. R. MCKEOWN. Automating the generation of coordinated multimedia explanations. In M. M. MAYBURY, editor, *Intelligent Multimedia Interfaces*, pages 117–138. AAAI Press, Menlo Park, CA, 1993.

[For95]   T. FORCADE. *3D Studio IPAS Plug-In Reference.* New Rider, Indianapolis, 1995.

[Fow89]   G. R. FOWLES. *Introduction to Modern Optics.* Dover Publications, New York, 1989.

[FPF88]   K. M. FAIRCHILD, S. E. POLTROCK, and G. W. FURNAS. Semnet: Three-dimensional graphic representation of large knowledge bases. *Cognitive Science and its Applications for Human Computer Interaction*, 1988.

[Frè88]   C. FRÈRE. *Verallgemeinerte Konfiguration der Rekonstruktions- und der Hologrammfläche in der digitalen Holografie.* PhD thesis, University of Essen, 1988.

[FS76]   R. W. FLOYD and L. STEINBERG. An adaptive algorithm for spatial grey scale. In *Proceedings of the Society for Information Display*, volume 17, pages 75–77, 1976.
[Fur86]   G. W. FURNAS. Generalized fisheye views. In *Proceedings of CHI '86, , Human Factors in Computing Systems*, pages 16–23. ACM SIGCHI, 1986.
[FvDFH90] J. D. FOLEY, A. van DAM, S. K. FEINER, and J. F. HUGHES. *Computer Graphics. Principle and Practice*. Addison-Wesley, Reading, MA, 2nd edition, 1990.
[FZ94]   G. W. FURNAS and J. ZACKS. Enriching and reusing hierarchical structure. In *Proceedings of CHI '94, Human Factors in Computing Systems*, pages 330–335. ACM SIGCHI, 1994.
[Gab48]   D. GABOR. A new microscopic principle. *Nature*, 161:777, 1948.
[GCEG93]   N. D. GERSHON, J. M. COGGINS, P. R. EDHOLM, and A. GLOBUS. How to lie and confuse with visualization. In *Proceedings of SIGGRAPH '93*, Computer Graphics Proceedings, Annual Conference Series, pages 387–388. ACM SIGGRAPH, 1993.
[GHJV95]   E. GAMMA, R. HELM, R. JOHNSON, and J. VLISSIDES. *Design Patterns. Elements of Reusable Object-Oriented Software*. Addison-Wesley, Reading, MA, 1995.
[GHM96]   S. GEITZ, T. HANSON, and S. MAHER. Computer generated 3-dimensional models of manual alphabet handshapes for the World Wide Web. In *Proceedings of ASSETS '96*, pages 27–31. ACM, 1996.
[Gil74]   J. M. GILL. Tactual mapping. *Research Bulletin of the American Foundation for the Blind*, 10(28):57–80, 1974.
[GN96]   D. GENTNER and J. NIELSEN. The Anti-Mac interface. *Communications of the ACM*, 39(8):70–82, 1996.
[God97]   L. S. GODWIN. Coordinating standards on data quality: An important ingredient for cartographers. In *Proceedings of the 18th ICA/ACI International Cartographic Conference*, volume 1, pages 533–540. Gävle, Stockholm, 1997.
[Gom84]   E. H. GOMBRICH. *The Sense of Order – A Study in the Psychology of Decorative Art*. Phaidon Press, London, 2nd edition, 1984.
[Gra90]   C. B. GRAFTON. *Trades and Occupations – A Pictorial Archive from early sources*. Dover Publications, 1990.
[Gri75]   H. P. GRICE. Logic and conversation. In P. COLE and J. L. MORGAN, editors, *Speech Acts*, pages 41–58. Academic Press, New York, 1975.
[GW86]   P. GOULD and R. WHITE. *Mental maps*. Allen & Unwin, 2nd edition, 1986.

[GW93] R. C. GONZALEZ and R. E. WOODS. *Digital Image Processing*. Addison-Wesley, Reading, MA, 1993.

[Hab95] P. HABERÄCKER. *Praxis der Digitalen Bildverarbeitung und Mustererkennung*. Carl Hanser Verlag, München, 1995.

[HCMM89] J. G. HOLLANDS, T. T. CAREY, M. L. MATTHEWS, and C. A. MCCANN. Presenting a graphical network: A comparison of performance using fisheye and scrolling views. In *Proceedings of 3rd International Conference on Human-Computer Interaction*, volume 2, pages 313–320. Elsevier Science Publishers, 1989.

[HDLM96] M. HUGHES, C. DIMATTIA, M. C. LIN, and D. MANOCHA. Efficient and accurate interference detection for polynomial deformation. In *Proceedings of Computer Animation '96*, pages 155–166. IEEE Computer Society Press, Los Alamitos, 1996.

[HE96] P. A. HARLING and A. D. N. EDWARDS. Hand tension as a gesture segmentation cue. In P. A. HARLING and A. D. N. EDWARDS, editors, *Progress in Gestural Interaction. Proceedings of Gesture Workshop '96*, pages 75–88. Springer-Verlag, Berlin, 1996.

[Hel75] J. HELD. Visualisierter Agnostizismus. Zum amerikanischen Fotorealismus der Gegenwart. *Kritische Berichte*, (5/6):1–6, 1975.

[HG94a] G. HAKE and D. GRÜNREICH. *Kartographie*. Walter de Gruyter Verlag, Berlin, 7th edition, 1994.

[HG94b] P. HECKBERT and M. GARLAND. Multiresolution modeling for fast rendering. In *Proceedings of SIGGRAPH '94*, Computer Graphics Proceedings, Annual Conference Series, pages 1–8. ACM SIGGRAPH, 1994.

[HHK92] W. M. HSU, J. F. HUGHES, and H. KAUFMANN. Direct manipulation of freeform deformations. In *Proceedings of SIGGRAPH '92*, Computer Graphics Proceedings, Annual Conference Series. ACM SIGGRAPH, 1992.

[HHRS98] K. HARTMANN, R. HELBING, D. RÖSNER, and T. STROTHOTTE. VisDok: Ein Ansatz zur interaktiven Nutzung von technischer Dokumentation. In P. LORENZ and B. PREIM, editors, *Proceedings Simulation und Visualisierung '98*, pages 308–321. SCS Europe, Erlangen, 1998.

[HHWM92] W. C. HILL, J. D. HOLLAN, A. WROBLEWSKI, and T. MCCANDLES. Edit wear and read wear. In *Proceedings of CHI '92, Human Factors in Computing Systems*, pages 3–10. ACM SIGCHI, 1992.

[HLH96] A. HOPPE, K. LÜDICKE, and R. HAUSMANN. Emphasis in rendered images using contrast information. In A. BEHROOZ, editor, *Proceedings of Knowledge Transfer '96*, pages 513–522. Pace, Pacific & Middle East Center for Research, London, 1996.

[HLW93] S. C. HSU, I. H. H. LEE, and H. E. WISEMAN. Skeletal Strokes. In *UIST: Proceedings of the ACM Symposium on User Interface Software and Technology '93*, pages 197–206. ACM, 1993.

[HMS95] J. HAMEL, R. MICHEL, and T. STROTHOTTE. Verfahren zur Generierung taktiler Routenkarten. In *Kolloquium Taktile Medien*, pages 67–73. Technische Universität Dresden, 1995.

[Hod89] E. R. S. HODGES. *The Guild Handbook of Scientific Illustration*. Van Nostrand Reinhold, New York, 1989.

[Hop96] H. HOPPE. Progressive meshes. In *Proceedings of SIGGRAPH '96, Computer Graphics Proceedings, Annual Conference Series*, pages 99–108. ACM SIGGRAPH, 1996.

[Hou92] S. HOUDE. Iterative design of an interface for easy 3D direct manipulation. In *Proceedings of CHI '92, Human Factors in Computing Systems*, pages 135–142. ACM SIGCHI, 1992.

[HPR+94] K.-H. HÖHNE, A. POMMERT, M. RIEMER, T. SCHIEMANN, R. SCHUBERT, and U. TIEDE. Medical volume visualization based on "intelligent volumes". In L. ROSENBLUM, R. A. EARNSHAW, J. ENCARNAÇÃO, H. HAGEN, A. KAUFMAN, S. KLIMENKO, G. NIELSON, F. POST, and D. THALMANN, editors, *Scientific Visualization. Advances and Challenges*, pages 21–35. Academic Press, London, 1994.

[HRI97] R. HELBING, M. RÜGER, and U. ILGENSTEIN. A flexible approach to modeling computer visualization using simulation traces. In K. REGER, editor, *Proceedings of Concurrent Engineering*. SCCS, 1997.

[Hud83] D. HUDELMAYER. Aspekte der taktilen Wahrnehmung für das Lesen von Blinden-Stadtplänen. In *First European Symposium on Tactual Town Maps for the Blind*, Annex K, 1983.

[HV96] B. L. HARRISON and K. J. VINCENTE. An experimental evaluation of transparent menu usage. In *Proceedings of CHI '96, Human Factors in Computing Systems*, pages 391–400. ACM SIGCHI, 1996.

[HvDG94] K. P. HERNDON, A. van DAM, and M. GLEICHER. The challenges of 3D-interaction. *SIGCHI Bulletin*, 26(4):36–43, October 1994.

[IBM95] IBM. *OS/2 Developer CD Documents*, 1995.

[Imm95] C. IMMLER. *Autodesk 3D Studio. Version 4*. Data Becker, Düsseldorf, 1995.

[Itt70] J. ITTEN. *Kunst der Farbe*. Verlag Otto Maier, Ravensburg, 1970.

[Jäg90] E. JÄGER. *Untersuchungen zur kartographischen Symbolisierung und Verdrängung im Rasterformat*. PhD thesis, University of Hannover, 1990.

[Jäh97] B. JÄHNE. *Digital Image Processing. Concepts, Algorithms and Scientific Applications.* Springer-Verlag, Berlin, 4th edition, 1997.

[Joã95] E. M. JOÃO. The importance of quantifying the effects of generalization. In J. C. MÜLLER, J. P. LAGRANGE, and R. WEIBEL, editors, *GIS and Generalization: Methodology and Practice*, pages 183–192. Taylor & Francis, London, 1995.

[JRV+89] J. JOHNSON, W. ROBERTS, W. VERPLANK, D. C. SMITH, C. H. IRBY, M. BEARD, and K. MACKEY. The XEROX Star: A retrospective. *IEEE Computer*, 22(9):11–29, 1989.

[JS91] B. JOHNSON and B. SHNEIDERMAN. Tree maps: A space filling approach to the visualization of hierarchical information structures. In *Proceedings of IEEE Visualization '91*, pages 284–291. IEEE, 1991.

[Kad75] N. KADMON. Data-band derived hyperbolic-scale equitemporal town maps. *International Yearbook of Cartography*, 15:47–54, 1975.

[Kah79] K. KAHN. *Creating Animations on the base of High-Level Specifications.* PhD thesis, AI Lab, MIT, 1979.

[Kam90] H. KAMP. On the representation and transmission of information: Sketch of a theory of verbal communication based on discourse representation theory. In E. KLEIN and F. VELTMAN, editors, *Natural Language and Speech, Symposium Proceedings*, Esprit Basic Research Series, pages 135–158. Springer-Verlag, Berlin, 1990.

[KE93] W. KAPIT and L. M. ELSON. *The Anatomy Color Book.* Harper Collins Publishers, New York, 2nd edition, 1993.

[KEH+96] T. KAMBA, S. ELSON, T. HARPOLD, T. STAMPER, and P. SUKAVIRIYA. Using small screen space more efficiently. In *Proceedings of CHI '96, Human Factors in Computing Systems*, pages 383–390. ACM SIGCHI, 1996.

[Ken80] J. M. KENNEDY. Blind people recognizing and making haptic pictures. In M. A. HAGEN, editor, *The Perception of Pictures*, volume 2, pages 263–303. Academic Press, New York, 1980.

[Ker96] I. V. KERLOW. *The Art of 3-D Computer Animation and Imaging.* Van Nostrand Reinhold, New York, 1996.

[KF93] P. KARP and S. K. FEINER. Automated presentation planning of animation using task decomposition with heuristic reasoning. In *Proceedings of Graphics Interface '93*, pages 118–127. Canadian Information Processing Society, 1993.

[KL73] W. KAMLAH and P. LORENZEN. *Logische Propädeutik – Vorschule des vernünftigen Redens.* BI Wissenschaftsverlag, Mannheim, 1973.

[KL89] M. KAISER and C. LIESS. *Perspektive als Mittel der Kunst.* Colloquium Verlag, Berlin, 1989.

[KLS96] R. KLEIN, G. LIEBICH, and W. STRA"SER. Mesh reduction with error control. In *Proceedings of IEEE Visualization '96*, pages 311–318, 1996.

[KM79] J. KEENAN and R. MOORE. Memory for images of concealed objects: a re-examination of Neisser and Kerr. *Journal of Experimental Psychology: Human Learning and Memory*, 5:374–385, 1979.

[Koc84] D. H. U. KOCHANEK. Interpolating splines with local tension, continuity and bias control. In *Proceedings of SIGGRAPH '84*, Computer Graphics Proceedings, Annual Conference Series, pages 33–41. ACM SIGGRAPH, 1984.

[Kof35] K. KOFFKA. *Principles of Gestalt Psychology.* Hartcourt Brace, New York, 1935.

[Kol92] D. KOLLER. *Detektion, Verfolgung und Klassifikation bewegter Objekte in monokularen Bildfolgen am Beispiel von Straßenverkehrsszenen.* infix, St. Augustin, 1992.

[KR97] T. A. KEAHEY and E. L. ROBERTSON. Nonlinear magnification fields. In *Proceedings of the IEEE Symposium on Information Visualization.* IEEE, 1997.

[KRS94] M. KURZE, L. REICHERT, and T. STROTHOTTE. Access to business graphics by blind people. In *Proceedings of the RESNA '94 Annual Conference*, pages 388–390, 1994.

[KS78] N. KADMON and E. SHLOMI. A polyfocal projection for statistical surfaces. *The Cartographic Journal: Journal of the British Cartographic Society*, 15:36–41, 1978.

[KS96] E. KANDOGAN and B. SHNEIDERMAN. Elastic windows: Improved spatial layout and rapid multiple window operations. In *Proceedings of the Workshop on Advanced Visual Interfaces, AVI '96*, pages 29–38. ACM Press, New York, 1996.

[KSP+95] M. KURZE, T. STROTHOTTE, H. PETRIE, S. MORELY, and F. DECONINCK. New approaches for accessing different classes of graphics by blind people. In I. PLACENCIA-PORRERO and R. P. de la BELLACASA, editors, *The European Context for Assistive Technology*, pages 268–271. IOS Press, Amsterdam, 1995.

[KY93] H. KOIKE and H. YOSHIHARA. Fractal approaches for visualizing huge hierarchies. In *Proceedings of the 1993 IEEE Symposium on Visual Languages*, pages 55–60. IEEE, 1993.

[Lan90] *Langenscheid Wörterbuch.* Langenscheid, 1990.

[Las87]   J. LASSITER. Principles of traditional animation applied to three-dimensional computer animation. In *Proceedings of SIGGRAPH '87*, Computer Graphics Proceedings, Annual Conference Series, pages 35–44. ACM SIGGRAPH, 1987.

[LBT96]   K. H. LIM, I. BENBASAT, and P. A. TODD. An experimental investigation of the interactive effects of interface style, instructions, and task familiarity on user performance. *ACM Transactions on Computer-Human Interaction*, 3(1):1–37, 1996.

[LE95]   P. LÜDERS and R. ERNST. Improving browsing in information by the automatic display layout. In *IEEE Symposium on Information*, 1995.

[Lei94]   W. LEISTER. Computer generated copper plates. *Computer Graphics Forum, Proceedings of Eurographics '94*, pages 69–77, 1994.

[Les87]   D. LESEBERG. Computer generated holograms: cylindrical, conical, and helical waves. *Applied Optics*, 26(20):4385–4390, 1987.

[LF87]   D. LESEBERG and C. FRÈRE. Free positioned and oriented focal lines from computer-generated holograms. *SPIE Proceedings*, 812:113–118, 1987.

[LG83]   A. LEROI-GOURHAN. *Gesture and Speech*. MIT Press, Cambridge, MA, 1983.

[LG95]   M. LUCENTE and T. A. GALYEAN. Rendering interactive holographic images. In *Proceedings of SIGGRAPH '95*, Computer Graphics Proceedings, Annual Conference Series, pages 387–394. ACM SIGGRAPH, 1995.

[LH95]   P. LORENZ and R. HELBING. *Tutorial Simulation and Animation*. Eurosim Congress Vienna, September 1995.

[Lic83]   W. LICHTNER. Computer-unterstützte Verzerrung von Kartenbildern bei der Herstellung thematischer Karten. In *Internationales Jahrbuch für Kartographie*, pages 83–96. 1983.

[Lie94]   H. LIEBERMAN. Powers of ten thousand: Navigating in large information spaces. In *UIST: Proceedings of the ACM Symposium on User Interface Software and Technology '94*, pages 15–16. ACM, 1994.

[LK95]   J. LEE and T. L. KUNII. Model-based analysis of hand posture. *IEEE Computer Graphics and Applications*, 15(5):77–86, September 1995.

[LKW95]   W. LAUTERBORN, T. KURZ, and M. WIESENFELDT. *Coherent Optics, Fundamentals and Applications*. Springer-Verlag, Berlin, 1995.

[Loc90]   J. LOCKE. *An Essay Concerning Human Understanding*, 1690. Reprint: A. D. Woozley, editor, Meridian Books, Cleveland, 1964.

[Low80]   B. LOWENFELD. Psychological problems of children with impaired vision. In W. M. CRUICKSHANK, editor, *Psychology of Exceptional Children and Youth*, pages 263–303. Prentice-Hall, Englewood Cliffs, NJ, 1980.

[LR94]   J. LAMPING and R. RAO. Visualizing large trees using the hyperbolic browser. In *UIST: Proceedings of the ACM Symposium on User Interface Software and Technology '94*, pages 13–24. ACM, 1994.

[LRP95]   J. LAMPING, R. RAO, and P. PIROLLI. A focus+context technique based on hyperbolic geometry for visualizing large hierarchies. In *Proceedings of CHI '95, Human Factors in Computing Systems*, pages 401–409. ACM SIGCHI, 1995.

[LS87]   J. H. LARKIN and H. A. SIMON. Why a diagram is (sometimes) worth ten thousand words. *Cognitive Science*, 11:65–69, 1987.

[LS95]   J. LANSDOWN and S. SCHOFIELD. Expressive rendering: A review of nonphotorealistic techniques. *IEEE Computer Graphics and Applications*, 15(3):29–37, May 1995.

[Luc93]   M. LUCENTE. Interactive computation of holograms using a look-up table. *Journal of Electronic Imaging*, 2(1):28–34, 1993.

[Lux88]   K. LUXTON. Computer-aided map production. In A. TATHAM and A. DODDS, editors, *Second International Symposium on Maps and Graphics for Visually Handicapped People*, page 126, 1988.

[Mar78]   G. S. MARMOR. Age at onset of blindness and the development of the semantics of colour names. *Journal of Experimental Child Psychology*, 25:267–278, 1978.

[Mar82]   D. MARR. *Vision: A Computational Investigation into Human Representation and Processing of Visual Information*. W. H. Freeman and Co., New York, 1982.

[Mea92]   S. MEALING. *The Art and Science of Computer Animation*. Intellect, Oxford, 1992.

[Mei96]   B. J. MEIER. Painterly rendering for animation. In *Proceedings of SIGGRAPH '97*, Computer Graphics Proceedings, Annual Conference Series, pages 477–484. ACM SIGGRAPH, 1996.

[Mit90]   D. A. MITTA. A fisheye presentation strategy: Aircraft maintenance data. In *Proceedings of IFIP INTERACT '90: Human Computer Interaction*, pages 875–880. Elsevier Science Publishers, 1990.

[MLW95]   J. C. MÜLLER, J. P. LAGRANGE, and R. WEIBEL. *GIS and Generalization: Methodology and Practice*. Taylor and Francis, London, 1995.

[MM33]   R. V. MERRY and F. K. MERRY. The tactual recognition of embossed pictures by blind children. *Journal of Applied Psychology*, 17:148–163, 1933.

[MO94]	H.-M. MEYER and K. OBERMAYR. *Objekte integrieren mit OLE2*. Springer-Verlag, Berlin, 1994.
[Mon89]	M. MONMONIER. Interpolated generalization: Cartographic theory for expert-guided feature displacement. *Cartographica*, 26(1):43–64, 1989.
[Mon95]	J. MONACO. *Film verstehen, Kunst, Technik, Sprache, Geschichte und Theorie des Films und der Medien. Mit einer Einführung in Multimedia*. Rowohlt, Reinbeck, 1995.
[Mon96]	M. MONMONIER. *How to lie with maps*. University of Chicago Press, Chicago, 1996.
[MRC91]	J. D. MACKINLAY, G. G. ROBERTSON, and S. K. CARD. The perspective wall: Detail and context smoothly integrated. In *Proceedings of CHI '91, Human Factors in Computing Systems*, pages 173–179. ACM SIGCHI, 1991.
[MRD94]	J. D. MACKINLAY, G. G. ROBERTSON, and R. DELINE. Developing calendar visualizers for the information visualizer. In *UIST: Proceedings of the ACM Symposium on User Interface Software and Technology '94*, pages 109–118. ACM, 1994.
[MRM+95]	V. MITTAL, S. ROTH, J. D. MOORE, J. MATTIS, and G. CARENINI. Generating explanatory captions for information graphics. In *Proceedings of IJCAI '95*, pages 1276–1283. Morgan Kaufmann, Los Altos, CA, 1995.
[MS97]	R. MICHEL and T. STROTHOTTE. Visualisierungstechniken zur computerunterstützten Erzeugung taktiler Karten: das System Map Wizard. *Technische Informatik/Informationstechnik*, 39(2):13–18, 1997.
[MWB97]	W. MACKANESS, R. WEIBEL, and B. BUTTENFIELD. *Report of the ICA Workshop on Map Generalization*. Gävle, Sweden, 1997.
[MWLS95]	J. C. MÜLLER, R. WEIBEL, J. P. LAGRANGE, and F. SALGÉ. Generalization: State of the art and issues. In J. C. MÜLLER, J. P. LAGRANGE, and R. WEIBEL, editors, *GIS and Generalization: Methodology and Practice*, pages 3–17. Taylor & Francis, London, 1995.
[Mye75]	A. MYERS. An efficient visible surface program. Technical report, National Science Foundation, Computer Graphics Research Group, Ohio State University, 1975.
[MZ92]	M. MCKENNA and D. ZELTZER. Three dimensional display systems for virtual environments. *Presence: Teleoperators and Virtual Environments*, 1(4):421–458, 1992.
[NDW93]	J. NEIDER, T. DAVIS, and M. WOO. *OpenGL Programming Guide: the Official Guide to Learning OpenGL*. Addison-Wesley, Reading, MA, 1993.

[Nie94]   J. NIELSEN. Enhancing the explanatory power of heuristics. In *Proceedings of CHI '94, Human Factors in Computing Systems*, pages 152–158. ACM SIGCHI, 1994.

[NK73]   U. NEISSER and N. KERR. Spatial and mnemonic properties of visual images. *Cognitive Psychology*, 5:138–150, 1973.

[Noi93]   E. NOIK. Exploring large hyperdocuments: Fisheye views of nested networks. In *Proceedings of ACM Hypertext '93*, pages 192–205. ACM, 1993.

[Noi94]   E. NOIK. A space of presentation emphasis techniques for visualizing graphs. In *Proceedings of Graphics Interface '94*, pages 225–233. Canadian Information Processing Society, 1994.

[Nor90]   D. NORMAN. *The Design of Everyday Things*. Doubleday, New York, 1990.

[Nug83]   G. C. NUGENT. Deaf students learning from captioned instructions: The relationship between the visual and the caption display. *Journal of Special Education*, 17(2):227–234, 1983.

[NW80]   J. NIEVERGELT and J. WEYDERT. Sites, modes and trails: Telling the user of an interactive system where he is, what he can do and how to get to places. *Methodology of Interaction*, pages 327–338, 1980.

[O'R95]   M. O'ROURKE. *Principles of Three-Dimensional Computer Animation*. W. Norton & Co., New York, 1995.

[oRAN94]   H. S. of ROYAL AUSTRALIAN NAVY. *Bowen to Cape Bowling Green (Australian chart series, 1:500,000)*, 1994.

[Par82]   F. PARKE. Parameterized models for facial animation. *IEEE Computer Graphics and Application*, 2(9):61–68, November 1982.

[PCS95]   C. PLAISANT, D. CARR, and B. SHNEIDERMAN. Image-browser taxonomy and guidelines for designers. In *IEEE Software*, volume 12, pages 21–32, March 1995.

[PE93]   I. PITT and A. D. N. EDWARDS. *Final Report on the Nuffield Project: Making Line Graphs Accessible to Blind Students*. Department of Computer Science, University of York, UK, 1993.

[PF93]   K. PERLIN and D. FOX. Pad: An alternative approach to the computer interface. In *Proceedings of SIGGRAPH '93*, Computer Graphics Proceedings, Annual Conference Series, pages 57–72, 1993.

[Pia37]   J. PIAGET. *La construction du réel chez l'enfant*. Delachaux & Niestlé, Neuchâtel, Switzerland, 1937.

[Pit96]   I. PITT. *The Principled Design of Speech-Based Interfaces*. PhD thesis, Department of Computer Science, University of York, UK, 1996.

[Pon94]   *Pons English-German Dictionary*. Klett, Stuttgart, 1994.

[Pow93] B. M. POWITZ. *Zur Automatisierung der kartographischen Generalisierung topographischer Daten in Geo-Informationssystemen*. PhD thesis, University of Hannover, 1993.

[PPR+94] A. POMMERT, B. PFLESSER, M. RIEMER, T. SCHIEMANN, R. SCHUBERT, U. TIEDE, and K.-H. HÖHNE. Advances in medical volume visualization. In *EUROGRAPHICS '94, State of the Art Reports*, pages 111–139, September 1994.

[PRS+95] B. PREIM, A. RITTER, T. STROTHOTTE, T. POHLE, D. R. FORSEY, and L. BARTRAM. Consistency of rendered images and their textual labels. In H. SANTO, editor, *Proceedings of CompuGraphics '95*, pages 201–210, 1995.

[PRS96] B. PREIM, A. RITTER, and T. STROTHOTTE. Illustrating anatomic models: A semi-interactive approach. In *4th International Conference on Visualisation in Biomedical Computing, Hamburg, September 22–25, 1996*, pages 23–32. Springer-Verlag, Berlin, 1996.

[PRS97] B. PREIM, A. RAAB, and T. STROTHOTTE. Coherent zoom of illustrations with 3D-graphics and text. In *Proceedings of Graphics Interface '97*, pages 105–113. Canadian Information Processing Society, 1997.

[RB95] M. RÜGER and T. BEHLAU. Create!: An object-oriented IDE for discrete event simulation. In C. ALEXOPOULOS, K. KANG, W. R. LILEGDON, and D. GOLDSMAN, editors, *Proceedings of SCS Winter Simulation Conference '95*, 1995.

[Rei80] S. REICH. Significance of pauses for speech perception. *Journal of Psycholinguistic Research*, 9.4:379–389, 1980.

[Rei95] E. REITER. Natural language generation versus templates. In *Proceedings of the 5th European Workshop on Natural Language Generation*, pages 95–195. University of Leiden, Leiden, The Netherlands, 1995.

[Ris95] T. RIST. *Wissensbasierte Verfahren für den automatischen Entwurf von Gebrauchsgraphik in der technischen Dokumentation*. PhD thesis, University of the Saarland, 1995.

[RK82] A. ROSENFELD and A. KAK. *Digital Picture Processing*. Academic Press, New York, 1982.

[RM93a] E. REITER and C. MELLISH. Optimizing the costs and benefits of natural language generation. In *Proceedings of IJCAI '93*, pages 1164–1169. Morgan Kaufmann, Los Altos, CA, 1993.

[RM93b] G. G. ROBERTSON and J. D. MACKINLAY. The document lens. In *UIST: Proceedings of the ACM Symposium on User Interface Software and Technology '93*, pages 101–108. ACM, 1993.

[RMC91]   G. G. ROBERTSON, J. D. MACKINLAY, and S. K. CARD. Cone trees: Animated 3D visualizations of hierarchical information. In *Proceedings of CHI '91, Human Factors in Computing Systems*, pages 189–202. ACM SIGCHI, 1991.

[RMC93]   G. G. ROBERTSON, J. D. MACKINLAY, and S. K. CARD. Information visualization using interactive 3D-animation. *Communications of the ACM*, 36(4):56–72, 1993.

[RPR96]   M. RÜGER, B. PREIM, and A. RITTER. Zoom Navigation: Exploring large information and application spaces. In *Proceedings of the Workshop on Advanced Visual Interfaces, AVI '96*, pages 40–48. ACM Press, New York, 1996.

[RR86]   J. R. ROSSIGNAC and A. A. G. REQUICHA. Depth-buffering display techniques for constructive solid geometry. *IEEE Computer Graphics and Applications*, 6(9):29–39, 1986.

[RR96]   A. RAAB and M. RÜGER. 3D-Zoom: Interactive visualisation of structures and relations in complex graphics. In H.-P. S. B. GIROD, H. Niemann, editor, *3D Image Analysis and Synthesis*, pages 125–132. infix, St. Augustin, 1996.

[SABS94]   M. P. SALISBURY, S. E. ANDERSON, R. BARZEL, and D. H. SALESIN. Interactive pen-and-ink illustration. In *Proceedings of SIGGRAPH '94*, Computer Graphics Proceedings, Annual Conference Series, pages 101–108. ACM SIGGRAPH, 1994.

[SALS96]   M. P. SALISBURY, C. ANDERSON, D. LISCHINSKI, and D. H. SALESIN. Scale-dependent reproduction of pen-and-ink illustrations. In *Proceedings of SIGGRAPH '96*, Computer Graphics Proceedings, Annual Conference Series, pages 461–468. ACM SIGGRAPH, 1996.

[SASW96]   V. SPITZER, M. J. ACKERMAN, A. L. SCHERZINGER, and D. WHITLOCK. The visible human male: A technical report. *J. Am. Med. Inf. Ass.*, 2(3):118–130, 1996.

[SB92]   M. SARKAR and M. H. BROWN. Graphical fisheye views of graphs. In *Proceedings of CHI '92, Human Factors in Computing Systems*. ACM SIGCHI, 1992.

[SB94]   M. SARKAR and M. H. BROWN. Graphical fisheye views. *Communications of the ACM*, 37(12):73–84, 1994.

[SB96]   A. SMITH and J. F. BLINN. Blue screen matting. In *Proceedings of SIGGRAPH '96*, Computer Graphics Proceedings, Annual Conference Series, pages 259–268. ACM SIGGRAPH, 1996.

[SC92]   P. S. STRAUSS and R. CAREY. An object-oriented 3D graphics toolkit. In *Proceedings of SIGGRAPH '92*, Computer Graphics Proceedings, Annual Conference Series, pages 341–350. ACM SIGGRAPH, 1992.

[SCC76] W. C. STOKOE, D. C. CASTERLINE, and C. D. CRONEBERG. *A Dictionary of American Sign Language*. Linstock Press, Silver Spring, 1976.

[Sch82] D. SCHOEN. *The Reflective Practitioner: How Professionals Think in Action*. Basic Books, New York, 1982.

[Sch84] D. SCHREIER. *Synthetische Holografie*. Physik-Verlag, Weinheim, 1984.

[Sch93] J. R. SCHIRRA. Connecting visual and verbal space – preliminary considerations concerning the concept 'mental image'. In M. AURNAGUE, A. BORILLO, M. BORILLO, and M. BRAS, editors, *Semantics of Time, Space, and Movement*, pages 105–121. Group "Langue, Raisonnement, Calcul", CNRS, and the universities *Paul Sabatier* and *Le Merail*, Toulouse, 1993.

[Sch94a] J. R. J. SCHIRRA. *Bildbeschreibung als Verbindung von visuellem und sprachlichem Raum – Eine interdisziplinäre Untersuchung von Bildvorstellungen in einem Hörermodell*. infix, St. Augustin, 1994.

[Sch94b] S. SCHOFIELD. *Non-photorealistic rendering: A critical examination and proposed system*. PhD thesis, School of Art and Design, Middlesex University, 1994.

[Sch95a] J. R. J. SCHIRRA. Understanding radio broadcasts on soccer: The concept 'mental image' and its use in Spatial Reasoning. In K. SACHS-HOMBACH, editor, *Bilder im Geiste. Zur kognitiven und erkenntnistheoretischen Funktion piktorialer Repräsentationen*, pages 107–136. Rodopi, Amsterdam, 1995.

[Sch95b] R. SCHLEICH. *Visualisierung abstrakter Objekte und Beziehungen in einem interaktiven Graphiksystem*. PhD thesis, University of Zurich, 1995.

[Sch97] H. SCHLICHTMANN. Functions of the map legend. In *Proceedings of the 18th ICA/ACI International Cartographic Conference*, volume 1, page 430. Gävle, Stockholm, 1997.

[SD94] R. SCHLEICH and M. J. DÜRST. Beyond WYSIWYG: Display of hidden information in graphics editors. In *Computer Graphics Forum, Proceedings of Eurographics '94*, pages 185–194, 1994.

[SDS+93] C. SCHONEMAN, J. DORSEY, B. SMITS, J. ARVO, and D. GREENBERG. Painting with light. In *Proceedings of SIGGRAPH '93*, Computer Graphics Proceedings, Annual Conference Series, pages 143–146. ACM SIGGRAPH, 1993.

[Sei93] H.-P. SEIDEL. An introduction to polar forms. *IEEE Computer Graphics and Applications*, pages 38–46, 1993.

[SF91a]   D. D. SELIGMANN and S. K. FEINER. Automated generation of intent-based 3D-illustrations. In *Proceedings of SIGGRAPH '91*, Computer Graphics Proceedings, Annual Conference Series, pages 123–132. ACM SIGGRAPH, 1991.

[SF91b]   D. D. SELIGMANN and S. K. FEINER. Automated generation of intent-based 3D-illustrations. In *Proceedings of SIGGRAPH '91*, Computer Graphics Proceedings, Annual Conference Series, pages 123–132. ACM SIGGRAPH, 1991.

[SG81]   S. SECHREST and D. P. GREENBERG. A visible polygon reconstruction algorithm. In *Proceedings of SIGGRAPH '81*, Computer Graphics Proceedings, Annual Conference Series, pages 17–27. ACM SIGGRAPH, 1981.

[SGD93]   F. P. SEILER, R. GRÜNFELDER, and H. DEISENHAMMER. Producing hardcopy graphics for blind and visually impaired persons using a special drawing program called relief. *Journal of Microcomputer Applications*, (16):301–306, 1993.

[SH97]   S. STAAB and U. HAHN. "Tall", "good", "high" – compared to what? In *Proceedings of IJCAI '97*, pages 996–1001. Morgan Kaufmann, Los Altos, CA, 1997.

[Sha82]   S. SHARFF. *The Elements of Cinema*. Columbia University Press, 1982.

[SHB93]   M. SONKA, V. HLAVAC, and R. BOYLE. *Image Processing, Analsysis and Machine Vision*. Chapman & Hall, London, 2nd edition, 1993.

[Shn92]   B. SHNEIDERMAN. *Designing the User Interface: Strategies for Effective Human-Computer Interaction*. Addison-Wesley, Reading, MA, 1992.

[SKS95]   J. SCHUMANN, E. KERNCHEN, and T. STROTHOTTE. Rendering CAAD models as preliminary drafts. In *Proceedings of the 6th International Conference on Computing in Civil and Building Engineering*, pages 791–797. A. A. Balkema Publishers, Rotterdam, 1995.

[SNTH96]   T. SCHIEMANN, J. NUTHMAN, U. TIEDE, and K.-H. HÖHNE. Generation of 3D anatomical atlases using the visible human. In R. F. KILCOYNE, editor, *Proceedings of CAR'96*, pages 62–67, 1996.

[Sny87]   J. P. SNYDER. "Magnifying-glass" azimuthal map projections. *The American Cartographer*, 14(1):61–68, 1987.

[Sob88]   J. SOBOTTA. *Atlas der Anatomie des Menschen*. Urban & Schwarzenberg, Munich, 19th edition, 1988.

[SP95]   S. SCHLECHTWEG and B. PREIM. Emphasising in linedrawings. *NORSIGD Info, medlemsblad for NORSIGD*, (1):9–10, 1995.

[SPR+94] T. STROTHOTTE, B. PREIM, A. RAAB, J. SCHUMANN, and D. R. FORSEY. How to render frames and influence people. In *Computer Graphics Forum*, pages 455–466. Blackwell, Oxford, UK, 1994.

[SS95] A. SAVIDIS and C. STEPHANIDIS. Developing dual user interfaces for integrating blind and sighted users: the HOMER UIMS. In *Proceedings of CHI '95, Human Factors in Computing Systems*, pages 106–113. ACM SIGCHI, 1995.

[SS97] C. STROTHOTTE and T. STROTHOTTE. *Seeing Between the Pixels: Pictures in Interactive Systems*. Springer-Verlag, Berlin, 1997.

[SSRL96] J. SCHUMANN, T. STROTHOTTE, A. RAAB, and S. LASER. Assessing the effect of non-photorealistic rendered images in CAD. In *Proceedings of CHI '96, Human Factors in Computing Systems*, pages 35–42. ACM SIGCHI, 1996.

[SSTR93] M. SARKAR, S. SNIBBE, O. J. TVERSKY, and S. P. REISS. Stretching the rubber sheet: A metaphor for viewing large layouts on small screens. In *UIST: Proceedings of the ACM Symposium on User Interface Software and Technology '93*, pages 81–91. ACM, 1993.

[ST90] T. SAITO and T. TAKAHASHI. Comprehensible rendering of 3-D shapes. In *Proceedings of SIGGRAPH '90*, Computer Graphics Proceedings, Annual Conference Series, pages 197–206. ACM SIGGRAPH, 1990.

[Str71] P. F. STRAWSON. *Logico-Linguistic Papers*. Methuen, London, 1971.

[Str86] S. STRASSMANN. Hairy Brushes. In *Proceedings of SIGGRAPH '86*, Computer Graphics Proceedings, Annual Conference Series, pages 225–232. ACM SIGGRAPH, 1986.

[SW75] A. SINOWJEW and H. WESSEL. *Logische Sprachregeln – Eine Einführung in die Logik*. Fink, München, 1975.

[SWHS97] M. SALISBURY, M. WONG, J. F. HUGHES, and D. H. SALESIN. Orientable textures for image-based pen-and-ink illustration. In *Proceedings of SIGGRAPH '97*, Computer Graphics Proceedings, Annual Conference Series. ACM SIGGRAPH, 1997.

[SZB+93] D. SCHAFFER, Z. ZUO, L. BARTRAM, J. DILL, S. DUBS, S. GREENBERG, and M. ROSEMAN. Comparing fisheye and full-zoom techniques for navigation of hierarchically clustered networks. In *Proceedings of Graphics Interface '93*, pages 87–96. Canadian Information Processing Society, 1993.

[SZG+96]   D. SCHAFFER, Z. ZUO, S. GREENBERG, L. BARTRAM, J. DILL, S. DUBS, and M. ROSEMAN. Navigating hierarchically clustered networks through fisheye and full-zoom methods. *ACM Transactions on Computer-Human Interaction*, 3(2):162–188, 1996.

[TB96]   G. TURK and D. BANKS. Image-guided streamline placement. In *Proceedings of SIGGRAPH '96*, Computer Graphics Proceedings, Annual Conference Series, pages 453–460. ACM SIGGRAPH, 1996.

[Tes81]   L. TESLER. The Smalltalk environment. *Byte*, 6(8):90–147, August 1981.

[The95]   THE GUIB CONSORTIUM. *Textual and Graphical User Interfaces for Blind People: Final Report on the GUIB Project*. Royal National Institute for the Blind, London, 1995.

[TJ81]   F. THOMAS and O. JOHNSTON. *The Illusion of Life: Disney Animation*. Hyperion, New York, 1981.

[Tug82]   E. TUGENDHAT. *Traditional and Analytic Philosophy: Lectures on the Philosophy of Language*. Cambridge University Press, Cambridge, UK, 1982.

[Tur95]   R. TURTSCHI. *Praktische Typographie*. Niggli, Sulgen, Switzerland, 2nd edition, 1995.

[TW83]   E. TUGENDHAT and U. WOLF. *Logisch-semantische Propädeutik*. Reclam, Stuttgart, 1983.

[TW90]   D. TERZOPOULOS and K. WATERS. Physically-based facial modelling, analysis, and animation. *Visualization and Computer Animation*, 1(2):73–80, 1990.

[vB95]   K. VAN OVERVELD and B. BARENBRUG. All you need is force: a constraint-based approach for rigid body dynamics in computer animation. In *Computer Animation and Simulation '95*, pages 80–94, September 1995.

[Vie91]   L. VIEU. *Sémantique des relations spatiales et inférences spatio-temporelles. Une contribution à l'étude des structures formelles de l'espace en Langage Naturel*. PhD thesis, Paul Sabatier University, Toulouse, 1991.

[VKPW82]   K. VOSSSCHULTE, E. KÜMMERLE, H.-J. PEIPER, and S. WELLER, editors. *Lehrbuch der Chirurgie*. Georg Thieme Verlag, Stuttgart, 1982.

[vS74]   E. v. SAVIGNY. Zeichen. In H. KRINGS, H. M. BAUMGARTNER, and C. WILD, editors, *Handbuch philosophischer Grundbegriffe*, volume 6. Kösel, München, 1974.

[WA77]   K. WEILER and K. ATHERTON. Hidden surface removal using polygon area sorting. In *Proceedings of SIGGRAPH '77*, Computer Graphics Proceedings, Annual Conference Series, pages 214–222. ACM SIGGRAPH, 1977.

[WAF+93] W. WAHLSTER, E. ANDRÉ, W. FINKLER, H.-J. PROFITLICH, and T. RIST. Plan-based integration of natural language and graphics generation. *Artificial Intelligence*, 63:387–427, 1993.

[Wan93] J. WANDMACHER. *Softwareergonomie – Mensch-Computer-Interaktion Grundwissen*. Walter de Gruyter Verlag, Berlin, 1993.

[Wat93] A. WATT. *3D Computer Graphics*. Addison-Wesley, Reading, MA, 2nd edition, 1993.

[Web90] *Dictionary of the English Language*. Random House, New York, 1990.

[Web95] G. WEBER. Reading and pointing – new interaction methods for braille displays. In A. EDWARDS, editor, *Extra-Ordinary Human-Computer Interaction: Interfaces for Users with Disabilities*, pages 183–200. Cambridge University Press, Cambridge, UK, 1995.

[Wei89] B. WEIDENMANN. Informative Bilder (Was sie können, wie man sie didaktisch nutzt und wie man sie nicht verwenden sollte). *Pädagogik*, pages 30–34, September 1989.

[Wer94] J. WERNECKE. *The Inventor Mentor*. Addison-Wesley, Reading, MA, 1994.

[WM92] A. WALDEYER and A. MAYET, editors. *Anatomie des Menschen*. Walter de Gruyter Verlag, Berlin, 1992.

[Woo83] S. WOODFORD. *Looking at Pictures – (Cambridge Introduction to Art)*. Cambridge University Press, Cambridge, UK, 1983.

[WS94] G. WINKENBACH and D. H. SALESIN. Computer-generated pen-and-ink illustration. In *Proceedings of SIGGRAPH '94*, Computer Graphics Proceedings, Annual Conference Series, pages 91–100. ACM SIGGRAPH, 1994.

[WS96] G. WINKENBACH and D. H. SALESIN. Rendering free-form surfaces in pen and ink. In *Proceedings of SIGGRAPH '96*, Computer Graphics Proceedings, Annual Conference Series, pages 469–476. ACM SIGGRAPH, 1996.

[WW92] A. WATT and M. WATT. *Advanced Animation and Rendering Techniques*. Addison-Wesley, Reading, MA, 1992.

[Yan94] N. YANKELOVITCH. Talking versus taking: Remote speech access to computers. In *Companion to the CHI '94, Human Factors in Computing Systems*, pages 275–276. ACM SIGCHI, 1994.

[ZBM96] S. ZHAI, W. BUXTON, and P. MILGRAM. The partial occlusion effect: Utilizing semi-transparency in 3D human computer interaction. *ACM Transactions on Computer-Human Interaction*, 3(3):254–284, 1996.

[Zel90]   D. ZELTZER. Task-level graphical simulation: Abstraction, representation and control. In N. BADLER, B. BARSKY, and D. ZELTZER, editors, *Making them Move: Mechanics, Control and Animation of Articulated Figures*, pages 3–33. Los Altos, CA, 1990.

[Zha95]   E. ZHANG. *Computer Holography: Theory, Algorithms, and Realization*. PhD thesis, University of Heidelberg, 1995.

[ZK83]   J. ZIMLER and J. KEENAN. Imagery in the congenitally blind: How visual are visual images? *Journal of Experimental Psychology: Learning, Memory and Cognition*, 9:269–282, 1983.

Index of Names

Aagedal H., 359, 361
Abmayr W., 127, 128
Ackermann G., 359
Ackerman M., 310
Agarwal P., 40
Aho A. V., 404, 405
Akutsu A., 124
Anderson S. E., 86
André E., 203, 217, 262, 308
Arman F., 124
Arvo J., 124
Atherton K., 72
Aumann G., 370

Banks D., 119
Barenbrug B., 260
Bartram L., 20, 24, 29, 56, 151, 152, 154, 161, 189, 216, 219, 234, 268
Barzel R., 86
Beard M., 42
Bederson B. B., 30, 282
Behlau T., 168, 283
Bergmann L., 359
Berk T., 212
Bernard R. M., 198
Beth T., 359, 361
Bizouarn E., 249
Blinn J. F., 124
Boddy M., 76
Booth K. S., 106
Bordegoni M., 210
Boyle R., 128
Brambring M., 342
Briscoe M. H., 219
Brooks F., 40

Brownstone L., 212
Brown M. H., 15, 24, 26, 141, 150, 161, 282
Bruderlin A., 124
Brugger R., 314
Bryngdahl O., 366, 367, 369, 376
Bury K. F., 29
Buttenfield B., 355
Butz A., 41, 262
Buxton W., 33

Calvert T., 24
Card S. K., 32, 33, 52, 62, 152, 228
Carenini G., 203
Carey R., 53, 54
Carey T. T., 20
Carpendale M. S. T., 32, 33, 36, 141, 149, 150
Carr D., 51, 52
Casterline D. C., 314
Catmull E., 106
Chiu M. Y., 124
Coggins J. M., 403
Cohen J., 40
Cournarie E., 249
Cowperthwaite D. J., 32, 33, 36, 141, 149, 150
Croneberg C. D., 314
Cruz-Neira C., 362
Culhane S., 245

Dahlberg M., 344
Dale R., 411
Darnell M. J, 29
Davis S. E., 29

Davis T., 372, 375
Dean T., 76
Deconinck F., 187
DeFanti T., 362
Deisenhammer H., 344
Depommier R., 124
Dill J., 20, 29, 56, 151, 152, 154, 161, 219, 268, 282
DiMattia C., 124
Dore J., 389
Dorsey J., 124
Douglas D. H., 344
Drucker S. M., 261
Dubs S., 20, 29, 151, 152
Durst M. J., 51, 52
Dyck M., 29, 152, 154, 161

Eades P., 31
Edholm P. R., 403
Edman P. K., 339
Edwards A. D. N, 315
Edwards A. D. N., 186
Eichler J., 359
Elson L. M., 4
Elson S., 39
Engelbart D., 286
English W. K., 286
Ernst R., 282

Faconti G., 210
Fairchild K. M., 36
Farin G., 91
Fauconnier G., 391
Feiner S. K., 8, 39, 41, 47, 65, 69, 203, 217, 250, 259, 261, 308
Fekete J. D., 249
Finkler W., 203, 217, 308
Floyd R., 112
Foley J. D., 8, 47, 65, 69, 250
Forcade T., 91
Forsey D. R., 68, 71, 106, 189, 216, 234
Fowles G. R., 359
Fox D., 161

Fracchia F. D., 32, 33, 36, 141, 149, 150
Frege G., 389
Frère C., 365–367, 369, 376
Furnas G. W., 15, 21, 23, 25, 36, 51, 52, 62, 152, 161, 216, 219, 281, 401

Gabor D., 359
Galas Th., 249
Galyean T. G., 361, 364
Gamma E., 302
Garland M., 40
Geitz S., 314
Gentner D., 281
Gershon N. D., 403
Gill J. M., 340
Gleicher M., 231
Globus A., 403
Godwin L. G., 352
Gombrich E. H., 197
Gonzalez R. C., 124
Gould P., 21
Greenberg D. P., 71, 76, 124
Greenberg S., 20, 29, 151, 152
Grice H. P., 391
Grünfelder R., 344
Grünreich D., 22

Haberäcker P., 127
Hahn U., 212
Hake G., 22
Hake R., 7
Hamel J., 342
Hanson T., 314
Harling P. A., 315
Harpold T., 39
Harrison B. L., 39
Hartmann K., 334
Hausmann R., 45, 129
Havens W. S., 29, 152, 154, 161
Heckbert P., 40
Helbing R., 271, 326, 329, 334
Held J., 380
Helm R., 302

Henigmann F., 56, 219, 268
Herdon K. P., 231
Hill W. C., 166
Hlavac V, 128
Hodges E. R. S., 80, 88
Hollands J. G., 20
Holland J. D., 30
Hollan J. D., 166, 282
Hopcroft J. E., 404, 405
Hoppe A., 45, 129
Hoppe H., 40
Houde S., 231
Hovy E. H., 411
Ho A., 56, 219, 268
Hsu A., 124
Hsu S. C., 68, 82
Hsu W. M., 43
Hudelmayer D., 339
Hughes J. F., 8, 43, 47, 65, 69, 250
Hughes M., 124
Höhne K.-H., 218, 307

Ilgenstein U., 326
Immler Ch., 52
Irby C. H., 42
Itten J., 124, 125

Johnson B., 30, 152
Johnson J., 42
Johnson R., 302
Johnston O., 246
João E. M., 352
Jäger E., 345
Jähne B., 129

Kadmon F., 24
Kadmon N., 140, 149
Kahn K., 261
Kaiser M., 384
Kak A. C., 108
Kamba T., 39
Kamlah W., 389
Kamp H., 391
Kandogan E., 30, 168

Kapit W., 4
Karp P., 261
Kaufmann A., 212
Kaufmann H., 43
Keahey T. A., 37
Keenan J., 179, 180
Kennedy J. M., 179
Kerlow I. V., 246, 251
Kernchen E., 5
Kerr N., 179
Klein R., 40
Kochanek D. H. U., 253
Koffka K., 393
Koller D., 393
Krüger A., 41, 262
Kunii T. L., 315
Kurze M., 187
Kurz T., 359–361, 364

Lagrange J. P., 201, 345, 346, 355
Lai W., 31
Lamping J., 23, 38, 52
Lansdown J., 70, 106, 124
Larkin J. H., 184
Laser S., 6, 14, 404
Lassiter J., 247
Lauterborn W., 359–361, 364
Lee I. H. H., 68, 82
Lee J., 315
Leister W., 106
Leroi-Gourhan A., 388
Leseberg D., 365–367, 369, 375
Lichtner W., 140
Lieberman H., 40
Liebich G., 40
Ließ C., 384
Lim K., 288
Lin M. C., 124
Locke J., 178
Lorenzen P., 389
Lorenz P., 271, 329
Lowenfeld B., 183
Lucente M., 361, 364
Luxton K., 344
Lüders P., 282

Lüdicke K., 45, 129

Mackaness W., 355
Mackey K., 42
Mackinlay J. D., 32, 33, 52, 62, 152, 228, 282
Maher S., 314
Manocha D., 40, 124
Marmor G. S., 181
Marr D., 394
Matthews M. L., 20
Mattis J., 203
Maybury M. T., 210
Mayet A., 199, 296
McCandles T, 166
McCann C. A., 20
McKenna M., 361
McKeown K. R., 203
Mealing S., 243
Meier B. J., 250
Mellish C., 209
Merry F. K., 183
Merry R. V., 183
Meyer H.-M., 162
Michel R., 7, 342, 354
Milgram P., 33
Misue K., 31
Mittal V., 203
Mitta D. A., 24
Monaco J., 263, 266
Monmonier M., 200, 202, 345, 352
Moore J. D, 203
Moore R., 179
Morely S., 187
Myers A., 106
Müller J., 262, 308
Müller J. C., 201, 345, 346, 355

Neider J., 372, 375
Neisser U., 179
Nielsen J., 213, 281
Nievergelt J, 28
Noik E. G., 15, 22, 24, 25, 29, 152, 161, 229, 281
Norman D., 282

Nugent G. C., 197
Nuthman J., 218

O'Rourke M., 246
Obermayr K., 162
Ovans R., 29, 152, 154, 161

Paeth A. W., 106
Parke F., 314
Perlin K., 161
Petrie H., 187
Peucker T. K., 344
Pflesser B., 218
Phillips R. L., 8, 65, 69
Piaget J., 393
Pirolli P., 23
Pitt I., 186, 193
Plaisant C., 51, 52
Pohle T., 189, 216, 234
Poltrock S. E., 36
Pommert A., 218, 307
Powitz B. M., 345
Preim B., 45, 68, 71, 106, 124, 189, 216, 224, 230, 234, 268
Profitlich H.-J., 203, 217, 308

Raab A., 6, 14, 33, 45, 57, 58, 68, 71, 106, 156, 216, 219, 226, 230, 404
Rao R., 23, 38, 52
Reich S., 194
Reiss S. P., 28, 30, 141, 150
Reiter E., 208, 209
Requicha A. A. G., 106
Riemer M., 218, 307
Rist Th., 22, 203, 210, 217, 222, 262, 308
Ritter A., 189, 216, 224, 234, 268
Robertson E. L., 37
Robertson G. G., 32, 33, 52, 62, 152, 228
Roberts W., 42
Roseman M., 20, 29, 151, 152
Rosenfeld A., 108

Rossignac J. R., 106
Roth S., 203
Ruggieri S., 210
Rösner D., 334, 411
Rüger M., 33, 57, 58, 156, 168, 219, 224, 226, 282, 283, 326

Saito T., 67, 70, 87, 106, 108, 119, 124, 128
Salesin D. H., 6, 68, 71, 86, 106
Salgé F., 355
Salisbury M. P., 86, 106
Sandin D. J., 362
Sarkar M., 15, 24, 26, 28, 30, 141, 150, 161, 282
Savidis A., 189
Schaefer C., 359
Schaffer D., 20, 29, 151, 152, 154, 283
Scherzinger A., 310
Schiemann Th., 218, 307
Schirra J. R. J., 389, 390, 392, 393, 401
Schlechtweg S., 124
Schleich R., 49, 51, 52
Schlichtmann H., 199, 200, 352
Schoen D., 293
Schofield S., 68, 70, 106, 124
Schoneman C., 124
Schreier D., 361, 363, 367
Schubert R., 218, 307
Schumann J., 5, 6, 14, 68, 71, 106, 404
Schwarzer H., 359, 361
Sechrest S., 71, 76
Seidel H.-P., 91
Seiler F. P., 344
Seligmann D. D., 39, 217, 259, 308
Sharff S., 266, 273
Shlomi E., 24
Shneiderman B., 20, 30, 51, 52, 152, 168, 281, 286
Simon H. A., 184

Sinowjew A., 389
Smith A., 124
Smith D. C., 42
Smits B., 124
Snibbe S., 28, 30, 141, 150
Snyder J. P., 141, 149
Sobotta J., 199, 215, 219, 233, 239, 269, 296, 308
Sonka M., 128
Spitzer V., 310
Spitzmüller K., 370
Staab S., 212
Stamper T., 39
Steinberg S., 112
Stephanidis C., 189
Stock O., 411
Stokoe W. C., 314
Strassmann S., 68
Strauss P. S., 53, 54
Strawson P. F., 391
Straßer W., 40
Strothotte C., 11, 42, 391, 392
Strothotte T., 5–7, 11, 14, 42, 45, 68, 71, 106, 187, 189, 216, 230, 234, 268, 334, 342, 354, 391, 392, 404
Sugiyama K., 31
Sukaviriya P., 39

Taillefer F., 249
Takahashi T., 67, 70, 87, 106, 108, 119, 124, 128
Teiwes S., 359, 361
Terzopoulos D., 314
Tesler L., 281
Thomas F., 246
Tiede U., 218, 307
Tonomura Y., 124
Trahanias P., 210
Tugendhat E., 389, 391, 393, 396
Turk G., 40, 119
Turtschi R., 204
Tversky O. J., 28, 30, 141, 150

Ullman J. D., 404, 405

van Dam A., 8, 47, 65, 69, 231, 250
van Overveld. K., 260
Varshnay A., 40
Verplank W., 42
Vieu L., 395
Vincente K. J., 39
Vlissides J., 302
von Savigny E., 388

Wahlster W., 203, 217, 308
Waldeyer A., 199, 296
Wandmacher J., 21
Waters K., 314
Watt A., 3, 69, 246, 406
Watt M., 246
Weber G., 190
Weber H., 40
Weibel R., 201, 345, 346, 355
Weidenmann B., 15, 197
Weiler K., 72
Wernecke J., 234, 270
Wessel H., 389

Weydert J., 28
White R., 21
Whitlock D., 310
Wiesenfeldt M., 359–361, 364
Williams L., 124
Wilson M., 210
Winkenbach G., 6, 68, 71, 86, 106
Wiseman H. E., 68, 82
Wolf U., 389
Woodford S., 121
Woods R. E., 124
Woo M., 372, 375
Wright W., 40
Wroblewski A., 166

Yankelovitch N., 189

Zacks J., 52, 62
Zeltzer D., 261, 361
Zhai S., 33
Zhang E., 361, 363
Zimler J., 180
Zuo Z., 20, 29, 151, 152

Index

3D fisheye techniques, 33–39
3D zoom, 58, 219, 226, 413

a priori importance, 24
a priori interest, 163 174
abstract data type, 404
abstraction
    continuity, 407
    definition, 14
    in cartography, 200, 201, 345
    in computer graphics, 40
    in interactive computer
        visualization, 13
    in medical illustrations, 296
    in non-photorealistic images,
        248
    in user interfaces, 42
    term, 13
accentuating, 125
adaptive graphical zoom, 226
ADT, *see* abstract data type
affordance, 282
AKZENT, 45
anatomical atlases, 199
animation, 243
    computer, 246
    content, 263, 325
    facial, 314
    freeform surfaces, 254
    gestures, 313
    intent-based, 259
    line drawings, 252, 313
    line styles, 255
    non-photorealistic, 248
    offline, 326
    online, 326
    painterly, 252
    polygonal models, 252
    problems, 122
    technical, 259
    traditional, 244
animation actions, 325
animation design, 325
    communicative goals, 262
    interactive fine-tuning, 263
    positional parameters, 275
    time parameters, 275
animation pipeline, 250
animation techniques
    camera motion, 265, 274
    camera position and
        direction, 264
    direct emphasis, 264
    indirect emphasis, 264
    master shot, 274
    multi-angularity, 274
    parallel action, 274
    separation, 273
    shots and cuts, 265
ANIPLUS, 271
annotation, 222
anytime algorithm, 76
AOI, *see* aspect of interest
APEX system, 41
API, *see* a priori importance
application space, 161
aspect of interest, 163–174, 189,
    282, 284

binocular disparity, 361
blind people
    graphics for, 177

bookmarks, 39
Braille, 183, 184
Braille display, 190

cam trees, 34
camera control, 261, 271
cartographic generalization, 200, 345
CATHI, 262
cluster deformation, 254
coherent zooming, 216, 239
color contrast, 124
COMET project, 203
communication theory, 388
communicative intention, 397
comprehension cues
    graphical, 412
    linguistic, 414
computational linguistics, 411
computational visualistics, 403
conceptual distance, 22, 163
cone trees, 33, 52
congenitally blind, 178
connectivity constraints, 159
context expert, 209
context view, 49
contextual information, 46, 47, 54
copper plates, 106, 117
core section, 143
corridor effect, 143
CREATE!, 168, 283
cut away views, 37, 217

damping section, 143
data mining, 20
decomposition tree, 261
degree of interest, 23, 51, 84, 163–174, 221, 224, 282
depth cues, 361
diagrammatic representation, 184
dialog systems, 11
didactification, 15
difference operator, 110
difference vector, 82
direct manipulation, 51

direction angle, 111
displacement vector, 140
distorted view, 60
distortion, 139–150
    direction dependent, 142
    focus line, 142
    hyperbolic, 140
    orientational, 145
    polyfocal, 140
document lens, 34
DOI, *see* degree of interest

educational illustration, 259
enrichment, 49
error diffusion, 107
ESPLANADE, 261
evenly spread meshes, 92

figure captions, 197–214, 414
    adaptable, 204
    content selection, 204
    descriptive, 198
    dynamic, 203
    for maps, 352
    instructive, 198
    interactive, 206
    invalid, 205
    object monitoring, 205
    structure, 202
film language, 266
fisheye techniques
    3D, 216
fisheye views, 19–44, 51, 141, 218, 282
    3D, 33–39
    applications, 25–30
        graphs and maps, 26
        hypertext structures, 28
        multiple foci, 28
        supervisory control, 29
        viewing source code, 25
        window management, 29
    comprehensibility, 30
    taxonomy, 24
focus

Index   451

linear, 141
multiple, 140
point shaped, 140
polygon shaped, 141
focus line, 142–150, 351
focus+context, 23
foveated vision, 21
frame-to-frame coherence, 249
freeform surfaces, 91

G-buffer, 67, 105–112, 128, 129
geometric information, 47
geometry view, 49
German film, 179
Gestalt factors, 393
gesture builder, 318
gestures, 313
graphical information, 47
graphics editors, 49
graphics vs. text, 184
gray-scale map, 107
GUIB project, 185, 188

half-toning, 106, 112–117
hand-drawing, 244
hardware, 105, 107
hatching, 98, 106
hatching lines, 112
hidden line removal, 71
hidden surface removal, 70
holography, 359
hyperbolic space, 38
hypertext, 28

IBIS system, 217
icons, 42
id-buffer, 108, 130, 135
illustration
    anatomical, 215, 218, 234
    interactive, 45, 216, 217
    line drawings, 80
    medical, 4, 88, 295
    scientific, 80, 114
    technical, 203
    text-driven, 298

image operator, 107, 108
image processing, 106, 127, 128, 249
image-text relation
    consistency, 216, 219
    Intelligent Voxels, 218
images
    computer generated, 3
    topographical / topological, 185
    vector-oriented, 65
inbetweening, 245
information exploration, 20
information hiding, 11
information retrieval, 19
information space, 9, 19, 161
information visualization, 19, 49
informationally equivalent, 185
insets, 22, 217
IntelliMedia, 217
interaction history, 39, 173
interaction tasks, 49
intersection lines, 114, 115
Iso-operator, 111
isoparametric net, 94

keyframes, 244, 316

label navigation, 216
labels, 215, 297
layout manager, 221
legends, 200
level of detail, 51, 161, 162, 164, 205, 224, 262, 284, 298, 320
lexical context, 391
line drawing, 78, 92, 106, 313
line style, 81, 106

magnification grids, 37
magnifying glass, 141
manual alphabet, 315
map fidelity, 201, 351
MAP WIZARD, 354
maps, 6, 139, 142

digitizing, 343
tactile, 339
media coordination, 203
media selection, 203
mediator, 302
mental imagery, 179
menus, 42
methodological background, 379
model, 3, 47
modeless interface, 281
Moiré pattern, 119
morphing, 141
motion parallax, 361
multi-dimensional interaction, 151

naturalism, 379
naturalistic residue, 397
navigation
    information and application space, 161
    zoom, 162
navigation techniques, 19
navigational affordance, 282
nominator, 389
non-photorealism, 106
non-rigid object treatment, 159
nonlinear magnification, 37
normal buffer, 108
normal coordinates, 25
normal view, 25

object constitution, 393
object hierarchy, 47
observer model, 400

pan and zoom, 20, 53, 151, 283, 288
part-whole relations, 395
peripheral vision, 21
perspective wall, 33
photography, 4
pinwall, 227
pixel-vector conversion, 114
plant ecosystems, 119
plants, 119

pliable surfaces, 36
pluggable zoom, 166, 169
plugin, 329
predicator, 389
presentation fidelity, 201
presentation parameters, 49
presentation space, 197
presentation techniques, 20
presentation variables, 200, 223
prioritized stroke textures, 68, 106
prosody, 193, 194

ray tracing, 106
realism, 379
recognition, 188
recognition constraints, 157
reference lines, 215, 228, 230, 231, 233
referential context, 391, 395
refinement view, 55
rendering, 3
    analytic, 69
    non-photorealistic, 67
    pixel-based, 105–119
representation
    diagrammatic / sentential, 184
representation matrix, 164, 165, 224
rondell, 229
rubber sheet, 141

screen real estate, 139, 281
scripting language, 263
sentential representation, 184
shadow, 99
shape constraints, 158
shower-door effect, 249
sign language, 313
silhouette, 41
situational context, 390
skeleton, 315
sketches, 5
SOBEL operator, 108

SOUNDGRAPH, 186
space filling properties, 155, 156
spatial distance, 163
speech synthesizer, 190
stereogram, 364
stereopsis, 361
stippling, 86, 98
structure browser, 48, 52
structure editor, 48
structure information, 47, 54, 267
structure view, 49
symbol displacement, 345

tactile display, 182
tactile images, 179
task-level specification, 261
tele-rendering, 387, 392, 400
templates, 208
text generation, 208
text vs. graphics, 184
TEXTILLUSTRATOR, 298
textual description, 186
topographical images, 185
topological images, 186
trace file, 331
transition constraints, 159
transparency, 159
    in user interfaces, 39
tunnel vision, 151

UIMS, 188
user, 4

variable zoom, 56
varying scale, 139
vector field, 119
verbal description, 186, 389

visibility information, 221, 267
visual access distortion, 37
visual complexity, 41
visual constraints, 157
visual object recognition, 393
visual perception, 21
visualization
    computer generated, 3
    non-computer generated, 4–9
visualization tasks, 49
visually impaired people
    graphics for, 177
volume texturing, 106
VOXELMAN, 218, 307

WIMP, 281
window management, 29
window placement, 51
WIP project, 203, 217
wireframe, 92

XEROX STAR, 42

z-buffer, 106, 108, 130, 132, 135
zoom
    continuous, 152
    dimension independent, 154
    intelligent, 161, 282
    pluggable, 166, 283, 286
    text, 224
    variable, 282
zoom navigation, 162, 168,
    281–293
ZOOMSTRUCTOR, 53–62, 220
ZOOMILLUSTRATOR, 169, 189,
    216, 269, 306, 388
ZOOMNAVIGATOR, 168, 283

Contributors

Oliver Deussen, born in Munich in 1966, holds a Ph.D. in Computer Science from the University of Karlsruhe. Since 1996 he has been working on his Habilitation degree in the Department of Simulation and Graphics at the University of Magdeburg. His research interests include modeling, visualizing, and animating complex biological objects. He is involved in the leadership of the special interest group "Graphical Simulation and Animation" of the Gesellschaft für Informatik (GI).

Frank Godenschweger, born in Magdeburg in 1965, studied Computer Science at the University of Magdeburg from 1988 to 1993, specializing in Simulation and Graphics. Subsequently, he worked as programmer, and since 1996 he has been research student holding a scholarship for doctoral studies in the Department of Simulation and Graphics at the University of Magdeburg. His research interests lie in the field of rendering line drawings for presenting gestures and facial expressions.

Jörg Hamel, born in Magdeburg in 1970, studied Computer Science at the University of Magdeburg from 1990 to 1995, specializing in Simulation and Graphics and earning a Diploma degree. In 1994 and 1995, he spent twelve months as an exchange student at the University of Uppsala, Sweden. He joined the research staff of the Department of Simulation and Graphics in 1995 where he worked for two years on a project funded by the European Community. Presently, he is holding a scholarship to work toward his doctorate. His research interests are in the area of distortions in pictures and the combination of different rendering styles in hybrid pictures.

Ralf Helbing, born in Burg in 1968, studied Computer Science at the University of Magdeburg from 1990 to 1995, with specialization in Graphics and Simulation, and earned a Diploma degree. In 1994, he spent six months as research scholar at the Virtual Reality Laboratory of the University of Michigan, Ann Arbor. Since 1995 he has been a member of the scientific staff in the Department of Simulation and Graphics at the University of Magdeburg and is working toward a doctorate. His research interests are in the area of realtime 3D animation and interfaces between simulation and animation.

Axel Hoppe, born in Halle (Saale) in 1968, underwent a vocational training as a mechanic for locomotives before studying Computer Science at the

University of Magdeburg from 1989 to 1994, specializing in Simulation and Graphics and earning a Diploma degree. From 1994 to 1998, Axel Hoppe carried out doctoral studies in the Department of Simulation and Graphics, graduating in June 1998. He currently works on virtual reality for a company in Munich.

Kathrin Lüdicke, née Weese, has been a member of the scientific staff at the Department of Simulation and Graphics of the University of Magdeburg since 1993. She was born and raised in Magdeburg, and studied Computer Science at the Technical University of Dresden, completing her Diploma degree in 1992. She was then the recipient of a Fulbright Fellowship for graduate studies at the University of Oklahoma at Norman. She has been on extended maternity leave since December, 1995.

Maic Masuch, born in Braunschweig in 1966, has been holding a scholarship for doctoral studies in computer science in the Department of Simulation and Graphics at the University of Magdeburg since 1995. He received his Diploma in genetic programming from the Technical University of Braunschweig. His current interest is in computer animation with an emphasis on non-photorealistic 3D computer animation.

Rainer Michel, born in Halle (Saale) in 1969, studied Computer Science at the University of Magdeburg from 1989 to 1994, specializing in Simulation and Graphics and earning a Diploma degree. He joined the scientific staff of the Department of Simulation and Graphics then and, from 1994 to 1997, worked on a research project funded by the European Union which aimed at developing a navigation aid for visually impaired people. After the successful completion of this project work, he is now working on his Ph.D. thesis. His research interests are in the area of creating customized maps, with particular emphasis on the creation of adapted maps for blind people.

Ian Pitt was born in Weston-Super-Mare in the South West of England in 1957. He graduated from Exeter University in 1982 with a BA in Music and Theatre Arts, and shortly afterwards moved to London where he worked for five years as a journalist. In 1987 he went to the University of York, first to take a master's degree in Music Technology, and subsequently to prepare a doctoral thesis on the design of auditory interfaces for blind computer-users (D.Phil, Computer Science, 1996). In June 1996 he moved to Magdeburg to take up a Research Fellowship funded by the Commission of the European Union. He is now working as a lecturer at University College Corck, Ireland.

Bernhard Preim, born in Magdeburg in 1969, studied Computer Science, specializing in Simulation and Graphics, at the University of Magdeburg from 1989 to 1994. He graduated with a Diploma thesis on computer-generated sketches and soon joined the scientific staff in the Department of Simulation and Graphics. His research interests include interactive illustrations and animations as well as 3D interaction. He finished his Ph.D. in this field in January 1998.

Andreas Raab, born in Rostock in 1968, came to the University of Magdeburg in 1989 to take up studies in Computer Science. He specialized in the fields of Simulation and Computer Graphics and earned his Diploma in 1994. From 1994 to 1997 he worked in the MoBIC research project funded by the European Community. He submitted his doctoral thesis in July, 1998 and then went to work for Disney Imagineering in Los Angeles.

Alf Ritter, born in Hohenmölsen in 1969, joined the scientific staff in the Department of Simulation and Graphics at the University of Magdeburg in 1995, after having successfully completed his studies in Computer Science there. During his studies he spent six months as a visiting researcher at the University of Michigan's Virtual Reality Laboratory. In July, 1998 he earned a doctorate at the University of Magdeburg for his research in 3D visualization techniques with an emphasis on synthetic holography. He now works as a CAD developer in Munich.

Michael Rüger, born in Bochum in 1958, studied Computer Science at the University of Dortmund from 1980 to 1988, specializing in object-oriented programming and earning a Diploma degree. Subsequently he worked at the Fraunhofer Institute for Material Flow and Logistics (IML) in Dortmund and Bielefeld. During this time, in 1992, he spent three months as a visiting researcher at the University of Canterbury in Christchurch, New Zealand. In 1994 he moved to Magdeburg to join the scientific staff in the Department of Simulation and Graphics at the University of Magdeburg, where he earned his doctorate in March, 1998. Since mid-1997, he has been working as a consultant at Ars Nova GmbH in Berlin.

Jörg R. J. Schirra was born in Saarland in 1960. He studied computer science, physics, psychology, and philosophy at the University of Saarland at Saarbrücken, where he also worked, after having received his Diploma in computer science, as a researcher in the Special Collaborative Project "Artificial Intelligence and Knowledge-Based Systems" of the German Research Council (DFG) until 1993. In 1994, he received his doctoral degree in computer science there. Subsequently, he worked as a researcher at the University of Bremen. During this time, he spent one year as a post-doc fellow at the International Computer Science Institute at Berkeley, California. At the University of Magdeburg, where he has been working since 1996, he is responsible for the organization of the undergraduate program for Computational Visualistics. His research interests are in the area of semantics and pragmatics of spatial expressions, argumentation-theoretic interpretation of cognitive science, and philosophical image theories in computational visualistics.

Stefan Schlechtweg, born in Bad Salzungen in 1971, took up studies in Computer Science at the University of Magdeburg in 1990, specializing in Simulation and Graphics. After graduating in 1995 he spent five months as a visiting researcher at the University of Michigan's Virtual Reality Laboratory. From 1995 to 1997, he worked on the research project "Adaptive Graphical Zoom" funded by the German Research Council (DFG). He now holds a scholarship to work toward his doctorate. His research interests are in the area of rendering line drawings for medical applications and the interactive creation and manipulation of scientific illustrations.

Martin Scholz, born in Neuss in 1963, is photographer by profession. He completed his studies with the Diploma degree in design at the BUGH Wuppertal. During 1989 and 1995, he held lectures in photography. In 1995, he joined the research staff in the Department of Simulation and Graphics at the University of Magdeburg. His main interests are in the fields of visualization in technical documentation, development, research of pictorial information, and esthetic theory.

Thomas Strothotte is Professor of Computer Science and head of the Computer Graphics and Interactive Systems Laboratory at the University of Magdeburg. He was born in Regina, Saskatchewan, Canada in 1959, was raised in Vancouver, and studied at Simon Fraser University (B.Sc. in Physics in 1980, M.Sc. in Computer Science in 1981). His graduate training was at the University of Stuttgart in Germany, the University of Waterloo in Ontario, and McGill University in Montreal (Ph.D. in Computer Science, 1984). Subsequently he worked in teaching and research at INRIA Roquencourt in France, the University of Stuttgart (where he earned a Habilitation degree in 1989), the IBM Scientific Center in Heidelberg, and the Free University of Berlin, before moving to Magdeburg in 1993. He has served as the Dean of his faculty, and as Vice-President and President pro tem of the University of Magdeburg.

Kornelia Ullrich, born in Korbach in 1968, studied Psychology at the Catholic University of Eichstätt specializing in Industrial and Organizational Psychology, completing her degree in 1993. During 1990, she was an exchange student at the Washington State University in Pullman, Washington State. Since 1995 she has been working on her Ph.D. in the Department of Pedagogy at the University of Magdeburg and collaborating with the scientific staff at the Departement of Simulation and Graphics. Her research interests include computer-aided learning and self-regulated knowledge acquisition by adults.

Hubert Wagener, born in Büren in 1956, studied Mathematics and Chemistry at the University of Bielefeld and received his Diploma degree in 1982.

He graduated at the Technical University of Berlin (Ph.D. in Computer Science, 1986). Subsequently, he worked in teaching and research at the Technical University of Berlin (1986–1992), at the University of Paderborn (1992–1994) and at the University of Magdeburg. He is currently completing his Habilitation degree. His research interests include computer graphics, computational geometry, and parallel algorithms.

Springer and the environment

At Springer we firmly believe that an international science publisher has a special obligation to the environment, and our corporate policies consistently reflect this conviction.

We also expect our business partners – paper mills, printers, packaging manufacturers, etc. – to commit themselves to using materials and production processes that do not harm the environment. The paper in this book is made from low- or no-chlorine pulp and is acid free, in conformance with international standards for paper permanency.

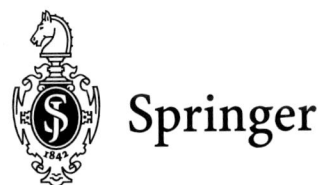

Printing: Mercedesdruck, Berlin
Binding: Buchbinderei Lüderitz & Bauer, Berlin